The Essential Guide to Group Practice in Mental Health

THE CLINICIAN'S TOOLBOX

A Guilford Series
Edward L. Zuckerman, Series Editor

Clinician's Thesaurus, 4th Edition:
The Guidebook for Writing Psychological Reports
Edward L. Zuckerman

Clinician's Thesaurus:
Electronic Edition, Version 4.2
Edward L. Zuckerman

Breaking Free of Managed Care:
A Step-by-Step Guide to Regaining Control of Your Practice
Dana C. Ackley

The Paper Office, 2nd Edition:
Forms, Guidelines, and Resources
Edward L. Zuckerman

Insider's Guide to Mental Health Resources Online
John M. Grohol

The Essential Guide to Group Practice in Mental Health:
Clinical, Legal, and Financial Fundamentals
Simon H. Budman and Brett N. Steenbarger

The Essential Guide to Group Practice in Mental Health

CLINICAL, LEGAL, AND FINANCIAL FUNDAMENTALS

Simon H. Budman

Brett N. Steenbarger

THE GUILFORD PRESS
New York   London

© 1997 The Guilford Press
A Division of Guilford Publications, Inc.
72 Spring Street, New York, NY 10012

Printed in the United States of America

This book is printed on acid-free paper.

Last digit is print number: 9 8 7 6 5 4 3 2 1

Library of Congress Cataloging-in-Publication Data

Budman, Simon H.
    The essential guide to group practice in mental health :
clinical, legal, and financial fundamentals / Simon H.
Budman, Brett N. Steenbarger.
        p.   cm. — (The Clinician's toolbox)
    Includes bibliographical references and index.
    ISBN 1-57230-254-2
    1. Group practice in clinical psychology.
2. Psychotherapy—Practice.   3. Managed mental health
care.   I. Steenbarger, Brett N.   II. Title.   III. Series.
RC467.95.B83   1997
616.89′0068—dc21   97-20098
                                                      CIP

Foreword

Many solo, independent clinicians view group practice as a threat to their autonomy. In this enlightening volume, Drs. Budman and Steenbarger illustrate, however, that the array of collaborative structures clinicians have invented in the past several years provides ways of satisfying needs for autonomy as well as marketability. Quite simply, the future of independent practice may lie in *inter*dependence.

So how do you begin to collaborate? If you have been considering joining or forming a group practice, you will find in this book all the information you need to hit the ground running:

- There are many possible legal structures for a practice. These are fully explained, along with their advantages and disadvantages.

- Many practices fail for financial reasons, like lack of capital or a realistic business plan. Here you'll find what you need to know about finances, salaries, and start-up costs.

- A business in this field cannot be run without computers, for both billing and management information systems. This book provides exactly what you need to make smart decisions in this area.

- A group practice may fail because of ineffective management of the complex interpersonal interactions among staff and clinicians. The best guidance I have seen anywhere on the subject is in this book.

If you are already running a group practice, you will also find invaluable information in this book:

- Recommendations for day-to-day management, based on real experiences by those who have done it and have the scars to prove it.

- Insights into current theory and future developments, so that you too can anticipate the directions the field is most likely to take.

- Inside information, which you cannot get from your competitors, on essential areas like marketing.

- Advice distilled from the authors' extensive experience consulting with all kinds of provider organizations.

This book offers several unique features. First, Budman and Steenbarger present and articulate a model of collaboration and integration flexible enough for any setting and practical enough for long-term organizational design. Then, they flesh out this model with examples and details, so that you will be able to actualize it in your setting. Last, they present frank and revealing interviews with a number of clinicians who have built successful group practices. These case studies illustrate the subtleties of program development and management in these difficult and sometimes chaotic times. You will benefit if you can build on the innovations of these clinicians as well as avoid their mistakes.

As the editor of The Clinician's Toolbox series, I have seen many books on the future of therapeutic practice. We have published a fine book on thriving outside of managed care (Dana Ackley's *Breaking Free of Managed Care*), and there are dozens of books on surviving within the ever-tightening confines of managed care. However, when it comes to building and managing the most common model of practice for now and for the future—a group of collaborating professionals—there is nothing out there that provides half the information or a tenth the practical guidance of this book.

EDWARD L. ZUCKERMAN, PHD

Preface

During the days when we were cast headlong into the arena of practice development and management, there were few guideposts by which we could steer our efforts. Our graduate programs certainly did not teach us how to form, market, and manage a mental health practice. In fact, the entire topic of private practice was a little bit like that of sex: It was on everyone's mind, but no one would acknowledge it or tell you how it was done.

Today, of course, the needs are ever more acute. The oversupply of behavioral health practitioners in many regions, combined with tightening managed care markets, has made it crucial to be good businesspeople as well as effective clinicians. Surprisingly, however, the guideposts are still few and far between. It is rare to find a newly graduating professional who knows what to look for (and avoid!) in a preferred provider contract, how to calculate a capitation rate, or how to communicate with a reviewer through an outpatient treatment report. No wonder some of the questions we hear most often from the graduate students, interns, and residents we teach is, What should I look for in joining a group practice? How can I form a group of my own?

This book is one of the very first that directly addresses these questions. In the following pages, we take you through the developmental process of conceptualizing your needs, interests, strengths, and weaknesses; evaluating opportunities in your regional marketplace; and identifying the practice structures that will most likely meet your needs while capitalizing on marketplace opportunities. The book's central theme is quite simple: **In a consolidating world, you cannot (and do not need to) go it alone.** Through multidisciplinary collaboration, you can join and form practice organizations that will be both personally and professionally rewarding—**even if your aim is to retain your independence as a self-employed clinician.**

A critical premise in our work is that the traditional system of managed care, which rigidly separates those who manage clinical services and those who deliver them, is facing fatal limitations. With the rise of public- and private-sector coalitions of benefits purchasers, states and corporations that shop for health insurance are becoming far more knowledgeable and concerned about *quality*. This is most clearly evidenced in the recent National Committee for Quality Assurance (NCQA) guidelines for behavioral health care organizations. Managed care organizations that manage cost alone will be left behind in this quality revolution. Those that wish to survive will be forced to form partnerships with practitioners who can deliver the quality. This dynamic will greatly influence the structure and content of mental health practice in coming years. In a word, it will fuel *collaborations*.

Although the two of us have been immersed in practice development, management, administration, training, and consultation for decades, we have been careful to avoid basing our findings on our experience alone. Our approach has been to identify practice organizations that are unusually successful and innovative and ask, How did they do it? Hence, throughout the book you will find interviews with leaders in the field as well as numerous references to cutting-edge publications. We have also included a wealth of "Reader's Resources" that help you explore topics in a hands-on fashion. Perhaps most helpful of all, we have included three expanded case studies in Chapter 7 that highlight key concepts in a "real world" fashion. As we state in our first chapter, our goal is to be *your* collaborator, helping you determine the kind of practice that will meet your personal and professional goals.

The book is organized according to the developmental process of thinking through a collaborative practice. The first chapters orient the reader to the idea of collaboration, trends in behavioral health care, and the planning process of assessing strengths, weaknesses, opportunities, and threats. Subsequent chapters detail the practical and legal hurdles of structuring and financing a multispecialty practice and developing a coherent mission and business plan. The final chapters identify the kinds of information systems and clinical services that are needed in an environment that demands cost and quality accountability. Throughout, we attempt to address the concerns of readers wishing to *join* group practices and networks, as well as those who seek to form new organizations. Indeed, we believe one of our most valuable contributions will be helping readers in solo practice understand how they can be part of the collaborative revolution while still retaining their offices and independence.

We are acutely aware of how much material we left out of this book. Indeed, our initial draft was close to 1,000 manuscript pages! Even after reading this text, it is likely that you will have questions regarding contracting, marketing, the organization of public- and private-sector delivery systems, and the assessment of quality. Toward that end, we have included a Resource List in the Appendix to help readers delve into topics in greater detail. We also invite readers to contact us with questions and comments at the e-mail addresses included in the Appendix. That's part of the collaboration!

Assembling a manuscript of this scope was no easy feat. We were blessed every step of the way with a wonderful set of collaborators, many of whom are named in our dedications. We also wish to acknowledge Kitty Moore, Anna Brackett, and the excellent editorial and production staff at The Guilford Press for their continued support, advice, and encouragement; our series editor, Ed

Zuckerman, for his very helpful feedback and enthusiasm; and the unwavering assistance provided by our home organizations: Innovative Training Systems and the Department of Psychiatry and Behavioral Sciences at the SUNY Health Science Center in Syracuse. Most of all, we want to acknowledge our interviewees, who graciously gave of their time to share their insights and help smooth the path for their colleagues. We have learned much from our case study participants, Bret Smith, Julie Bigelow, and Jeff Zimmerman.

To you, our readers: Best of luck in your professional development. This is a very difficult economic and practice environment. It is not an impossible one, however. Figure out what you do well and where your passion lies, find others who share in your dreams, and make the collaboration happen. The interview and case research behind this book show that it *can* be done. We hope that these pages will be of help in guiding the way.

SIMON H. BUDMAN, PHD
BRETT N. STEENBARGER, PHD

Contents

The Essential Guide to Group Practice
in Mental Health

CHAPTER ONE

Collaborative Practice: Key to the Future of Mental Health

This is the one true joy in life, the being used for a purpose recognized by yourself as a mighty one; the being thoroughly worn out before you are thrown on the scrap heap; the being a force of Nature instead of a feverish selfish little clod of ailments and grievances complaining that the world will not devote itself to making you happy. And also the only real tragedy in life is being used by personally minded men for purposes which you recognize to be base. All the rest is at worst mere misfortune or mortality. . . .

—George Bernard Shaw, *Man and Superman*

THE FUTURE OF YOUR PRACTICE

This book was inspired by three simple questions we posed to our colleagues and workshop attendees:

- What will your professional practice in mental health look like in 10 years?

- What is your plan for success in this rapidly changing economic environment?

- How will you realize the rewarding career you anticipated when you first entered professional school?

Though we have posed many questions in recent years, we have received few answers. If you're not sure of *your* answers, this book may prove quite helpful.

Your Career Investment

Let's begin with a brief exercise.

First, add up the number of years of professional education and training you have undertaken in a mental health profession. This would include time spent in graduate, practicum, internship, and residency training, as well as continuing education and specialty certification programs. Next, write down the cost of that education. Include direct costs—amounts spent on tuition, fees, books, and living expenses—as well as indirect, or opportunity, costs. The latter consist of income that you decided to forgo by attending professional school. For example, if you attended a training program for 4 years at $12,000 a year and could have used that time to earn $30,000 a year, the *real* cost of your education was $168,000.

Finally, estimate the amount of time you have invested in your professional practice to date, including office space, equipment, and clerical services. Calculate the amount of unreimbursed time you have devoted to building and maintaining your practice, performing such administrative chores as billing, paperwork, marketing, and record keeping. Try to place an hourly value on your time and calculate the magnitude of your investment in your practice. If, for example, you have spent $50,000 equipping and running your practice and have worked 10 unreimbursed hours a week for 5 years and your time is worth $70 an hour, you have invested more than $225,000 in your career.

Now let's put it all together. **How much have you invested in your career?** Chances are, if you've been in business a little while and have an advanced degree, your career investment runs well into six figures.

We strongly suspect you have purchased insurance for any assets that approach the size of your career investment: your car, for example, or your house. No doubt you have also purchased malpractice insurance to protect your career from professional liability. When it comes to the very real threat of changes in health care economics, however, **most of our careers remain at risk**. The minimal response to the questions we posed earlier suggested to us that our professional investments are at risk in a way that we would never tolerate with our life savings. This vulnerability in no way reflects an absence of concern. Rather, our training simply has not provided us with the models or tools needed to master a shifting practice environment.

The Birth of This Text

We decided that the best way to study the future of mental health practice would be to examine success. How *were* professionals succeeding in those difficult "oversupplied" markets? What are the ingredients shared by thriving, innovative, quality-oriented practices? As we began an 18-month exploration, to our surprise—and delight—not only were there success stories, but they were very creative ones at that. Forms of practice never before seen were springing up to secure the futures of participants. They combined practitioner autonomy with tight integration. They melded cost-consciousness with quality-consciousness. They created cultures based on teamwork yet allowed individuals to maintain their own offices, hours, and specializations. Different markets developed different structures, based on the regional needs of clients and referral sources. It was as if we had discovered one of those "punctuated equilibria" of evolutionary biology: a sudden, sweeping shift in adaptation.

Although each market developed its own unique models, **in every case the new, successful practice structures we observed were collaborative.** They created ways for mental health professionals to join forces and secure their futures. Others had already discovered the value of collaboration: Purchasers of insurance benefits were forming coalitions; insurers were merging into managed care conglomerates. Now, behavioral practitioners were aligning in groups, networks, joint ventures, and alliances. What's more, those collaborations were succeeding.

The conclusion seemed inescapable: **Collaboration is the key to the future of mental health.** Strength in numbers, combined with unity of purpose, was central to success and security in each of these markets. Our mission was set: Capture the essence of this evolutionary and revolutionary development.

How You Can Use This Volume

We recognize that readers will be coming to this book with a variety of needs and interests. Perhaps you already belong to a group practice and are looking to expand your services and meet future challenges. You may be a practitioner thinking of forming a collaborative entity, such as a multispecialty group practice without walls. Alternatively, you might be a newly graduating professional or solo practitioner seeking an affiliation with a larger delivery system. In each case, you are contemplating a significant career move and a major investment of time and money. This book has one practical aim: to walk you through the process of joining and forming a multispecialty practice in an enjoyable, understandable, and comprehensive manner. (See Table 1.1.)

We think of this book as **our collaboration with you.** In the coming pages, you will encounter interviews with national leaders in behavioral health, a wealth of hands-on exercises, and as much clinical, legal, and financial information as we could pack into several hundred pages. Our goal is to provide a meal, not just a menu: a set of useful insights and tools that will enable you to tap into the very real opportunities that are present in the mental health professions. Most of all, through these chapters, we hope to share in the excitement of your next stage of professional development, as you design an exciting, rewarding, and fulfilling career.

We begin in this chapter by examining the factors driving the demand for multispecialty groups, so that you can appreciate *why* the future of mental health lies in multispecialty collaboration. We also review the variety of collaborative forms dotting the practice landscape and integrate these into a model that can guide your thinking about joining and forming groups. With this conceptual

TABLE 1.1. What You Can Get from This Book

What you'll find in:	YOUR PRIMARY INTEREST		
	Affiliating with a practice	Expanding an existing practice	Starting your own practice venture
Chapters 1–2	Market trends and opportunities. Tools for planning your career direction and matching a practice to your professional needs.	Identifying opportunities for expansion in a market. Exercises to uncover unmet needs in a marketplace and adapt a practice to these.	Tools for gauging the need for new practices in a region. Evaluating your strengths and weaknesses as a practice leader/manager.
Chapters 3–4	Strategies for evaluating a practice and its potential for success. How to create a match between your professional needs and the structure of the practice.	Understanding and obtaining the financial and information resources needed for expansion. Tools for developing a basic strategy and business plan.	Creating a legal structure for a start-up practice. Steps for developing a core strategy and business How to obtain financing and other start-up resources.
Chapters 5–7	Strategies for assessing and improving cost and quality of your clinical services. Participating in team-based service delivery. Examples of successful collaborations.	Use of online communications and information systems to expand your practice. Tools for organizing and delivering programmatic clinical services.	Building a team-based organizational culture. Organizing integrated clinical services. Successful collaborations and their ingredients of success.

framework under your belt, you will be better prepared for the nuts-and-bolts work of determining the type of practice most likely to meet your personal and professional needs.

☆ IN THIS CHAPTER

- Quality: The force driving collaboration
- Forms of collaboration: Ways of linking services to create success
- The Collaborative Cube model
- Avoiding collaborative pitfalls

THE PROMISE OF COLLABORATION

A collaborative practice is an alternative structure for the delivery of mental health services in which a multidisciplinary collection of professionals coordinates and integrates its services. Through this shared enterprise, the participating professionals create a whole that is greater than the sum of its parts, with distinct benefits to clients, insurers, and clinicians. A collaboration is *not* a collection of individuals operating in isolation. It is a novel structure created by the interdependent union of practitioners.

Collaboration in Behavioral Health Care

For years, the health care professions—including the mental health fields—were largely solo enterprises. This is rapidly changing, as practitioners recognize the benefits of affiliation. By linking to other professionals, they can create convenience for customers and professional and financial synergies for themselves. Consider the Professional Affiliation Groups (PAGs) described by Pomerantz, Liptzin, Carter, and Perlman (1996). These are clusters of solo private practices yoked to psychiatric practices (also solo) for the purposes of case consultation, cross-referral, marketing, and contracting. Participants in the PAGs can offer a wide array of services to clients and referral sources, generating increased business. They also enjoy enhanced professional communications and innovative mechanisms for case management and cost control.

Note, moreover, that the PAG participants do not surrender their personalized forms of service. In the past, collaboration among health care professionals necessarily meant the creation of centralized groups in which all solo practice is abandoned. Although this is one way to organize, it is far from the only model. Solo practices can be melded into shared enterprises with no relocation whatsoever. **The glue supporting the collaboration is not a physical structure but structures of communication and information, supported by well-articulated, shared values.** Traditional groups establish linkages through physical colocation. The new breed of collaborative practice is just as often joined by pagers, computer networks, and fax modems.

> ### ☞ LOOKING AHEAD
>
> The marketplace for behavioral health services is changing rapidly.
>
> Monica Oss, President of Open Minds, shares her perspectives at the end of this chapter (Reader's Resource 1.1).

Although economic trends have no doubt hastened the arrival of collaborative practice structures, we believe that the major influence has been the explosion in communication technology. Just a few years ago, one could not have imagined wireless modems connecting users to the World Wide Web, networked workgroups, and a host of electronic mail (e-mail) services. The maturing of these technologies has made possible practice connections across vast distances.

With expanded communications comes the potential for enhanced collaboration. For example, prior to 1994, the mental health services offered at the SUNY Health Science Center at Syracuse (in Dr. Steenbarger's academic department) consisted of the onsite solo practices of approximately 20 psychiatrists and psychologists. Recognizing that such services were losing their attractiveness to insurers and primary care referral sources, the department of psychiatry established a management services organization called PrimeCare of Central New York, which links the academic faculty to more than 50 community-based social workers, psychologists, psychiatric nurses, and psychiatrists.

With centralized billing, a single point of referral and triage, and an aggressive marketing campaign to the medical community, PrimeCare has created several synergies: (1) greater coordination of behavioral and primary care services, (2) greater access to practitioners and rapid availability of appointments, and (3) new sources of referrals for member clinicians, who now can be competitive for managed care contracts without having to abandon their solo private practices. Indeed, PrimeCare has been asked by insurers to extend its network to other regions—a request that would have been inconceivable in the earlier days. Now, it can be accomplished by recruiting practitioners and integrating them into the larger network through a central computer and communications system.

Collaboration and the Crisis of Quality in Behavioral Health Care

To be sure, collaborative undertakings such as the PAGs and PrimeCare offer multiple synergies, benefiting practitioners, insurers, community referral sources, and clients. A more profound reason, however, underlies the demand for collaborative models: **Traditional models of managed care are not working**.

Managed care primarily arose as a response to alarming escalations in the cost of health care. According to Health Care Financing Administration (HCFA) data cited by Levit et al. (1994), health care expenditures have risen steadily since 1960, from slightly more than 5% of gross domestic product to 13.9%. Adjusted for general inflation in the economy, per capita health care expenditures during that span rose nearly threefold, with those in the public sector exceeding their private counterparts by 50%. Mental health care expenditures rose even more dramatically, doubling the rate of medical inflation during the 1980s (Melek, 1993). The cost of mental health insurance further skyrocketed from the late 1980s to the early 1990s, rising nearly twofold to $318 per employee (Patricelli & Lee, 1996).

State governments and private employers, burdened by these mushrooming costs, embraced managed care as a solution. Unlike indemnity coverage, which passed inflation through to purchasers on a year-by-year basis, managed care limits the cost of health care coverage to a single, fixed dollar amount per insured person (capitation). In so doing, utilization-based financial risk is passed from the benefits purchaser to the insurer, who may in turn attempt to pass it

☞ LOOKING AHEAD

Managed care is only one of the challenges facing mental health professionals.

Our exercise at the end of this chapter (Reader's Resource 1.2) illustrates the growing supply of providers and what it means to your practice.

along to provider organizations. As we shall see, this transfer of risk is one of the major attractions of group practices to insurers. Groups can absorb a sufficient referral flow to predict and manage financial risk. Solo practitioners cannot.

Although it appears that managed care has had a slowing effect on health care inflation (Levit et al., 1994), concerns have mounted that capitated financing rewards the withholding of treatment and compromises quality of care. Comparisons between prepaid and fee-for-service settings, for example, suggest that psychiatrists are more likely to identify and treat depression in the latter (Rogers, Wells, Meredith, Sturm, & Burnam, 1993). There is also evidence that primary care physicians, the traditional gatekeepers of health maintenance organizations (HMOs), are much less effective than psychiatrists in accurately detecting and adequately treating depression (Wells et al., 1989; Sturm & Wells, 1995). Studies of dose–effect in psychotherapy (Howard, Kopta, Krause, & Orlinsky, 1986) call into question the effectiveness of abbreviated treatments for mental health problems of high severity, creating an enhanced likelihood of relapse (Steenbarger, 1994). This conclusion was underscored by the National Institute of Mental Health (NIMH) Treatment of Depression Collaborative Research Program (Elkin, 1994), which found high relapse rates among patients receiving brief psychotherapeutic and pharmacological treatments. Such work raises significant questions as to whether clients with chronic mental health problems are adequately treated at health plans that aggressively attempt to constrain services.

Surveys of mental health professionals reflect this unease. Miller (1996) cites several studies in which an overwhelming majority of practitioners reported that patient confidentiality and quality of treatment were compromised by compliance with managed care policies. In a national survey of more than 700 psychologists, for example, Tucker and Lubin (1994) found that 90% reported incidents in which reviewers interfered with treatment plans and 49% reported adverse outcomes due to treatment delays or denials.

Nor are these concerns limited to practitioners. Two recent surveys of patient experiences strongly suggest that managed plans vary widely in the quality of the services they offer. An investigation commissioned by *U.S. News and World Report* ("Rating the HMOs," 1996) examined the degree to which managed plans met five prevention goals established by the U.S. Public Health Service (PHS), including immunizations, prenatal care, mammographies, Pap tests, and cholesterol screenings. Using data collected by the National Committee for Quality Assurance (NCQA), the report rated 132 HMOs and found that 21 of these exceeded the PHS goals by a full standard deviation or more. Another 23 fell short of those goals by more than a standard deviation. Altogether, 52 of the 132 HMOs failed to live up to PHS standards, including *all* rated HMOs in the states of California, Ohio, Kansas, and Kentucky.

Perhaps the most troubling evidence regarding cost containment and quality was contained in a recent survey of managed health plan enrollees conducted by Consumers Union ("How Good Is Your Health Plan?," 1996). More than 20,000 individuals rated their satisfaction with their health plans on a 100-point scale. There were wide differences in access to care, denials of care, service satisfaction, and physician performance between the top- and bottom-rated plans. Especially noteworthy was the finding that the 10 top-rated plans were organized on a nonprofit basis; of the bottom 10-rated plans, 9 were for-profit. This suggests that a tension may indeed exist between the maximization of profits in managed care and the delivery of quality services.

From Managed Care to Collaborative Care

This crisis in health care quality is of great concern to public and private purchasers of insurance benefits, who face hidden, future costs if illnesses are not adequately treated. Their response has been to form coalitions to demand greater accountability among managed health plans. This is most clearly seen in the accreditation criteria for managed behavioral health care organizations established by the NCQA (1996). To become accredited, managed plans must demonstrate that they have ongoing programs of quality assurance, research-based practice guidelines for triage and clinical care, and evidence of patient satisfaction and service quality. By demanding accreditation as part of the bidding process for contracts, purchasers place quality on a more even footing with cost as a priority.

This trend is not lost on managed care organizations (MCOs) and consumers of health services. The American Managed Behavioral Healthcare Association (AMBHA), a trade association of behavioral MCOs, has recently developed a standardized report card for its members that addresses access, satisfaction, quality, and outcomes (Panzarino, 1995). Called PERMS (performance measures for managed behavioral healthcare programs), it contains such detailed information as access to care based on age and diagnostic category, cost data for severe and persistent mental illness, consumer satisfaction with service and clinical outcome, and effectiveness measures for major affective disorders and substance abuse (AMBHA, 1995). A recent coalition of purchasers and consumers of health care, the Foundation for Accountability (FACCT) has taken a proactive role in developing standardized outcome measures for health care organizations so that the quality of actual clinical care can be determined and compared.

Such efforts are also under way in the public sector (Nelson, Hartman, Ojemann, & Wilcox, 1995), reflecting state governments' concerns that managed Medicaid dollars be used effectively as well as efficiently. In New York, for example, nonprofit organizations such as IPRO (1996) are conducting medical case reviews and quality measurement among managed health plans working under Medicare, yielding programs that both save money and improve health outcomes.

We believe the implications of this development are profound. **The days of adversarial managed care, in which payers lean on providers for ever tighter cost containment, are numbered.** Purchasers of health benefits are no longer simply interested in managing care and its costs; **they want the best possible quality for their money.** Increasingly, a health plan with low cost and low quality is viewed with suspicion. What is saved up front is subsequently lost in needed repairs. This is nicely illustrated in the Medical Outcomes Study of Sturm and Wells (1995). Treatment of depression by mental health specialists (as compared to treatment by general medical practitioners) was twice as expensive in their study but yielded significantly better patient functioning. Overall, the use of specialists *reduced* the cost of achieving a given level of functional improvement by approximately 40%. This is not lost on purchasers, who pay as much in absenteeism and reduced productivity due to depression as they do in direct treatment costs (National Institute of Mental Health, 1994).

This shift in priorities toward quality promises to restructure care every bit as much as the prior shift toward cost containment. This is a result of two fundamental realities:

1. MCOs and purchasers can unilaterally cut costs, but they cannot unilaterally provide quality.

2. Solo practitioners and small groups lack the financial, technological, and personnel resources to meet the quality mandates of purchasers.

These are two of the most important ideas in this book. The provision of superior care requires collaboration between insurers and providers, creating a more interdependent relationship. This collaboration, in turn, necessitates the creation of new practice structures that can engage in large-scale data collection, coordinate and integrate various clinical services, and ensure ready access and availability to clients. **Demands for quality are fueling the need for collaboration.** (See Table 1.2 and Cummings, Pallak, & Cummings, 1996.)

A perfect example of this shift toward collaboration is the clinical group program begun by Value Behavioral Health, Inc. (VBH) and highlighted as one of our case studies in Chapter 7. VBH is a specialty manager of behavioral health services and conducts most of its business in this mode, administering managed mental health services for employers and state governments. In its new program, however, it leaves the administration of clinical services—including authorizations for care—up to collaborative groups of clinicians. Instead, VBH assists these groups in the assessment of quality, using many of the HEDIS (Health plan employer data and information set) and PERMS criteria. Under this arrangement, the clinicians are the managers of care; the managed care company now func-

TABLE 1.2. Why Group Practices Represent the Future of Mental Health

- Group practices can readily coordinate various helping services, such as individual therapy, group work, and psychopharmacology.
- Group practices can offer rapid availability of appointments in easily accessed locations.
- Group practices can invest in the information infrastructure needed to document performance with respect to cost effectiveness and quality.
- Group practices can handle the number of clients needed to participate in risk-bearing contracts.
- Group practices can offer 24-hour crisis coverage and programmatic alternatives to inpatient hospitalization.
- Group practices have the staffing power to assemble ongoing programs of utilization management and quality improvement.
- Group practices have the marketing power to sustain referral flows in a competitive marketplace.
- Group practices offer clinicians the potential of a collegial, collaborative culture and a secure flow of referrals.
- **Most of all, group practice is flexible.** It can be implemented in a way that allows practitioners to retain their solo practices or it can offer a highly integrated, team-based approach to the delivery of services. It can allow clinicians to practice outside of managed care, or can make them more competitive for managed contracts.

tions more as a quality management organization. And, most important, adversarial relations are now replaced with collaboration; instead of ratcheting down reimbursements, VBH offers a quality-based bonus to clinicians.[1]

Designing the Perfect Practice: An Exercise

So far, we have advanced the argument that a new health care revolution is afoot, as managed care becomes collaborative care. It is important, however, that you appreciate these developments for yourselves and achieve a firsthand understanding of their implications. Toward that end, we propose a fantasy exercise.

Imagine that you have a solo behavioral health practice. You are contacted by a representative of a federal grant agency that will make up to $200,000 available to you so that you can design the perfect practice: one with superior service, clinical quality, and cost-effectiveness. What's more, your practice will be reimbursed by clients entirely in cash; no insurance will be involved. (As we said, this

---

[1]Lest we appear Pollyannaish, we must indicate that we have also consulted to a number of group practices that have had very painful and difficult experiences with the managed care companies for which they offer services. On several occasions, group practitioners have described situations to us where the better the group practice did in keeping down costs and maintaining quality the *more* their capitation rates were cut back. Because most managed care organizations are experiencing enormous pricing pressures, it is not at all surprising that this pressure is frequently "pushed down" to the providers, regardless of quality.

is a *fantasy* exercise!) The only catch is that the system you design must be able to *document* its virtues *objectively*. You need to demonstrate that clients receive prompt attention and service and effective care—all at a price they can afford.

Take a moment to jot down some of your ideas. How would clients access services in this practice? How would you ensure that they obtained care that was truly needed according to the best research: no more and no less? How would you address the needs of clients with severe presenting problems, so as to maximize their functioning in vocational and household settings? How could you objectively evaluate the quality of the services that you offered? The outcomes of your interventions? How would you ensure that there is superior coordination of medical, psychotherapeutic, and chemical dependency services?

Many of the coming chapters are devoted to answering precisely these questions. Suffice it to say right now that regardless of your professional affiliation or approach to care, three inescapable conclusions emerge:

1. **You cannot go it alone**. A solo practitioner cannot simultaneously staff a triage phone (for prompt, personal service), meet with clients in routine treatment, and handle emergent situations as they arise. Nor is it likely that any one provider could handle the variety of behavioral health needs that a group of clients are likely to bring in: needs for medication, child therapy, chemical dependency treatment, and so on. An integrated, multi-specialty team of professionals would be necessary to meet the multiple needs of families.

2. **You cannot practice in a vacuum**. The ideal practice would have to be able to address such complex presenting issues as child abuse, eating disorders, and substance abuse. Such problems do not merely touch on the emotional and relationship functioning of clients but have much broader social and medical ramifications. Accordingly, our practice would coordinate services with social services agencies, hospitals, medical providers, and rehabilitation facilities. Close linkages between the practice and these entities would ensure a coordination of treatment plans and an integrated approach to care.

3. **You will need dedicated management**. If the ideal practice is to collect data pertaining to cost and quality and use these data to improve the ongoing performance of professional staff, at least one individual in a managerial role will need to be entrusted with the responsibilities of data collection, maintenance of data collection systems, feedback, and oversight of quality. Moreover, this manager would need a measure of authority within the practice to ensure that the practice patterns of clinical staff take into account conclusions drawn from cost and quality data.

Note that meeting the demands of perfection requires the solo practice to become a collaborative one. As the solo practice becomes responsive to the need to provide and coordinate multiple services, it quickly mushrooms into a shared effort. Further note that this movement is entirely independent of the managed care penetration within the region. It doesn't matter whether the payer is the client, the government, or an MCO; whether we have single-payer health reform, managed competition, or a client-driven system of medical savings accounts. **The very best, accountable care that can be provided requires a shift from fragmented service delivery to coordinated, integrated forms of practice.** This is the single most important reality affecting the future of your practice. Those that succeed in the future of mental health will make the transition away from the mind-set of competing with other disciplines toward a collaborative framework that integrates the best of all specialties (Cummings et al., 1996).

☞ LOOKING AHEAD

What are the 10 critical indicators of quality and how does *your* practice stack up?

Take the Practice Index of Quality (IQ) test at the end of this chapter (Reader's Resource 1.3) and check out your Practice IQ!

FORMS OF COLLABORATION

Perhaps the most fascinating aspect of collaborative practice is its diversity. Every time we think we have exhausted the possibilities of structures, another creative alternative emerges. As a way of organizing our thinking about these forms, we have identified three dimensions of collaborative structure: *scope*, *integration*, and *governance*. We have described them in detail and then combined them into a useful heuristic model. (See Figure 1.1, later.)

Dimension 1: Scope of Collaboration

Scope refers to the breadth of domains covered by the shared enterprise. A collaboration among five mental health professionals, for instance, is narrower in scope than a venture linking a state government to a network of community mental health centers, hospitals, and insurers. In assessing scope, we differentiate *first-*, *second-*, and *third-order* undertakings.

First-Order Collaborations

A first-order structure is the simplest form of practice integration. It is a cooperative venture of professionals from two or more behavioral health disciplines: a multidisciplinary practice. There are three basic models of first-order collaboration: cooperatives, network-model groups, and staff-model groups:

Practice Cooperatives. Practice cooperatives consist of individual, self-employed providers from differing specialties and/or disciplines sharing space and overhead and establishing (usually informal) patterns of cross-referral and coordination of services. Participants in cooperatives cannot hold themselves out to the public as a distinct entity without incurring the shared legal liabilities of a group. Hence, the arrangement is thus primarily one of convenience for providers and patients. This maximizes the autonomy of the participants but limits their ability to collaborate in marketing and contracting.

Network-Model Practices. A network is a decentralized, federated practice in which self-employed professionals supply and occupy their own space and connect to one another through distance technologies. The dispersed nature of the network makes it more difficult to coordinate integrated programs of treatment but allows the providers to flexibly cover wide geographic areas. Participants can conduct their professional practices both within the federated structure and outside, as solo providers.

Staff-Model Practices. Professionals from different professions and specialties are employed by the group and link their services to provide greater integration of care. Such practices feature care for children, adolescents, adults, and families; psychopharmacology, chemical dependency, and psychotherapeutic services; individual and group therapy; and so on. The clinical staff share office space in one or more buildings and draw on their specialties to create integrated programs of treatment.

Satellite-Model Practices. A satellite practice is a hybrid of the network- and staff-model forms: a hub-and-spokes structure. A centralized, multispecialty group creates wider geographic coverage by establishing smaller, satellite practices or by effecting alliances with other provider organizations. These satellites can be as small as a solo office, creating a true melding of staff and network models.

These first-order forms are the basic building blocks of collaborative practices. Each can be formalized, staffed, and managed in a variety of ways to create distinctive strengths (see Chapter 3). A large portion of this book is devoted to the process of evaluating and structuring first-order collaborations, so that practitioners can determine which are most promising for their marketplace and professional needs.

Second-Order Collaborations

First-order structures are multispecialty efforts (typically outpatient) within the mental health disciplines. They create *horizontal integration* by uniting similar professionals. Second-order forms are created by the linkage of these first-order entities with other health care-related enterprises. Such linkages create *vertical integration* by joining organizations in a comprehensive structure that offers programs of treatment across a range of client needs. Let's look at examples of second-order alternatives.

Medical Collaborations. A medical collaboration is a service delivery structure created by the alignment of a multispecialty behavioral practice with a medical practice. For example, a multispecialty group practice might create an alliance with a primary care practice to coordinate the health care needs of clients. The venture may be as informal as the provision of mutual consultation and cross-referral or as comprehensive as merged, colocated services.

Facility Collaborations. When a multispecialty behavioral practice joins with a facility, such as an inpatient psychiatric hospital or a residential treatment facility, new possibilities are created. Such an organization can link levels of care to provide a fuller continuum of services, with cost savings to insurers and patients. The linkage can be structured as an informal alliance or formalized as a separately incorporated joint venture.

Insurance Collaborations. The simplest collaboration with an insurer is a contract between a multispecialty practice and a managed care organization to provide a defined range of services. More elaborate ventures include provider networks or groups owned and funded by an insurer or established to exclusively service a covered population. Such alliances guarantee a referral flow to practitioners and comprehensive services for insurers.

Governmental Collaborations. A governmental collaboration features an alliance between a local, state, or federal government and a multispecialty entity. The most common example occurs when the government is the insurer via Medicaid and Medicare programs. Multispecialty practices might also contract with governments to provide social services and consultative assistance, as with disability evaluations or child abuse programs.

Second-order collaborations tend to be complex endeavors, linking organizations that may have very different operations, cultures, priorities, and missions. A key to their success is the development of a shared mission that meets the needs of all participants. Such projects can also be complex from a legal and an accounting perspective, requiring a high degree of management skill and expertise. For instance, if a multispecialty practice contracts with a business to provide employee assitance program (EAP) services, these services will almost certainly be reimbursed on a per-employee/per-year (capitated) basis. Such reimbursement requires new systems of accounting and careful management of overhead to ensure that the contract is financially advantageous to the practice.

Third-Order (and Higher) Collaborations

Even more intricate from an organizational and management vantage point are third-order collaborations, which feature the integration of a second-order venture with yet another provider, payer, or purchaser of services. Some of these linkages are referred to in the medical literature as *integrated delivery systems (IDSs)*. Often, they synthesize mechanisms for payment/reimbursement with those for comprehensive service delivery. Such systems allow professionals to serve as managers as well as providers of care.

Comprehensive Medical Systems. This third-order alternative features an integrated outpatient health–mental health system linked to one or more facilities. The resulting integrated system can then provide the fullest continuum of services to private patients, MCOs, and recipients of governmental health benefits.

Provider-Model HMOs/MCOs. Here the second-order health/mental health practice entity is utilized as a preferred or exclusive referral option by an HMO or perhaps even purchased by the HMO. The resulting entity is thus both an insurer and a provider of health care. In the reverse model, an integrated health care system could organize as an insurer and contract directly with governmental and private purchasers of health benefits. Such provider care organizations (PCOs) allow professionals to manage their own services without a separate MCO serving as intermediary.

Governmental Systems of Care. These are second-order, multispecialty entities that contract with the government under managed Medicaid or Medicare programs. For instance, community mental health centers might form a statewide coalition and link with a specialty manager of behavioral health care. This entity could then contract with a state government to provide Medicaid services across the state. Alternatively, a governmental program (e.g., CHAMPUS) might contract with a network of provider-model MCOs to deliver in-network health services to employees.

Third-order collaborations are *systems of care.* They are comprehensive entities operating at multiple levels of client need and across health and mental health domains. They are to health care what ABC, CBS, and NBC are to television: complex systems that link local outlets in a comprehensive network.

Dimension 2: Integration

In addition to categorizing collaborations as first-, second-, and third-order, we can arrange these forms along a continuum of integration running from *loose* to *tight.* A loose level of integration is one that does not embrace the total practice of the participants. Tight integration creates an organization that supersedes the preexisting structures of the participants. In large measure, the level of integration determines the degree of commitment each of the participants makes to the new venture.

Loose Integration

Practice within loosely integrated collaborations tends to be highly elective, even on a case-by-case basis. For instance, a therapist could join a practice network and participate in one of the network's contracts but not others. Similarly, a group practice could contract with an HMO but also sign contracts with other insurers. In loose arrangements, clinicians can belong to multiple networks and facilities can participate in multiple IDSs—even ones that compete.

Loose structures do not employ the participants and thus have more limited control over their practices. They often set guidelines and may even monitor adherence to those but have somewhat limited options in terms of dictating practice patterns, policies, and procedures. Loose structures may be perceived as a weakness by practice managers, who find them to be relatively unresponsive to the needs of the enterprise. Because a small amount of a provider's total practice may be conducted within the shared framework, managers have fewer carrots and sticks to offer and less control over the venture's fate.

Looseness, however, is often perceived as a strength by clinicians, who enjoy greater freedom of choice and autonomy in such arrangements. Self-employment is a major attraction of the mental health disciplines for practitioners, including the ability to control one's own working conditions and schedule. Accordingly, professionals may not be motivated to become employees of a large, tightly organized, and potentially more rigid enterprise. A loose degree of integration allows providers to continue practicing within their own frameworks while capturing many of the benefits of interprofessional affiliation.

Tight Integration

Tight structures embrace much or all of the practice of the participants. Not infrequently, tight forms supersede the initial structures of participants through mergers, purchases, or joint ventures. For instance, each department in an academic health center may have its own practice plan, each operating in relative isolation from one another and only loosely affiliated. In a tighter arrangement, the various plans might be merged into a central provider organization with a single source of billing and contracting. The contracts entered into by the provider organization would be binding on all departments and members, creating a tighter linkage. Such a structure is much more maneuverable than a loose practice confederation, a distinct advantage in highly competitive markets. A tight organization, with a high level of commitment from participants, is also apt to maximize the collegial benefits of affiliation. What might be lost in terms of individual autonomy is gained in terms of teamwork, affiliation, and the rewards of being part of a larger cause.

Note that the scope of a collaboration is entirely distinct from its tightness of integration. This is very important. Third-order collaborations can be loose; first-order collaborations can be quite tight. A coalition of community mental health providers that contracts with MCOs, facilities, and state governments is quite large, integrating many entities. It might be a loose confederation, however, with limited control over the caseloads, practice patterns, and evolution of the participants. Conversely, it could be very tight, exercising considerable standardization in the definition and delivery of services.

The degree to which collaborations will be loose or tight will depend on the needs and interests of participants and the demands of the marketplace. **The beauty of collaboration is that it allows participants to choose their levels of integration and commitment**. A practitioner may simply decide to affiliate with a network to augment referrals. Alternatively, he or she may seek new horizons by spearheading a far-reaching venture with a local hospital or an MCO. In taking advantage of the unusual flexibility of collaborative formats, professionals can find the blend of teamwork and autonomy that will best fit their career objectives.

☞ LOOKING AHEAD

What are some of the challenges of finding the right blend of scope and integration in a highly managed environment?

Our featured interview with Bruce Cappo, PhD, at the end of this chapter (Reader's Resource 1.4) offers a first-hand look!

Dimension 3: Governance

A final dimension by which we organize our thinking about collaborations concerns their governance. Governance refers to the day-to-day management of the enterprise, as well as its long-range planning. A *vertical* governance structure, if drawn as an organizational chart, is tall and thin. There are a limited number of individuals at the top, entrusted with the duties of ownership and management, and many lines of authority running downward. A *horizontal* governance structure is relatively short and wide, with leadership roles and responsibilities dispersed among members. The degree to which a collaboration is structured along horizontal or vertical lines plays an important role in determining its management style and organizational culture.

Vertical Governance Structures

Imagine a corporation with a leadership group comprised of several officers and a board of directors setting all policies, procedures, and strategic plans. Many middle managers would be entrusted with coordinating and implementing these plans among employees at multiple sites. Such a vertical structure strives for lean-and-mean leadership and the efficiency of leaving decision making in the hands of a core group of seasoned individuals. It offers the founders of the corporation the greatest degree of control over their venture.

The governance structure also tends to dictate the profit- and equity-sharing characteristics of the firm. Vertical organizations tend to centralize ownership as well as authority, maximizing incentives for those at the top tiers of the organizational hierarchy ("management"). Risk and reward are minimized for frontline employees ("labor"), who are not compensated with stock (shares of ownership) that might become very valuable—or worthless—depending on the firm's fate. This sharp division between management and labor gives the vertical structure a distinctive organizational flavor and can make it difficult for collaborations of professionals to adequately motivate those in employee/staff (nonequity) roles.

Although vertical governance structures can sound authoritarian and noninclusive, they capture an important reality. When one or more individuals place the time, money, effort, and emotion into forming a collaborative enterprise, they are taking significant risks. Such risks will not be prudent unless they can yield meaningful rewards. Centralizing ownership and decision making in the hands of principals is a way of ensuring that risk taking can be adequately controlled and rewarded.

Horizontal Governance Structures

In horizontal governance structures, leadership is much more dispersed among participants than in vertical systems, with considerable decision making and even ownership vested in employees. Good examples of horizontal structures would be many membership organizations in which dues-paying members (or their designated representatives) take the role of shareholders and vote on all major shifts in policy and procedure. The leadership of officers is often augmented by a broad committee structure that has meaningful input into the directions taken by the organization. Here the priority is not lean-and-mean management but shared governance and collegiality.

The culture of a horizontal structure can be highly democratic and participative, which brings advantages and disadvantages. Members can feel more directly connected to—and invested in—organizational objectives, creating greater levels of commitment and motivation. Shared ownership and governance can also become excellent tools for collaborations to attract high-quality talent. Highly democratic organizations, however, can easily bog down in decision making, creating managerial nightmares. If every decision requires full consensus, it is unlikely that many decisions will be made.

Most collaborations seek to balance the advantages of vertical and horizontal structures. Accordingly, there are an infinite degree of intermediate forms, combining elements of vertical and horizontal governance. A matrix structure, for instance, might have an overall leadership format that looks quite vertical. Individual clinical programs within the practice, however, might be coordinated by a cross-section of practitioners acting as a workgroup, creating a horizontal structure for that particular project. Flexible organizations find ways of creating varying degrees of vertical efficiency and horizontal participation for their various undertakings.

It is common to equate integrative looseness or tightness with the horizontal or vertical nature of its governance. However, doing so is a mistake. The defining element of a loose/tight structure is the degree to which the collaboration covers, governs, and controls the entire professional practices of participants. A horizontal/vertical structure, alternatively, is defined by the degree to which participants have an active voice in setting the policies, procedures, and plans that govern the venture and directly share in the venture's success. If broad, multidisciplinary committees of professionals establish a set of practice guidelines that define the practice patterns for all work performed by participants, the result would be a tight structure with a horizontal governance. Conversely, a single owner of a network group practice could establish a vertical governance in a loose structure if network members were free to conduct much of their practice outside the network.

In all, it is our experience that collaborations tend to start small (first-order), loose, and horizontal and evolve toward greater scope, tighter integration, and more vertical leadership over time. This is not unlike romantic relationships, which begin as casual dates and then move through phases of "going steady," "engagement," and "marriage." The earlier, limited, and loose stages facilitate a "feeling out" that helps participants feel sufficiently secure to expand their commitments. The degree to which ventures will so evolve, however, will depend on the challenges posed by the marketplace and the needs of the participants.

The Collaborative Cube

Professional counselors are familiar with the cube concept (Morrill, Oetting, & Hurst, 1974), which defines counselor roles as a function of three intersecting dimensions. Similarly, we can conceptualize any collaboration along the three intersecting dimensions depicted in Figure 1.1. The X axis of the Collaborative Cube describes the scope of the venture: first-, second-, third-, or higher-order. The Y axis captures the degree to which the enterprise is loose versus tight in its level of integration. The third, Z axis depicts the governance structure of the organization along a dimension running from horizontal to vertical. If we imagine that each of these axes traverses an arbitrary scale from 0 to 10, we can see that the point (0, 0, 0) captures a collaboration that is small (first-order), loose, and horizontal. The point (10, 10, 10) describes a broad undertaking (third-order) that is tightly organized and vertically administered. There are many possibilities between these extremes, each with its particular appeal to practitioners and referral sources.

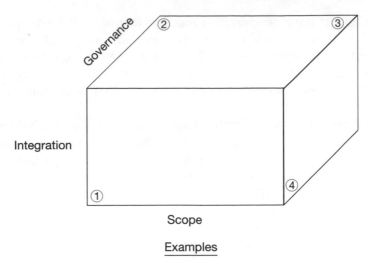

Scope

Examples

Membership Model Network:

1 = A first-order scope, loose integration, horizontal governance

2 = A staff-model group practice: first-order scope, high integration, vertical governance

3 = An integrated medical delivery system: high-order scope, high integration, vertical governance

4 = A multispecialty medical/mental health independent practioner association (IPA): high-order scope, low integration, horizontal governance

FIGURE 1.1. The Collaborative Cube.

The Collaborative Cube is a useful heuristic for the conceptualization of new practice forms. In a single graphic, it captures the essence of how a shared project has been implemented. Following the comprehensive presentations of Kongstvedt (1996) and Korenchuk (1994), we can identify major practice structures at various points on the cube, including:

- **Group practices without walls (GPWWs).** This is a network-model variant in which amalgamations of independent practitioners are linked by a central management entity, often called a management services organization (MSO), for the purposes of marketing and contracting. The network participants may form their own MSO to facilitate billing, contracting, and marketing or may contract with an external MSO for these functions.

- **Independent practice associations (IPAs).** These are multispecialty provider organizations established by clinicians (usually) for the purpose of engaging in at-risk contracts with managed care organizations (especially HMOs). Clinicians are both members and owners of the IPA and participate in its governance.

- **Provider–hospital organizations (PHOs).** Known as physician–hospital organizations in the medical literature, these are higher-scope ventures created when an outpatient provider organization links with an inpatient facility to cover a broad range of behavioral services. The PHO structure may be of relatively low integration, as when a group practice creates an informal alliance with a hospital, or may be highly integrated, in which the facility becomes the owner of the outpatient group.

- **Integrated delivery systems.** Multispecialty medical organizations such as the Mayo Clinic are excellent examples of high scope, high integration delivery systems, in which the full range of behavioral services is joined with a full menu of medical/surgical services. This is becoming a dominant model in regions that have well-known teaching hospitals, medical centers, and hospital systems.

In this book, we focus primarily on the evaluation and creation of first-order collaborations: network-, satellite-, and staff-model groups. This is because the majority of behavioral practitioners are organized in solo and small, single-specialty group formats and need to join or form broader collaborations that can meet the challenges of the quality revolution.

As the cube suggests, there are many ways for practitioners and practice organizations to join forces and share in one another's strengths and expertise. Collaborations can be large or small. They can operate inside or outside managed care. **There is no one best model of collaborative practice**. The key is finding the model that (1) best fits your distinctive strengths and interests and (2) best addresses the needs of the local and regional marketplace. As we shall see in the next chapter, **success in group practice comes when structure fits strategy**.

THE DARK SIDE OF COLLABORATION

We have gone to great lengths to illustrate the diversity and great potential of collaboration. Not all network or group efforts succeed, however. Indeed, an important function of this book is to help readers identify initiatives that are promising and avoid ones that are likely to fail. A poor collaboration is no less shattering than a poor marriage. Before sharing your career with another professional or organization, it is important to know what you're getting into.

How Collaborations Fail

Let's now draw a composite sketch of the Collaboration from Hell (we'll call it CFH Health Care). No single organization possesses all these flaws, but some deserve an A for effort. Indeed, we've seen some collaborations that give new dignity to the French alignment with the Axis powers in World War II.

Consider the plight of a group of solo practitioners in a large urban area. They read in their local paper that HMO enrollment is now exceeding 20% of the privately insured population in the region. Another 20% of the pie has been carved out to preferred provider organizations and specialty managed care organizations. Reimbursement rates are falling and referrals are becoming tighter. Equally alarming, the practitioners see that competition is rising, with medical facilities in the region becoming much more aggressive in their marketing of outpatient behavioral services. Though they enjoy solo practice, they are worried that they will not survive these trends. So they decide to collaborate.

Several of the professionals act as a leadership committee, raise several hundred dollars from each participant, and hire an attorney to set up a group practice. The group is loosely structured, with a horizontal governance. Each provider has one vote and all decisions are made collaboratively. The group maintains itself by charging an administrative fee against all referrals generated by the group. Member providers, however, are free to accept and service their own referrals outside the group structure.

Within several months, what one of our national leaders once called the "deep doo-doo" hits the proverbial fan. Internal squabbling creates significant rifts among the membership, as medical and nonmedical providers differ as to the proper triage of referrals. Those referrals are slow in coming, and the group quickly runs out of start-up capital. Worse still, the members are busy with their own practices and find little time or energy for their unpaid committee/governance responsibilities. Hence, decisions are made by an activist few, only to be challenged and countermanded later at general meetings. This greatly disenchants the activist leadership and bogs down the enterprise. Adding insult to injury, most group members refuse to take referrals generated by the group because these referrals are assessed a fee for administrative overhead whereas nongroup referrals are not.

What went wrong? **CFH Healthcare made the three most common mistakes in collaboration**. Specifically, CFH suffered from the following:

1. **Lack of vision**. The group had no overarching mission or culture. It was an arrangement of convenience and desperation. It failed to plan—and might as well have planned to fail.

2. **Lack of resources**. The group lacked money and time from its members. Because members had no financial incentive to participate in the group's leadership and did not adequately fund dedicated management, governance became a secondary priority.

3. **Lack of know-how**. Even broken clocks are right twice daily, but that doesn't mean that you should remove the battery from your watch. CFH's leadership was well meaning but started without a full appraisal of the needs of the marketplace and participants. The venture was a shot in the dark.

Most collaborations collapse because they are not built on an adequate foundation. Like CFH Health Care, they lack funding and expertise and show little forethought as to the selection of partners and the development of business plans. It is like an impulsive marriage of two individuals desperately seeking to change their circumstances. Such unions rarely last.

The Cost of Poor Collaborations

The several hundred dollars that CFH Health Care members will lose if their group collapses are probably the least of the costs that will be borne. Much more significant are the following:

- **Lost time.** While the group has muddled about, the marketplace has further tightened and opportunities have been unrecognized and lost.

- **Egg on the face.** A dismal venture taints its participants. If CFH does not live up to its obligations to referral sources and insurers, its bad reputation may survive its demise, haunting members for quite a while.

- **Lost momentum.** This is perhaps the least visible but most significant cost. The bitter disappointment of a failed effort can sour the participants on any future form of affiliation, leading to future lost opportunities.

- **Possible catastrophe.** As we shall see in coming chapters, new practice structures have significant legal and financial ramifications. If they are not organized properly, they can lead to catastrophic antitrust and malpractice liabilities lawsuits and IRS obligations. These obligations can pass through to the individual members, creating significant liabilities.

Are we outlining these grisly possibilities just to frighten you? Absolutely. We firmly believe that the future of mental health practice lies in creative collaboration. We have seen the dark side, however. Poor collaborations are like cheap insurance policies. They make you feel secure—until you read the fine print and discover the exclusions.

We encourage you to return to the beginning of this chapter and take another look at your investment in your profession. The choices you make about the future—to affiliate or not to affiliate—put that investment on the line. We encourage you to make your decisions carefully, armed with information and a road map that can guide you to your desired future.

WILL WE HANG TOGETHER . . . OR HANG SEPARATELY?

We conclude this chapter with a short graphic comparing the old, noncollaborative paradigm with the new one (Table 1.3). Successful collaborations create multilevel win-win scenarios. Clients win when they can enjoy convenient, well-integrated services of uniform, high quality. Insurers and benefits purchasers win when those high-quality services can be provided accessibly and affordably. Practitioners win when they can create supportive structures that succeed in the marketplace. The collaborative mind-set is a shift from win-lose, zero-sum games to inclusive, synergistic alternatives.

Much of our training, however, has been locked in a guild mentality in which

TABLE 1.3. Collaborative and Noncollaborative Paradigms

	Collaborative	Noncollaborative
Membership	Multidisciplinary and multispecialty; broad range of services within a single practice.	Unidisciplinary; each practice has a limited number of services for a limited clientele.
Clinical services	Tightly integrated; the work of different specialists is coordinated through the creation of treatment programs and formal practice guidelines.	Unintegrated; providers operate in relative isolation and have their own informal and idiosyncratic patterns of practice.
Culture	Teamwork; a strong emphasis on linking the distinctive contributions of different professionals and learning from one another.	Autonomy; a strong emphasis on the independence of the practitioner and the value of solo practice.
Finances	Risk assumption; group practice is able to accept prepayment for services for a defined population and manage the cost and quality of services in a prepaid environment.	Fee-for-service; practitioners cannot handle the volume of clients or invest in the computer/management resources to undertake financial risk.

disciplines battle one another for turf and attempt to stake out their exclusive positions. Few professional training programs offer meaningful, ongoing experiences in multispecialty care. Collaboration begins with the recognition that each specialty has its value and that this value can be multiplied when professionals join forces to create organizations that are truly accountable for the quality of their efforts. It is not easy to transcend years of fragmented service delivery. As we have seen in this chapter, however, the rich array of collaborative models makes it possible even for solo practitioners to actively participate in the creation of multispecialty efforts. We *can* chart a new course and secure our futures but only by breaking with the past and reaching out to our colleagues. **Those who would lead the orchestra must be willing to turn their backs to the crowd.**

✔ SUMMARY

- Benefits purchasers are driving the demand for accountability for cost and quality.
- Multispecialty group practices are able to provide the level of integrated care, service, and financial management needed to meet these demands.
- Collaborations can occur at various levels of scope and integration to meet the needs of different markets and practitioners.

READER'S RESOURCE 1.1
Conversation with Monica Oss

"We're all struggling with the same problems."

Monica Oss is the president of Open Minds, a provider of information and consultation services to managed behavioral health consumers, providers, purchasers, and payers. She is the editor of two newsletters, *Open Minds—The Behavioral Health Industry Analyst* and *The Open Minds Practice Advisor.* She also is executive editor of the magazine *Behavioral Health Management,* which she views as a potential *"Harvard Business Review* of the mental health field." One of the original founders of American PsychManagement (now Value Behavioral Health), Ms. Oss coordinates a wide range of professional education and consultation services to behavioral health providers and group practices. In a recent interview, she generously shared her perspectives on the field with Brett Steenbarger. A segment of that conversation appears below.

STEENBARGER: Tell me a little bit about your recent experience at Open Minds.

OSS: In our consultation practice we find everyone from the solo practitioner to the largest of hospital chains to the largest of specialty managed behavioral health firms all struggling with the same problems: the integration of the provision of care and risk and the need for better financial and management information systems. It's interesting to me how the problems are the same. Different scale, different applications, but everyone in the field is really grappling with the identical issues.

[The need for timely information regarding cost and quality is a major challenge for both insurers and provider organizations. It underlies much of the need for collaboration between these groups.]

STEENBARGER: What do you see as the major trends affecting behavioral groups in coming years?

OSS: The biggest one when we work with group clients—small or large—is: What is the likely impact of this whole backward integration trend going to be on their practice? For many practices, they are going to be unable without additional capital and organization to overcome the effects of most of the specialty players becoming providers. I see that as the single biggest competitive threat to the independent group.

STEENBARGER: Perhaps you could talk a little more about "backward integration."

OSS: Backward integration is the classic business school development where a large provider of service, rather than purchase the component parts,

(cont.)

READER'S RESOURCE 1.1 (*cont.*)

starts to manufacture them. GM buys Delco Battery. What we're seeing is the large specialty managed behavioral health firms are backward integrating and they're contracting with their networks less and developing their own practices, buying practices, doing joint ventures with practices, and using the independently contracted groups less. They're doing this because they feel that from a price/competition point of view, they need to be competitive.

[This is a fascinating perspective. Many MCOs have been burned when attempting to form or purchase outpatient groups or networks. The potential for collaboration between wholly owned practices and insurers can't be ignored, however. This was one of the pressures encountered by Bruce Cappo's group in Kansas (see Reader's Resource 1.4).]

STEENBARGER: You mentioned an issue that I've often encountered with groups: the matter of adequate capitalization.

OSS: An absolutely critical issue. For groups that decide that they're going into an emerging market like New York City . . . we see all of the major payers moving to managed care models. If people in private practice there . . . want to start a significant group, their issue is: How do they develop a delivery system that is capable of doing risk-based contracting in a geographic distribution area that's large enough to be attractive? It could be anywhere—depending on how the group is organized and structured already—from a $250,000 to $2 million project.

When you're looking at those numbers, there are only a few options available to groups. They can borrow the money, use lines of credit, factor their receivables, or look at other ways they can get commercial credit to finance that. Their second option is some kind of joint venture and sell part of equity in a joint venture group to some larger, better financed organization. It can be one of the specialty firms, a hospital or insurance company, a TPA [third-party administrator], any sort of institution with capital. A third option, and what I've seen an increasing number of groups do, is sell. Sell your group and become part of Apogee, CMG, Merit, Greenspring, or VBH. So I think behavioral health professionals are really struggling with their own identity and what to do to become part of an integrated delivery system.

[Some of the organizations mentioned by Ms. Oss have attempted to form national networks of wholly owned group practices as parts of integrated delivery systems. The notion of a "chain" of collaborative practices with a brand identity is interesting but not yet fully realized in the current marketplace.]

(cont.)

STEENBARGER: Maybe you could talk about future directions for Open Minds and behavioral health.

OSS: I would say the two biggest changes we're seeing are, first, where Medicaid and Medicare were relatively insignificant foci of our practice, that has changed completely in the last 6 months. We've done more capitation models for Medicaid beneficiaries than I ever would have thought possible.

We've also really expanded our scope. It's really interesting, there are different predictions. Some people see the behavioral health field moving to become more medical. I'm seeing some of that, but I'm seeing . . . more integration with child welfare and other human and social services. So we're doing more work with providers of MR/DD [mental retardation/developmental disability] services, foster care programs. That's been very interesting. We're seeing states look at solving these problems by rolling funding streams together and people who never collaborated before suddenly have to collaborate. . . . Many people on the medical side may see it as the demedicalization of the mental health field. . . . That has created some new challenges for being in the information business. People want and need different information than they did even 5 years ago.

[This may be one of the most prescient observations in the book. The shift toward privatization of public-sector services will create vast collaborative enterprises between "wraparound" social services and behavioral health care].

READER'S RESOURCE 1.2
The Provider Explosion:
An Exercise

With a record number of licensed mental health professions, an increasing share of psychopharmacological care provided by primary care physicians and nurse practitioners, tightening controls over utilization, and thousands of new graduating mental health professionals each year, the forces and supply and demand will help to keep reimbursement rates down. Fink (1996) estimates that there are 250,000 licensed/certified mental health professionals in the United States at present: approximately one for every 1,000 Americans. If we assume that 7% of the population utilizes behavioral health services annually for an average of 9 sessions per client (Freiman, Cunningham, & Cornelius, 1994), that amounts to roughly 12 hours of work per week per clinician! **With such an oversupply only becoming more acute as training programs graduate record numbers of new practitioners, the enhanced services offered by collaborative groups become increasingly important in garnering a steady referral flow.**

But how many behavioral health practitioners can *your* market support in a managed marketplace? Here's an exercise that can provide a very rough guideline:

1. Write down the population of your city and the suburban areas within 15 miles. This is the marketplace.
2. Take 7% of this number. This is the number of privately insured persons in the region likely to access behavioral health care in a managed environment.
3. Assume that the average number of sessions per privately insured patient is six. Multiply six times the figure in (2) above. This is the number of sessions provided to the marketplace.
4. Assume that the average provider sees 20 patients per week or 1,000 visits per year. Divide (3) above by 1,000 to arrive at the number of providers sustainable in the market.
5. Of those providers, about 20% will need to be seen by a psychiatrist for medical or psychopharmacological evaluation. Divide (4) above by 5. This is the number of psychiatrists sustainable in the market.
6. Subtract (5) above from (4) above. This is the number of nonmedical providers sustainable in the market.
7. Divide (1) above by 1,000 and multiply by 20. This is the number of inpatient psychiatric days per year within the privately insured marketplace.

(cont.)

8. Divide (7) above by an average length of stay of 7 days. This is the number of privately insured patients requiring inpatient care within the market.
9. Compare (5) and (6) above to the number of providers listed in the Yellow Pages of your phone book.
10. Compare (7) above with the number of bed-days currently available within psychiatric units of hospitals in the marketplace.

Note that these calculations assume a rather tightly managed marketplace. You can adjust the assumptions by using different figures for number of sessions per patient, number of inpatient days per 1,000 in the population, and average length of stay. Even a relaxation of these assumptions will yield figures that result in large-scale underemployment among providers and significant closures of inpatient psychiatric beds in many urban markets. It is our contention that well-managed collaborative practices will be best positioned to thrive in this highly competitive marketplace by offering superior levels of accountability for cost and quality to benefits purchasers.

READER'S RESOURCE 1.3
The Practice Index of Quality (IQ) Test

How does your practice stack up to the quality criteria being established by accreditation bodies such as the NCQA? This test will help you determine how competitive you are at present.

Instructions: Please answer "yes," "sometimes," or "no" to the following questions. Score 20 points for each "yes" answer, 10 points for each "sometimes" response, and 0 points for every "no." Your score is the total number of points.

ACCESS AND SERVICE

1. Does your practice offer multidisciplinary and multispecialty care, with easy access to psychiatric consultation, chemical dependency treatment, and services for children, adolescents, and families?
2. Can a new client with routine needs reach a triage staff person with a single phone call and receive an appointment that is within 5 business days of the initial call?

CLINICAL CARE

3. Does your practice utilize formal, written guidelines for triage and treatment planning?
4. Does your practice have formal mechanisms for interdisciplinary case consultation and peer review?

COST CONTAINMENT

5. Does your practice offer 24-hour crisis intervention as a means for containing problems and keeping clients out of the hospital?
6. Does your practice keep regular statistics pertaining to the utilization of services as a function of diagnostic, treatment, and demographic variables?

QUALITY IMPROVEMENT

7. Does your practice formally assess patient satisfaction with services that are offered and use this information to improve clinical and administrative practices?
8. Does your practice formally evaluate the effectiveness of its clinical

(*cont.*)

services (e.g., treatment outcomes) and use this information to improve treatment planning?

COORDINATION AND APPROPRIATENESS OF CARE

9. Does your practice have formalized mechanisms for facilitating communications and coordinating treatment among mental health providers, between mental health providers and primary care professionals, and between outpatient providers and inpatient facilities?

10. Does your practice ensure that clients with chronic chemical dependency problems, schizophrenia, major depression, bipolar disorder, and psychosis are evaluated and treated by appropriate medical specialists?

SCORING KEY

0–80: Fragmented practice. Few programmatic efforts at cost containment or quality improvement; little multidisciplinary integration of care. This is where most solo and small group practices stand.

80–120: Coordinated practice. Moderate degree of multispecialty integration and some efforts at cost containment and quality assessment. This is the status of most traditional group practices operating under managed care contracts.

120–200: Truly collaborative practice. High degree of multispecialty, programmatic service delivery. Ongoing efforts at maximizing value by improving quality and maximizing efficiency.

READER'S RESOURCE 1.4
Interview with Bruce Cappo, PhD,
Clinical Associates, P.A.

"[We want to] try to be big enough to handle everything in house."

Bruce Cappo, PhD, is the founder and owner of Clinical Associates, P.A., a major behavioral multispecialty satellite practice in the Kansas City area. Dr. Cappo has been innovative in branching out to underserved areas and growing his practice. But, as he details, competitive pressures are increasing. He kindly gave of his time to talk with Brett Steenbarger about the growth of his group, the collaborative strategies he has employed to this point, and the challenges of a consolidating market. Note how the issues of scope and integration have played a major role in the planning of the group practice.

STEENBARGER: Maybe you could give me a little background on yourself, how you became involved in group practice originally, and how your group has evolved.

CAPPO: When I was in the second year at Kansas University and had completed my master's degree, I had started working at the mental health center in Leavenworth. . . . A psychiatrist was there. I became very interested in his private practice. He had a large practice. He was doing a lot of rural stuff as well as work based out of Shawnee Mission near Kansas City. Then I went away, finished up my internship, came back, and ended up being the clinic administrator at that mental health center. He asked me if I was interested in joining his group. He had himself, another psychiatrist, a PhD psychologist, and a woman who was a nurse and a psychologist. The other psychiatrist died and it was the four of us. Then we started expanding a little more, adding people, some of them who had worked at the mental health center previously and had gone on to get their advanced degrees and were interested in the private practice world. . . .

STEENBARGER: This was back when? What year?

CAPPO: 1987, 1988. Then we started branching out a little more into the community there in Leavenworth as well as some of the outlying communities. As we grew bigger and people knew us because of the mental health center—it was because of the small towns where everybody knows you—then they would just call us. As people we had contact with spread out to further and further places, they would call us to further and further places. We started going to a lot of nursing

(cont.)

homes—I think we were covering nine nursing homes at one point—and in a lot of those we were the only nonphysicians to come in and offer services. . . .

[This is a great example of using a niche strategy to secure a base from which subsequent expansion can occur. See Chapter 2 for a discussion of core strategies.]

STEENBARGER: As you were expanding, how was that expansion taking place? Was everyone in the same physical locale or were you expanding in a network?

CAPPO: We were all based out of an outpatient office in Shawnee Mission. It really started as more of a billing office because the psychiatrist was more inpatient-based initially and would just see outpatients at the hospital. We also had another hospital in Leavenworth where they gave us offices. So we didn't have a huge need for an outpatient office. As the practice started growing more, we did move across the street into nicer, larger offices. Then in the smaller communities we would just find the local physician for the hospital and say, "Hey, we want to rent space a half day a week," and that worked out very well. The physicians loved to have us in there, because they could funnel their patients to us. . . .

[Note how Dr. Cappo's group kept start-up costs down by renting space cheaply and using independent contractors, even as it positioned itself nicely with hospitals, nursing homes, and medical practices.]

STEENBARGER: So you were really going after the medical practitioners, renting some space near them, facilitating referrals. Were you working from a staff model for your group at that point? . . . Were people added to the group employed on a salaried basis?

CAPPO: No, this was all on a percentage. . . . I think it was 30% would go back to the practice and that would include all overhead. You'd cover your own testing expenses, travel, and that sort of thing.

STEENBARGER: So the folks joining the practice were independent contractors.

CAPPO: Yes . . . and then when that started getting so big that it was difficult to manage, the psychologists were handling all the paperwork and the reports and had more demands for office staff in the outpatient area. The psychiatrists weren't experiencing that and didn't want to pay for it . . . so I ended up splitting off down the hall, let's see, 3 or 4 years ago, and I took some of the folks with me, including unlicensed assistants. It changed a bit in the last few years, but you could have comparable physician extenders in unlicensed assistants with a psychologist.

(cont.)

READER'S RESOURCE 1.4 (*cont.*)

So I could have PhDs [who weren't] finished with their supervision or hadn't completed all their requirements.

STEENBARGER: And they could bill under your name?

CAPPO: Right. Managed health care has pretty much put a stop to that!

STEENBARGER: Yes. In most areas, they're not too happy when people do that!

CAPPO: But you used to be able to do that. So I had those people as employees, because I was obviously supervising them. And now they've gone on to get their degrees and we have them as independent contractors.

So I split off down the hall . . . and started growing a little bit more there. I set up my own P.A. and I'm the only owner of it still. I brought in the unlicensed assistants who were employees at that time and the other people were independent contractors. We started growing with people who wanted to start a private practice and were doing something else part-time and were moving to the full-time aspect of things. Then there were a couple of people who just wanted part-time work to supplement. . . .

STEENBARGER: What market were you going after at that point? Were you sticking with the old strategy of going after the medical groups or were you expanding into managed care? How were you marketing yourself?

CAPPO: We were marketing toward managed health care. We had gotten on early. The psychiatrist's pull was very much an early force in managed care locally. . . . We joined everything in the beginning and then dropped most of them after a year, because they didn't pay, or weren't run right, or whatever. We were doing a lot of things for HealthNet, which is one of the bigger managed care organizations in town, and we're very open to any of the out-of-town folks. . . . So we started getting into those early on.

The second thing we were doing was contract work. We got into the federal prison system. They have a drug and alcohol prevention services program that was run by the federal government. But I actually started back in Leavenworth. Leavenworth has six prisons now, five back then, and they were looking for people to provide outpatient services to folks who were leaving the penitentiary and were staying in that area, who had gone in for drug problems. Well, the mental health center didn't really want to do it and I thought it would be a great idea. . . . So we started getting in there on a sort of fee-for-service basis. Every 3 years it comes up for cycles and so it started to come up for an actual contract award. We bid on that and also bid on some

(*cont.*)

surrounding areas . . . and eventually we were able to retain the Kansas City area.

[The work with nursing homes and prisons is an excellent example of collaborative practice. Dr. Cappo's practice has been fueled by forming effective partnerships with solid referral sources.]

STEENBARGER: And how much volume was that accounting for?

CAPPO: That was probably at its highest about $8,000 a month. And now it's fallen off, to only a few thousand a month because of the mandated minimum sentences coming into place. All the people who were getting out after one-third of their sentence are no longer getting out! Eventually down the line, there's going to be this huge bump in the snake, so to speak, when the minimum sentences come due.

The other thing we did was get into the Medicaid arena. There were not many private practice folks doing Medicaid, especially not in Johnson County and higher-income areas. So we had that area, where, if you were doing the volume, you could handle the lower fees. We were basically seeing everybody's patients, because we were the only ones doing it.

STEENBARGER: In doing Medicaid, were you doing it through managed care organizations or were you just working straight with the Medicaid system?

CAPPO: Straight with the Medicaid system. It's now coming out . . . there's going to be an RFP [request for proposal] to turn [Medicaid] mental health into managed health care.

STEENBARGER: And with the Medicaid folks, were you doing this through a clinic entity or through the private practice?

CAPPO: Through the private practice group. . . . It eventually became 20 to 25% of our business. Then we started saying, "Gee, this is getting too big. We need to back off on it." But then there started downward pressure on the rates. . . . By going out to the nursing homes—a lot of the people in the nursing homes had Medicaid—we could be on site and have a lot of people available to us. We knew people were not going to not show up. So it turned out to be economically feasible.

STEENBARGER: Did you find many differences between the public-sector clientele and the ones in the commercial insurance pool?

CAPPO: In the rural areas, not a lot. In the suburban areas . . . there were some difference there, obviously. Although we've had much better luck collecting patient payments from people in the lower-to-middle-income groups than we have from the millionaires!

(cont.)

READER'S RESOURCE 1.4 (*cont.*)

STEENBARGER: What kind of growth were you experiencing then?

CAPPO: We were doing about $4,000 a month in billings early on and got up to about $50,000 a month.

STEENBARGER: And in terms of practitioner numbers?

CAPPO: We have 13 now and . . . probably 6 of those are part-time.

STEENBARGER: How many total locations do you have?

CAPPO: Right now we just have this office and the Lawrence office, and we have three other places where we can see people.

STEENBARGER: How have you found the managed care business evolving for your group over the last few years? Is it accounting for more of your volume?

CAPPO: Much more of the volume. And we were in the negotiations more, early on. We were much more partners in bringing these changes about: "What can you do to help?" and so on. Now . . . they're setting more of the rules. "Are you willing to come on?" If they don't get enough people to come on with those rules, they modify the rules only slightly and see what they can get. And it's become much more adversarial. I think they're feeling the squeeze as well.

STEENBARGER: Are those mostly HMOs or the big carveouts also?

CAPPO: We have not worked with the big carveouts yet. We've had negotiations, all of which have fallen through.

STEENBARGER: Why did they fall through?

CAPPO: Well, in the two cases we've had, there have been simultaneous negotiations going on with different people that we were unaware of at the time. The negotiating entity stated that they were unaware that people in their organization were negotiating with different groups as well. But it's been a "whoever can cut the best deal fastest" kind of thing and I think that we were probably not willing to give in as much.

STEENBARGER: And where were they trying to cut deals? What kinds of conditions were they imposing?

CAPPO: Wanting to share the risk, some capitation. Also just super-discounted fees in terms of their holdbacks, where you didn't have control over whether the company would make a profit. If they take a 15% holdback, you're really counting on them to run their organization lean enough . . . and that just seemed like giving up too much control over things.

(*cont.*)

STEENBARGER: Let me get it straight. The withhold is based on *their* performance, not yours?

CAPPO: Well, it's based on the performance of the whole thing overall. They're saying, "We'll sell these contracts and we want a 15% holdback. And if there's a profit at the end, then you guys share in that profit to the extent that you paid into that pool."

STEENBARGER: I see. So it's not just based on your performance as a practice group. . . .

CAPPO: The whole organization. Right. . . .

STEENBARGER: So you're the exclusive provider under that contract?

CAPPO: No, we're in the exclusive provider group, which is less than 10% of their network. Our group is not the only psychologists, but we're probably one of three groups in the entire county. It's pretty limited but not totally exclusive.

STEENBARGER: So if they're doing a withhold, it's not only based on the managed care organization's performance and your performance but on the performance of the other groups as well.

[This is not an ideal arrangement. If a contract requires that a percentage of clinical revenues be withheld and placed at risk based upon cost-effective performance, one wants to be as much in control over the return of the withheld dollars as possible. Under the arrangement described, Dr. Cappo's group could practice very efficiently and still lose the withheld funds.]

CAPPO: Yes.

STEENBARGER: So you're taking multiple levels of risk, it seems.

CAPPO: Yes.

STEENBARGER: Maybe you could talk a little bit about the dilemmas you faced in deciding whether to go with a contract, not go with a contract . . . were those tough decisions for you?

CAPPO: We have, for the most part, been willing to give people a try for about 1 year. It wasn't until the last 1½ to 2 years that things really seemed to take a turn. As of now, we're not as willing to go in for 1 year on things. The one group, through a series of purchase buyouts and mergers, has over 300,000 lives just as a start. They were not willing to cover any psych testing, wanting to pay very low rates, wanting a holdback on the rates they were paying. And they had a ton of lives. And they had a ton of work. So it was a real tough decision in terms of, "Gee, you know they're not going to make money" [as a result of un-

(cont.)

READER'S RESOURCE 1.4 (*cont.*)

derbidding to get the contracts]. So you know you're not going to get that 15% back, if they're cutting deals like that.

STEENBARGER: I see. And what sort of rates were you looking at without the 15%?

CAPPO: In the $63–70 range. Seventy was the highest.

STEENBARGER: And they'd take the 15% out of that.

CAPPO: Correct.

[Note: This would create an approximately $42 reimbursement to an independent contractor, after the 30% overhead deduction.]

STEENBARGER: Wow! They really cut down on the reimbursement. It would almost be worth it to move toward a capitation basis with them.

CAPPO: It would, except that . . . the demand for services in the area we're in is pretty high. . . . We're dealing with a lot of kids, we see a lot of ADD [attention-deficit disorder], behavioral problems in adolescence. The parents are real interested. They're open to psychological services. That's an area they search out. A second group we deal with is the Medicaid types of population, even though they may not have Medicaid. There's just a lot of problem families that would be high utilizers of services. And that's what scared us a little.

STEENBARGER: That would be a tough one. They had 300,000 lives and you decided to pass that up. . . . Who decided to take on that business?

CAPPO: Older people who had not been in the managed health care arena and it was kind of a way to get in the door. Their practices had gone way down.

STEENBARGER: Were these groups or individuals in a network?

CAPPO: Individuals. The other were new people coming up. It was all they could get and they were willing to sell their soul to do it. The other thing that they have said to people is that they want an exclusive group. So they would be willing to let in a large group, but then they want to take over a majority of your business and would somewhat own you. A great deal for no one but them! Especially when next year comes around and it's like, "Gee, things are tighter. We need to increase that 15% to 20%" or whatever it is. So eventually I think what they're moving toward is owned practices without the risk of owning the practice.

STEENBARGER: It seems as though it puts pressure on you if there's a relative glut of practitioners who have to take fees in the $50 range.

(cont.)

CAPPO: Yes.

STEENBARGER: Because if you don't take the business, someone else will. As a result, it ratchets everything down. Have you noticed that in the Kansas City market?

[This is what happens when cost, independent of quality, becomes the central priority. It will be interesting to see how this market is affected by the continuing push for quality, including the need for accreditation among managed behavioral health care organizations and the drive for parity between mental health and medical coverage.]

CAPPO: It has. In fact, I was talking with the psychiatrists. Income is down about $20,000 this year each. Our billables have increased [i.e., hours billed], our collection rate has increased, and our receivables [i.e., cash received] have decreased. So we're getting less per unit served. Mostly because of managed health care. The rates have just snaked down, as you're saying.

STEENBARGER: Looking out into the future, the next five years, how are you as a group practice thinking about dealing with this trend?

CAPPO: The thing that we're talking about, that we haven't taken action on yet is that we would get bigger and add more specialties and try to be big enough where we could handle everything in house. We all know each other, we can provide savings by doing that, and then they [managed care organizations] would be more inclined to deal with us directly and more willing perhaps to not pressure us as much on price, because we have internal controls in house.

[Note how the managed care trend is pushing Bruce's group toward even greater levels of integration and collaboration. Note below also that greater collaboration allows the group to maximize its operations apart from the major managed insurers in the region.]

STEENBARGER: When you say "add specialties," what specialties do you currently have and what would you think about adding?

CAPPO: We have just psychiatry, psychology, and social work. Somebody should be into gerontology, perhaps to cover a lot of the nursing home and older dementia kinds of things that we have. We have an adult psychiatrist and a child psychiatrist, but just expanding that, adding more people, and possibly even down the road further a child-based model, going into pediatrics, something like that.

STEENBARGER: What do you foresee with the 1115 waiver [i.e., statewide waiver from Medicaid regulations allowing for demonstration projects re-

(cont.)

READER'S RESOURCE 1.4 (*cont.*)

garding cost-savings] going through and the Medicaid recipients being enrolled in the managed plans?

CAPPO: We could come out fine on that. The way the state has done it so far—they've done it with the medical end here last year—they've allowed three or four HMOs to cover the various areas. So if they do that same thing with mental health, there are enough players that we are probably going to be in on one of them that gets the contract.

In terms of being able to manage that, the costs are so escalated now because of the mental health centers that it would probably be quite easy to cut some fat and come out looking pretty good, at least the first few years.

STEENBARGER: Would you be partnering with the mental health centers? Would you be taking business from them?

CAPPO: The latter. . . . They've asked to talk with us. . . . I doubt that marriage is going to work. There's such different philosophies.

STEENBARGER: So all of this is creating tremendous competition for the community mental health centers.

CAPPO: The mental health centers in Kansas have formed their own private organization called the Consortium that can then go out and bid against the private practitioners for private business—you have to be a mental health center to join it—while maintaining the advantage of being able to have master's-level people call themselves psychologists and offer services without licenses.

STEENBARGER: Whoa!

CAPPO: That's been the big thing with the mental health centers that we've fought for years. They go out and they say, "Gee, we'll take that state contract from Blue Cross/Blue Shield. We can offer psychologist services for $30 an hour." Well, they can because they get to call their master's-level people psychologists.

STEENBARGER: So it's not a level playing field, from your vantage point. . . . That's a significant development. Sounds like it could be a significant volume.

CAPPO: Especially in certain areas. The way Kansas is set up, as you know, there are areas where there's just nobody out there. They have only the mental health center to deal with. That's their big advantage and that's what they can sell: "We can blanket the state."

[Note here the opportunities for collaborative practices that can cover wide ge-

(cont.)

ographic regions and offer high-quality, cost-effective services to the public sector.]

STEENBARGER: Sounds like you do have some capacity in the rural areas. Is that something you're looking to grow?

CAPPO: We do and we are looking to grow it, but we're also very hindered. The only way you can get psychologists out to some areas is by plane, unless you're living out there. . . . It's very expensive.

CHAPTER TWO

Planning Your Ideal Practice

Being unconquerable lies with yourself; being conquerable lies with the enemy.

—Sun Tsu, *The Art of War*

INTRODUCTION

Imagine, for a moment, going on a European vacation without a map or coaching a major football contest without a game plan. Chances are you wouldn't get very far. Success in any complex endeavor—business, family life, or politics—requires planning.

Strategic planning is the process by which individuals and organizations allocate limited resources to achieve desired ends. A solid plan takes into account one's strengths and weaknesses, as well as environmental opportunities and pitfalls. The cardinal question of planning is, "How can I best apply my distinctive strengths to existing opportunities?"

In this chapter, we take you through the process of planning a collaborative group practice. We help you evaluate your own strengths and weaknesses as well as the opportunities in your marketplace. Further, we help you translate this assessment into a core mission that can guide future collaborative efforts. The process that we describe will assist those starting or growing their own multispecialty practice structures, as well as those evaluating organizations that they

---

☆ IN THIS CHAPTER

- Identifying the resources you need to start a multispecialty group practice
- Making the decision to join versus forming a group
- Assessing the needs of your marketplace
- Developing a core strategy and mission for your practice

might join. With a near infinite number of collaborative formats available to you, how can you know which ones might be right for *your* practice? This chapter should help.

THE RISKS AND REWARDS OF COLLABORATIVE PRACTICE

Because of the marketplace dynamics outlined in the previous chapter, it is our contention that the lion's share of helping services over the next decade will be delivered within accountable, multispecialty structures. This means that your first decision concerns whether you wish to form or expand a collaborative venture versus affiliate with an existing one. There are distinctive risks and rewards inherent in running a complex organization. An honest self-appraisal is necessary to determine where you are apt to find your greatest personal and professional fulfillment.

The Business of Behavioral Health

Self-assessment is difficult. Most of us like to think well of ourselves. We don't enjoy dwelling on our shortcomings. It is rare to find a behavioral health professional who would describe his or her therapeutic or interpersonal skills as "average," even though not all of us can better our peers. Perhaps Oscar Wilde was right: to some degree, we are all self-made individuals in love with our creators.

Before you risk thousands of dollars, scores of hours, and considerable emotional energy, you need to decide whether you have the tools to make a new venture succeed. You don't enter a marathon race unless you have training, considerable motivation, and proper gear. Your collaboration's start-up requires no less.

Whether your initial effort is a small, informal multispecialty group practice near the zero points on Chapter 1's Collaborative Cube (see Figure 1.1) or an integrated system of care, one fact is paramount: **Any practice venture is a business**. A practice is a commercial organization with risks and responsibilities that transcend those of its individual members. As a business, the practice must be managed—and it must bring in more revenue than it expends if it is to survive.

The business nature of professional practice comes as no surprise if you have been engaged in full-time practice. You know all too well the challenges of covering rent, secretarial services, and billing costs. If, however, you are new to practice or engage in part-time private work, you may not think of yourself as a businessperson. Indeed, the very concepts of profit and enterprise may leave you cold.

A recent graduate of a psychology internship—we'll call him Bill—complained bitterly to us about the starting salaries at group practices and insisted that he was being gouged. His reasoning went something like this: I will be expected to schedule 30 hours a week of therapy for which the group will bill in excess of $70 an hour. At that rate, I can bring more than $100,000 of income to the group yet receive a salary of only $40,000. "They're taking advantage of me," insisted Bill, decrying the greed of those who enter the business world.

So we walked Bill through the numbers. True, he was going to schedule 30 hours a week, but how many of those hours would ultimately be billable, given cancellations, no-shows, and problems with collections? And who would be covering his salary during his break-in period with the group, when his referrals are few and far between? In addition to the $40,000, how much would his fringe benefits cost the group? When we figured out what the group would need just to (1) cover overhead, (2) meet plans for future growth, and (3) provide the founders with a reasonable return on their investment, it turned out that Bill needed to generate more than twice his salary to keep the group healthy. A bit more sensitive to the plight of practice owners, Bill took the position.

When you enter the realm of practice development, you are foregoing the safety of a salary and the control of a solo practice for the risks and rewards of owning a business. The first question you must answer in your professional planning process is: Do you want to be Bill, with a salary and a predictable workweek, or do you want to be his employer? Are you looking to build a new venture, or is your desire to see patients? The development of new practice structures is not for those who would shun competition and enterprise. As J. Paul Getty pointed out, the meek may inherit the earth, but not the mineral rights.

The Challenges of Practice Development

With the proliferation of mental health professionals achieving licensure, there is increasing competition for a relatively static clientele. Ten years ago, it was not unusual to open the Yellow Pages in a major town and see only line listings for clinicians. Now it is unusual if you do not encounter large display ads. Competition has increased.

We firmly believe that collaborative practice is a key strategy for success in the years ahead, but we also recognize that it is a perilous endeavor with many hazards.

Financial Risk

Even a small start-up requires an investment of approximately $100,000 in a medium-size market, given initial rent, office, computer, legal, and salary expenses. (see Reader's Resource 1.1, an interview with Monica Oss). Assuming that aspiring founders are able to raise or borrow this money, many cannot tolerate the financial pressures. Pledging your family home as collateral for a business loan takes an unusual level of confidence and risk tolerance.

Uncertainty of Referral Flows

An oft-overlooked hazard in today's practice environment is the fluidity of referral flows. It used to be the case that referrals were largely self-guided and greatly influenced by word of mouth. This created a measure of stability for practices that developed solid reputations within a community. With the increasing influence of managed care organizations, referral flows can change overnight if a major employer switches carriers.

Uncertainty of Pricing

As MCOs undercut one another to build a book of business in your area, they may attempt to maintain their profit margins by cutting reimbursement rates to providers and groups. It would stand to reason that multispecialty practices could command higher reimbursement rates than individual practitioners because they are providing more services to the payer and assuming greater responsibilities. That is not always the case, however. The reward for collaboration is the securing of a referral flow, not necessarily a premium reimbursement. (We have seen in some areas the rapid fall in pricing for capitated and case rate contracts. In some parts of California, where most bad and good trends begin, capitated rates have fallen as low as 25 cents—yes, you read that right—per member per month for outpatient behavioral healthcare. This compares to a more typical range of $1.75–$2.50 per member per month elsewhere.)

Personnel Pressures

The practice manager of a behavioral organization is in the position of reconciling the demands of clinical staff with those of referral sources and insurers. Not uncommonly, the manager is the messenger who is shot for the bad news. Providers are apt to vent their frustration with managed care and business trends to the manager and place unrealistic demands on the manager to wring concessions from insurers. This can produce significant interpersonal conflict within the workplace.

Time Demands

To a person, the practice leaders we interviewed indicated that the job could not be done in a 40-hour workweek. (This is not atypical in any business in which you are responsible for your own livelihood and often that of others as well. Both of us [S.H.B. and B.N.S.] had parents who were self-employed businesspeople who worked long, often unremunerated hours.) Daily schedules are frequently interrupted by late-breaking developments, evening crises, computer breakdowns, and billing problems. Rarely can the start-up venture afford to pay for a full-time administrator. As a result, practice managers often have to maintain an active caseload, adding to time demands.

In sum, leaders of practice enterprises are exposed to considerable wear and tear. The current business environment is highly unstable, with rapid change the norm. At the same time, there is considerable conflict that must be managed with providers, purchasers, referral sources, and insurers. Practice management thus consists of an unusual blend of aggressiveness and patience: an ability to eagerly pursue opportunity but not become discouraged by adversity.

☞ LOOKING AHEAD

Competition in behavioral health is perhaps fiercest in California.

Greg Alter, PhD, of Pacific Applied Psychological Associates offers his observations at the end of this chapter (Reader's Resource 2.1).

The Rewards of Practice Development

Developing a practice venture is a bit like raising a child. There are so many headaches and expenses that the uninitiated are apt to wonder, "Why would I want to go through all of that?" Balanced against these negatives, however, is the very real satisfaction of being a formative part of a growing entity. For many professionals, practice development is a meaningful response to the Eriksonian challenge of generativity.

A colleague with whom we spoke put it this way:

"Before I began this group practice, I worked for the State. It was a regular paycheck, but not very interesting. I did the same thing all the time. Things were always getting jammed up in the bureaucracy. Things would happen and I would have very little say over them. Since starting this group practice, I work 70 hours a week, don't have any real clarity about how much I will make next month and I love it. I am more excited and enthused by this than anything I have ever done in the past. I can be creative and problem solve. I can be seeing patients one hour and going out getting business the next. I'm very anxious about making a go of it, but I can't imagine *not* doing this."

Collaborative practice also offers the rewards of collegiality. As many solo practitioners can attest, private practice can be an intensely isolating experience. In our professional training, we became accustomed to the stimulating interchange of ideas and research. That can be recaptured in multidisciplinary practice. Many of the practices described in this text have explicitly built case conferencing and staff training into their routines, allowing for stimulating, lifelong learning.

Not least of the rewards of collaborative practice are its strategic advantages.

Because integrated structures can provide superior access to care, coordination of services, data collection for accountability, and capacity for risk assumption, they are eligible for a range of referrals that are not open to solo and small group providers. This directly translates into dollars and cents for professionals. As an individual provider, your income is limited to the number of hours you practice times the billable rate minus your overhead. As the principal of a shared practice, you have the potential to earn a meaningful rate of return from the practices of many professionals. In essence, you are making a deal with your clinical staff: You will provide them with a stable income, a positive work environment, and an ongoing flow of referrals in exchange for a portion of the income they generate. By assuming the risk of their overhead, you open yourself to enhanced financial rewards.

STRENGTHS AND WEAKNESSES: DETERMINING YOUR RESOURCES

Our interviews with successful multispecialty groups have convinced us that it takes a unique blending of resources to make a successful practice work. While each organization is unique, there are several elements that we have observed in every one of the stellar practices we've studied.

Resource 1: Leadership

Although there is no single formula for success among practice developers, one common trait stands out: the capacity for sustained, focused effort. The successful practice leader is immersed in his or her work. The group represents a career and a calling. (Remember the old commercial for the U.S. Army? "It's not just a job, it's an adventure.")

This means that many of the elements needed for practice success are identical to those demanded of any entrepreneur operating in a competitive environment, including long hours, a tolerance of risk, a drive to learn new skills and technologies, and a high level of achievement motivation. One challenge for successful practice developers is that their very success takes them away from the clinical work that initially drew them to their profession. It is not at all unusual for the leader of a growing venture to spend at least half of his or her time on administrative and business matters. Such a change is only possible if the entrepreneurial challenge is as meaningful as the clinical activities being replaced.

Blended with this work ethic is an equally strong emotional investment in the success of their staffs. Much as good coaches are devoted to the growth and development of their players, the heads of collaborative practices demonstrate an abiding concern for their clinical and administrative colleagues. This concern is neither authoritarian nor paternalistic; it very much has the flavor of dedication, nurturance, and mentorship.

We have written elsewhere (Steenbarger, Smith, & Budman, 1996) of the similarity between the new breed of collaborative practice structures and the "learning organizations" described by Senge (1990). In such organizations, the ongoing collection of information is used to catalyze the personal and professional development of all participants. The creation of dynamic learning environments was graphically illustrated in our case study of CPG Behavioral Health Resources, a Connecticut-based decentralized group practice (see Chapter 7). Strategic planning for the group was accomplished by a set of committees, each entrusted with a specific aspect of the organization's work: marketing, administrative services, and so on. Fully half of the members of the practice were directly involved in this team-based management. The key to successful leadership for CPG has been the creation of teamwork and the organizational cohesion accompanying a shared vision and effort. In such an organization, the leader is thought of as "coach," not "boss."

Resource 2: Teamwork

There are no hall-of-fame coaches without all-star players. The most talented practice management requires a dedicated staff of administrative and clinical talent. We have had the pleasure of interviewing stellar staff members of thriving collaborations and have noticed numerous underlying similarities:

- **Commitment to care.** Amidst the business pressures of group practice, the all-star clinicians we have observed have not lost their commitment to doing what's right for patients. This sometimes takes the form of going the extra yard to keep a patient out of the hospital or meet the urgent need of a referral source even when your schedule is "filled."

- **Intrapreneurship.** Successful members of collaborative practices are intrapreneurs: entrepreneurs within their own organizations. They actively seek opportunities within the practice and look for ways to develop new and better services. They welcome bonus compensation arrangements that reward productivity and quality.

- **Marketing mentality.** Jeff Zimmerman, the practice director profiled in Chapter 7, made this point effectively. Successful staff members look at everything they do as marketing, whether it is responding to a referral, talking to a patient over the telephone, or participating in a community event. A commitment to service permeates their work.

- **A capacity for work.** There is a saying in Congress that lumps members into two categories: showhorses and workhorses. Successful collaborators fall into the second category. It is not at all uncommon in a thriving practice for members to spend 30 hours per week in direct service and other chunks of hours in paperwork, staff meetings, and other administrative tasks.

Perhaps most outstanding among our observations is that the truly indispensable members of innovative practice organizations describe their work as a career, not a job. Their interest in their work goes far beyond punching a clock and even transcends laudable concern for client welfare. They feel connected to a broader organizational mission that has quality client service and care at its base. As one staff clinician related to us with pride, "We're doing things that have never been done in this region. We're on the cutting edge!" Beyond money and helping, a large part of his motivation was the sense of sharing ongoing learning and professional development with a set of valued colleagues. Stellar staff clinicians believe in what they are doing and are doing what they believe in.

☛ LOOKING AHEAD

Do your personality and needs fit the profile of a practice developer/coach or all-star clinician?

The Practice Temperament Assessment (PTA) at the end of this chapter (Reader's Resource 2.2) may help you decide whether you want to form or join a collaborative group!

Resource 3: Finances

It has been said of warfare that the Lord is on the side of the large cannons. Similarly, fate smiles on collaborations with considerable financial backing. It is a common observation that most small businesses fail because they are undercapitalized. Underestimates of start-up costs and overly rosy projections of first-year revenues combine to produce cash flow crunches and eventual insolvency. A common rule is that start-ups should begin with a cash reserve at least equal to 6 months of operating expenses. This provides some cushion during the initial period when referrals are slow and marketing costs are high. When you consider the expense of simply forming a legal entity; obtaining, equipping, and furnishing a location; and conducting initial marketing, it is easy to see that practice ventures require a substantial initial investment. Once the doors open, fixed costs—including rent, advertising, insurance, and computer maintenance—add to the budget burden.

One group practice we observed started with almost no spare capital, assuming success from day 1. The group, which ultimately succeeded because of fortunate circumstances, came within days of closing on more than one occasion. The stress on the owners was overwhelming. Looking back on the "bad old days," one of the owners of this practice recalled numerous payless Fridays for himself, disagreements and tension with his partners caused by his worry about the practice, and the onset of a terrible colitis problem. Although the practice was now very successful, even thinking about these early, undercapitalized days caused him to wince.

How much money is needed for a successful start-up? As Table 2.1 makes clear, the start-up of a collaborative enterprise is a major financial proposition. Simply furnishing a practice and adequately equipping it with computers, software, and office equipment can run well in excess of $50,000–$100,000. Lazarus (1995) details a start-up plan for a four-clinician group that leases 1,750 square feet of space and employs one and a half full-time equivalent administrative staff. (This, in our experience, would be a very typical start-up.) The group requires $100,000 in initial capital and will incur more than $80,000 of nonsalary, administrative expense in the first year (rent, equipment, insurance, etc.). Clearly, if such a practice cannot generate a steady referral flow in the first year of its existence, it will quickly dig itself a financial hole.

Not surprisingly, new practice ventures often try to get off the ground by cutting corners on these costs, especially in the area of information systems. As a result, these ventures begin their lives severely handicapped in their ability to monitor and document the efficiency and effectiveness of their services. Practices that are technologically challenged are perilously undercapitalized for the present market environment. They cut corners in the very areas that support accountability and collaboration, losing considerable strategic advantage.

Several creative strategies can help reduce the financial challenges of a start-up:

- **Reducing overhead.** Obtaining inexpensive office space, sharing space, using the home offices of practitioners as satellite locations, building word-of-mouth marketing, establishing Internet-based communications systems.

- **Retaining security.** Beginning work in the practice part-time, while holding a secure full-time job. Developing sources of revenue to supplement the practice (consultation, teaching, etc.).

- **Spreading risk.** Beginning with more than one principal and spreading the initial investment (and eventual rewards) across multiple participants, reducing the financial exposure of any one professional.

- **Do-it-yourself.** Creating your own marketing materials, staffing business and administrative functions yourselves, networking with knowledgeable professionals rather than hiring consultants.

Occasionally, practice developers attempt to spread risk broadly by creating a large network-style enterprise at the outset. Such entities are quite difficult to administer, with frequent governance nightmares. Rarely do they have the comput-

TABLE 2.1. Summary of First-Year Expenses, Group Practice Start-Up (4 Full-Time Equivalent Clinical Staff/Owners, 1.5 Full-Time Equivalent Office Staff)

Furniture and Fixtures ($4,000/year on lease basis)
    Office desks and chairs
    Carpeting
    Waiting-room furniture
    Window treatments
    Wall and other decorations
    File cabinets
    Lighting

Office Supplies and Equipment ($6,000/year on lease basis)
    Business stationery and cards
    Paper
    Pens, pencils, clips, staplers, files, etc.
    Fax machine
    Copier
    Phone system
    Pagers
    Mailing

Information System ($9,000/year on lease basis)
    "Server" computer for data processing
    "Client" computers networked to server for data entry
    Integrated clinical/administrative/financial software
    Scanners and software for data entry and document management
    Modems and software for electronic communications (e-mail)
    Installation, service/maintenance
    Word processing and business software

Consultation ($5,000+ for first year)
    Legal
    Accounting
    Information systems
    Clinical training
    Practice development

Initial Marketing ($5,000 for first year)
    Yellow pages and local media advertising
    Announcements
    Design and production of promotional materials
    Travel and conference

Move-in Costs ($21,000/year)
    Rent/Lease payments
    Utility/Phone payments
    Office/Building/Grounds maintenance

Insurance ($10,000/year)
    Commercial liability insurance (theft, fire, accident)
    Professional liability insurance

Personnel ($340,000/year)
    Administrative and clinical salary and compensation payments
    Fringe benefits (life insurance, health insurance, etc.)
    Payroll taxes

TOTAL FIRST-YEAR EXPENSES: $400,000

Note. Expense figures adapted from Lazarus (1995).

er and communications systems in place to adequately create the advantages of collaboration. They also require considerable management talent and effort, given their highly decentralized structure. At their worst, mega-networks are designed more to raise capital than to meet needs defined by strategic planning.

In our research, we have found that successful large collaborations evolve from smaller, successful collaborations. Although there are tremendous advantages to well-designed integrated delivery systems, these advantages rarely pertain to start-ups. If someone approaches you with an offer to invest in a technologically challenged, lightly capitalized, informally managed startup mega-network, our advice, paraphrasing Dorothy Parker, would be to not toss the idea aside lightly. Instead, hurl it with great force. The best predictor of future success is past success.

Resource 4: People

In choosing colleagues and business partners for a start-up practice, it is helpful to have a well-rounded team. A group of five general adult psychotherapists is much less attractive to a referral source than a diverse group of specialists. Were we to start a multidisciplinary practice in a medium-size market at present, we would look to assemble a group of all-star practitioners with superior reputations, established referral bases, and strong motivation to affiliate. We would seek at least one all-star from each of the following areas:

- **Psychiatry**, with strong background in psychopharmacology (preferably child/adolescent as well as adult).

- **Child/adolescent therapy**, with experience working with families, schools, medical, and social service systems.

- **Chemical dependency**, with strong group therapy and program-building skills.

- **Adult psychotherapy**, preferably with some experience with geriatric populations and/or behavioral medicine.

All of our all-star founders would be committed to the team concept. This would be expressed by the intention to conduct all of their practice within the new structure (tight integration) and by their willingness to invest significant time and/or money into the start-up. The founders would also have considerable experience in practice, with strong referral bases and roots in the community. They would have highly ethical characters, impeccable professional records, and demonstrated abilities to work well with others in a team. They would also have a practice philosophy that is compatible with cost-effective approaches to treatment and an interest in documenting the quality of their practice through systematic data collection.

Furthermore, we would try to make sure that some of the previously mentioned individuals (1) differed from the others in gender (and race, especially if seeking a diverse clientele); (2) had significant managerial and marketing background and/or experience; and (3) had significant experience with information systems and the collection of clinical data.

With respect to managerial expertise, most successful practice networks and groups have at least one person designated as Mr./Ms. Inside and one person as Mr./Ms. Outside. It is a happy circumstance when one individual can ably serve both of these roles. Mr./Ms. Inside is the internal practice manager, overseeing everything from hiring and firing to billing, scheduling, budgeting/accounting, and employee complaints. The inside manager usually possesses strong computer skills and experience with data collection, claims filing, and financial management.

Mr./Ms. Outside, conversely, handles external relations with referral sources and clients. The outside manager handles marketing, contracting, and relations with primary care physicians, MCOs, and employers. As the practice's face to the world, the outside manager fills all sales and marketing roles, engages in contract negotiations, and cultivates contacts for referrals. In short, the outside manager sells the service; the inside manager makes it work.

Unless the start-up is going to start large, so that it can support a full-time manager, several people may have to fill the inside/outside roles. Inside managers are good at attending to details and bottom-line issues. They need to be able to work well with clinical and administrative staff. Outside managers typically are friendly and sociable, with a superior ability to communicate the vision of the group to the outside world. When evaluating a group that you may wish to join, take a look at its leadership. Who is Mr./Ms. Inside and Outside? If you cannot envision any of your prospective partners or colleagues in these roles, you may need to rethink your affiliation. To paraphrase the Hart, Schaffner, & Marx commercial, the right collaborators won't guarantee success, but the wrong ones will certainly guarantee failure.

Resource 5: Technology

As we suggested earlier, one of the first things we look for in sizing up a multidisciplinary practice is its technological sophistication. In the old days, groups were built out of bricks and mortar. Today, with flat and even declining reimbursement rates and growing demands for wide geographic coverage, collaborations cannot afford such overhead. Accordingly, they create satellites and networks and link these to the core practice electronically. Computers are the bricks and mortar of the high-IQ practice.

The unsuccessful collaboration is a conglomeration of individuals, each practicing in his or her own way with minimal awareness of the rest of the system. Such systems have little or no idea of the cost or quality of their services.

They lack a coherent identity and mission. Successful collaborations create and maintain much of their sense of team electronically by linking providers for the following functions:

- **Communications.** Through e-mail systems and computer networks, clinicians can readily communicate with each other, facilitating professional consultation and coordination of care. Groups can grow by adding practitioners at sites far from the main office, linking the providers electronically, for low-cost expansion and broad geographic coverage.

- **Billing and financial management.** Centralized billing is attractive to payers, who now can reimburse and adjudicate claims with a single entity rather than scores of individual providers. Computerized systems also allow practices to capture critical information concerning the number of patients seen, types of problems, treated and average duration of treatment. Such systems greatly assist practice managers in financial and clinical management.

- **Service.** Electronic systems can speed and simplify the scheduling of patients through an online master schedule that covers providers at all locations. It is thus possible for a client in the west end of town to call the practice's central location and receive an appointment with a provider in his or her neighborhood—all with one call. Such systems can track the openings of providers, their participation in managed insurance plans, and their practice specializations to best match patients to professionals.

- **Accountability.** It is extremely time-consuming and inefficient to administer, score, and analyze questionnaires concerning quality by hand. Computers can be used to speedily process and summarize a variety satisfaction and outcome measures. This allows managers to identify and correct problems promptly and supports the ongoing professional development of staff members.

To achieve these ends, most collaborative practices need, at the very least, to have easily accessible phone, fax, and copier systems, networked computers for billing and administrative staff, and communication systems that link practice management and providers (see Chapter 5). With such a system, managers should be able to access clinical, financial, and administrative information on a timely basis. **Note: If a variable is not part of the information system, it cannot be monitored and managed**. An information-poor practice cannot be an accountable one.

It is quite common for network-model practices to be linked by separately incorporated management services organizations (MSOs) that handle all billing, clinical data collection, financial report generation, marketing, and contracting on behalf of clinician members. The MSO must be tightly connected to clinicians' offices—usually through a computer network—to facilitate the transfer of scheduling, billing, and clinical data, as well as to maintain a smooth flow of communications among staff and management. The MSO is then reimbursed either on a flat-fee, annual basis (membership fee) or as a percentage of clinical revenues. (We have seen fees as low as 15% for data collection, billing, marketing, and contracting and as high as 60% when the MSO is providing space and equipment, as well as the other services.)

The advantage of an MSO is that it frees providers to do what they do best: provide clinical care. It promises specialized, experienced management and access to technological resources that might be outside clinicians' affordability. The disadvantage of an MSO is that it places much of the venture's leadership outside clinicians' hands and can be quite expensive. Readers contemplating joining a network should carefully examine the technological capabilities of its MSO and its track record of attracting and retaining important contracts. The ultimate acid test, of course, is that the MSO should bring in far more business to clinicians than it charges in administrative fees and save clinicians considerable time with respect to billing, paperwork, and claims adjudication. The MSO should also be sufficiently financed to allow it to periodically upgrade its computers and grow with the group's needs. An MSO that is just breaking even on its current operations will lack such flexibility.

Summary: Your Strengths and Weaknesses

Let us summarize thus far. Your first step in planning to join or form a collaborative group is to identify your strengths and weaknesses with respect to key resources. At this point, you should be able to determine—in a general sense—whether you have the following building blocks:

- The drive, temperament, and commitment to run a successful business.

- The teamwork skills needed to join a successful collaborative practice.

In addition, you should be able to determine whether the practice entity you're thinking of joining or forming has the following:

- Adequate financial resources to begin and/or maintain successful operations.

- The key personnel to lead clinical and business functions.

- The technological expertise needed to create an information-driven system of service delivery.

Many of the mistakes we've seen in joining and forming new practices could have been avoided by engaging in such a basic assessment. It is vital that any practice you affiliate with be capable of surviving and thriving in the long run.

Most of the resources needed for success can be acquired by hiring the right talent, raising funds through investors or lenders, outsourcing needs (billing, etc.) that cannot be provided in-house, and forming alliances/joint ventures with other practice organizations. The one resource that cannot be readily acquired is determination. A recent cartoon in *The New Yorker* showed a darkened storefront with a large sign in the window reading, "Lost our motivation. Everything must go." If the practice is to succeed, passion and determination are vital ingredients **and must begin at the top.**

☞ LOOKING AHEAD

Thinking of joining a multispecialty group in your region? How can you evaluate its prospects for success?

Our Practice Assessment Checklist at the end of this chapter (Reader's Resource 2.3) may prove helpful!

OPPORTUNITIES AND THREATS: ASSESSING THE PRACTICE ENVIRONMENT

Once you have evaluated your strengths and weaknesses and those of your potential colleagues, strategic planning requires an outward turn of attention to promises and pitfalls in the environment. The group you join, expand, or form should fit with the needs of the surrounding community. We would not establish the same group structures in Los Angeles, Buffalo, and Miami Beach. Each of these communities has its own demographic distinctiveness, payer mix, health care infrastructure, and level of competition. In this section, we help you focus on crucial environmental variables that may influence the practice structures you form or join.

Defining Regions of Opportunity

In the first chapter, we outlined trends in mental health care and their accompanying challenges and mandates. Although it is true that these changes are creating great competitive pressures for behavioral health professionals and payers, they have also opened areas of opportunity. Purchasers and insurers alike *need* to work with providers who can deliver and document high-quality services at affordable rates. The changing national picture creates opportunities for entities capable of meeting this challenge. There are several especially important needs created by this development, including the integration of clinical services across specialties (linking child, family, psychotherapeutic, psychopharmacological, and substance abuse services) and the integration of services across levels of care (outpatient, intensive outpatient, residential, inpatient).

Nonetheless, the overwhelming majority of practices have not made the transition to delivering care in ways that can be shown to be convenient, affordable, and effective. Most are located where they always have been, conducting business in much the usual manner. In the terms of our Practice Index of Quality test, they are low-IQ structures. **This creates significant opportunities for visionary collaborations.**

Why do so many low-IQ practices exist? Because they are primarily established to meet the needs of clinicians, not clients or referral sources!

A little experiment might help make the point. On the day we were writing this, it was a national holiday. Many businesses and all government offices were closed. One of us brought the laptop over to the phone and dialed a group practice at random from the Yellow Pages, pretending that he was a patient with an urgent problem. Here is the outcome of the call: *a recorded message.* It said the following:

"You have reached [practice name]. Our offices will be closed from Friday [date] through Monday [date]. If you have an emergency, please go directly to the emergency room."

This is a word-for-word transcription taken from an answering machine from a well-known practice in a major urban area. It appears that the group's manner of handling calls accomplishes two things: It allows practitioners to enjoy their holiday weekends and it minimizes overhead. Meanwhile, it stands in the way of any early intervention with clients with urgent needs. It also routes those with acute, resolvable crises to the most expensive and restrictive forms of care. This is the essence of low-IQ practice. It is the bane of purchasers, and a source of considerable opportunity for you.

Finding Opportunity in Behavioral Health Care Trends

When evaluating the national picture, it is important to recognize that managed care itself is in a considerable state of ferment. For years it was assumed that staff-model HMOs would be the inevitable end point in the development of managed care, as such organizations can exercise the greatest control over cost. This outcome has failed to materialize. As the public's desire for choice among providers has become evident, point-of-service health plans have begun to eclipse more limited options, creating new organizational forms. As a result, managed care today looks quite different than it did just a few years ago.

Such fluidity has rippled through behavioral health as well. At present, several national trends are creating major changes for MCOs and opportunities for multispecialty practices:

1. **Changing antitrust regulations.** The Federal Trade Commission has recently indicated that it would be relaxing its antitrust guidelines regarding

practitioner organizations. In the past, concerted provider efforts to negotiate reimbursements were considered anticompetitive and, hence, a violation of antitrust law. Now, however, in the interest of spurring competition between provider organizations (IDSs) and managed care
organizations, the former group will enjoy greater latitude in negotiating
contracts with purchasers. This promises to create significant opportunities for provider groups that learn the business skills needed to manage
their own care. At present, these provider care organizations (PCOs) will
find the greatest latitude in the Medicare market. If, as anticipated, the result yields cost and quality benefits to Medicare recipients, it is likely that
restrictions on the activities of PCOs will be relaxed in the private insurance arena as well (Gunter & Abbey, 1996).

2. **Carve-in versus carve-out.** Until recently, specialty management firms
   have made the case that behavioral health is different from medical–
   surgical care, requiring separate funding and administration. This, however, has tended to isolate behavioral health from general medicine at a time
   that research in primary care supports the notion of greater integration.
   As a result, an increasing number of behavioral MCOs are looking for
   ways to work with medical organizations and HMOs to carve behavioral
   health care back into the medical system. This promises to create opportunities for collaborations involving medical institutions and primary care
   practices. It also indicates that behavioral practices with consultation/liai-
   son skills will find worthwhile niches (see Cummings, 1996).

3. **Health care reform.** Although the ambitious agenda proposed by President Clinton failed to win congressional approval, health care reform proceeds apace in statehouses. The use of waivers from Medicaid regulations
   to create opportunities for the privatization of governmental insurance
   programs is one of the most dramatic national trends at present. Under
   this arrangement, states are captitating the medical and behavioral health
   benefits of Medicaid recipients and allowing those funds to be administered by private entities. In several states, community mental health systems are banding together to form their own PCOs for the delivery of services under prepaid Medicaid. This is greatly blurring traditional lines, as
   PCOs compete with MCOs for the administration of public insurance
   funds and community mental health PCOs battle private collaborations
   for this business. In addition, there is an increasing push to mandate insurance coverage for behavioral health at parity levels with medical care,
   potentially expanding services under managed plans.

4. **Standardization of practice patterns.** There are meaningful differences
   in the practice patterns of behavioral professionals as a function of geography (Zablocki, 1995) and specialty affiliation (Sturm & Wells, 1995).
   One health care organization with which we worked found patterns of diagnosis and treatment to be widely discrepant between upstate New York

and Downstate New York sites, despite no seeming differences in the demographics of the populations served. Downstate providers were far more likely to diagnose and treat Axis II conditions than were their upstate counterparts, which leaned toward Axis I labels. Purchaser coalitions and insurers are increasingly emphasizing the use of research-based practice guidelines as a means of standardizing care across sites and providers. Indeed, this has become a cornerstone of NCQA accreditation among managed behavioral health care organizations.

These trends suggest that the turbulence of the past decade will continue well into the next. Amidst the threat of change, great opportunities are being created for practices that can do the following:

- Cover large geographic regions.

- Integrate their services with those of medical providers.

- Address the needs of public- and private-sector clientele.

- Manage and standardize their own clinical services.

- Manage increasing levels of financial risk.

Our experience, as well as the feedback we've received from others, suggests that fewer than 1% of all practices are currently capable of meeting these challenges. Groups we have interviewed that are delivering accessible, affordable, high-quality services (see Chapter 7) are expanding rapidly and winning an increasing share of business in their regions.

Opportunities and Threats in the Local Environment

Your assessment of opportunities begins with the recognition that your business has many customers. Clients certainly are customers, but so are insurers, local agencies, school systems, medical professionals, hospitals, and other referral sources. Your practice will thrive if it can address the needs of *all* consumers. This requires a multidimensional assessment.

Whereas the national picture of cost containment sets the overall tone of the marketplace, the dynamics of the local environment tends to shape the specific directions that groups take. A medium-size urban area with ample medical resources, such as Raleigh–Durham, North Carolina, will develop a very different behavioral health care delivery system than an urban area with an extensive public-sector clientele, such as Newark, New Jersey, or a small town setting such as Lawrence, Kansas. Your potential referral sources are perhaps the best source of information regarding your region's needs. These sources are easier to approach than one might think, as they too are looking for solutions in this changing environment. In your planning, you will want to poll several groups of referral agents:

- Directors of EAPs.

- Directors of provider relations for MCOs operating in the region.

- Physicians, especially in primary care (family medicine, general medicine, obstetrics–gynecology, and pediatrics).

- School counselors, school psychologists, teachers, and parent groups.

- Discharge planners and treatment coordinators at inpatient psychiatric and chemical dependency facilities.

To begin your assessment, you might introduce yourself, indicate that you will be joining or establishing a new and innovative multispecialty practice, and ask for the referral source's candid assessment of the local mental health market. In particular, you want to find out the specialty areas within mental health that are in short supply (and hence in need of referrals). You also want to find out the weaknesses of the mental health services currently offered in the community. Your general question to these individuals should be, "What could I provide that would make your job easier?" In addition, it is important to ask *where* services are needed. The MCO may not need another provider in a particular urban or suburban area, but may have enormous needs in a nearby rural area. As Yogi Berra was supposed to have said, "There's a lot you can hear by listening."

You will be surprised by the depth of the responses that you receive. Not uncommonly, referral sources have specific gripes that they are only too happy to share. After all, if you can offer a distinctive service, it can remove some real headaches for those making referrals. Here are a few of the comments we have heard in regional markets:

"It is difficult to find referrals for young children needing therapy."

"We can't find therapists whose strengths lie in working with multicultural populations."

"It's impossible to get someone seen promptly. Sometimes we have people who need to be seen right away."

"It is difficult to work with the psychiatrists in town. They don't seem to understand managed care."

"Once we make the referral, we never hear back from the therapist. It's like a black hole!"

"We have real problems getting prompt psychopharmacology consults."

"The therapists in town only want to work with well-adjusted cases. If a patient has a borderline personality disorder, everyone's practice suddenly becomes full."

"They don't provide any services on an urgent basis. As soon as a crisis arises, they send the patient to the emergency room."

☞ **LOOKING AHEAD**

Collaboration is sweeping the field of chemical dependency treatment.

Paul Curtin of Alcohol Services, Inc., shares his views at the end of this chapter (Reader's Resource 2.4).

Each of these complaints identifies an area of potential opportunity. Your task will be to discern general themes from various referral sources and construct a strategy that will address the identified needs. It is not enough to duplicate services already being offered; you must offer something distinctive to the local marketplace.

Finding Opportunity in Geography

Trends in health care are dependent on the region of the country. For example, it is estimated that 90% of all HMO enrollment is in urban areas ("HMO Enrollment Continues to Grow," 1995). According to Umland (1995), carve-out behavioral health plans are common in the Northeast, utilized by 24% of large employers, but are more rarely encountered on the West Coast, where HMO enrollment is typical. Carveouts are also most common among large employers (35%) but uncommon among small employers (3%). The ways in which your practice deals with managed care and the types of MCOs that you will encounter will depend in part on where you are locating. As a rule, cost pressures will be tightest in regions dominated by HMOs (which generally have limited benefit plans), while quality pressures may be greatest in regions dominated by carveouts (which tend to be more expensive and need to justify the value of that added cost).

Local geography also dictates the distribution of providers within a region. One area may be glutted with practitioners while an adjacent region may be underserved. Such maldistribution often can become a focal point for opportunity.

We suggest a simple exercise to assess the distribution of providers in your area. Purchase a local map and obtain the most recent issue of the area's Yellow Pages. On your map, draw a dot corresponding to the location of each licensed mental health professional in the pages and an × corresponding to the location of each group, hospital, or network practice. In a major urban area, this will take a bit of time and requires a map that includes suburban areas. Nonetheless, take the time. It will give you a picture of the forest beyond the individual trees.

What you will find in many regions is that mental health professionals clump together, with a surfeit of providers in some areas and a near complete absence in others. You'll also find that there may be many therapists within a metropolitan area, but just a few miles out into the country, there are few referral options. When we have talked with mental health professionals about their reasons for choosing a location, we've been surprised to hear that they chose the site not because of its attractiveness to the marketplace but because of its convenience for the provider. As one therapist told us, "I didn't want to have to drive across town to work." One of us started a group practice a number of years ago and, after discussions with insurers, located it 50 miles from the original site!

Geographic dispersion is important because it provides ready access for clients, an important facet of quality for purchasers of health benefits. An insurer with a wide, diverse network is apt to be much more attractive to an employer than one concentrated in a single region. In some cases, this can mean the difference between winning and losing a contract, especially as statewide efforts at privatization demand statewide coverage.

The issue is location . . . location, location, location. Indeed, in our experience, geographic location has been one of the best ways of getting on closed panels for behavioral health preferred provider organizations. It is not at all unusual to have a panel closed in one town but open in a region just minutes away. Not infrequently, the open region is less populated and less affluent than the more popular locations. By observing the clusters of dots and ×'s on your map, you will become aware of areas of potential opportunity.

While mapping provider distribution, keep your eye on areas in which there is a great deal of new-home construction. Many of these areas will be located on the outskirts of major urban centers in locales that are making the transition from rural to suburban. Typically, services do not enter such areas until after a critical mass of families has established residence. This can offer the group practice a ground-floor opportunity to be part of a growing community. Similarly, areas of urban renewal can attract an expanding population and create openings for a conveniently located practice.

Governmental and Insurance Initiatives

Many mental health initiatives emerge on a state-by-state basis and can create special opportunities for practices. Professionals who are well-connected to trade organizations and state governments can learn of new programs and place themselves in a position to benefit from changes. For example, a state might allocate funds for assistance programs designed to address the needs of abused children or families of displaced workers. By teaming up with appropriate social services agencies, it is possible for a multispecialty practice to deliver some of the services included in the assistance programs.

The most extensive statewide initiative at the present time is the transition of public-sector health programs to managed care frameworks. Given the explosion of health care costs in many states, there is growing interest in enrolling traditional Medicaid populations in prepaid health plans. This trend has very important implications for practitioners. Specifically, it suggests that collaborations with social services, community health, and other "wraparound" programs might be in an unusually strong position to build a base of public-sector business. It also suggests new practice opportunities and challenges for existing community mental health providers, who will be pushed to market their services more aggressively and to demonstrate value.

It is also worthwhile to stay in touch with the major insurers in a region and keep an eye on developments regarding plan designs. For instance, we have noted, in some areas, a growing trend toward insurance plans for small employers that place mental health benefits in a separate, optional rider. In those areas, the overwhelming majority of employers do not opt to purchase the rider, leaving employees without coverage. This creates a potential cash market, which could be attractive to groups of professionals seeking a niche outside managed care. Although this niche is likely to be limited in size and profitability, because it will be highly price sensitive, it can provide an important foothold in a community and lead to word-of-mouth referrals of other, higher-margin cases.

Another insurance trend involves the movement away from closed-panel HMOs to more flexible point-of-service (POS) options. In the staff-model HMO, clients are required to receive services from a provider who is an employee of the HMO. Although this gives the HMO control over utilization and cost, it limits the choices of consumers and becomes a frequent target of complaints. In response to the concerns of employers, many HMOs have moved to more flexible arrangements in which the HMO will cover out-of-network services at a higher levels of client out-of-pocket expense. The POS model allows individuals to make the choice of staying in network or going out of network **at the time that services are accessed**. This allows consumers choice but also provides incentives for efficiency. Practices can take advantage of this trend by marketing themselves directly to HMOs as in-network options or by marketing themselves to the public as worthy out-of-network alternatives.

Threats: Assessing Your Competition

No practice planning would be complete without a thorough assessment of the local competition. Clients can access assistance other than your own. Referral sources already have their preferred options. Managed care organizations have built their panels and perhaps already have awarded group contracts. Why should they consider you?

It is vitally important that you identify and assess every collaborative practice operating in your region. This includes group practices, networks, and outpatient practices connected to hospitals, clinics, and multispecialty medical groups. In a small market, this is a simple task. In major urban centers, it requires a concerted effort. Your assessment should not just cover groups in your immediate locale but should extend to those organizations that could plausibly move into your territory. A smalltown practice 30 miles from an urban location may feel like protected turf today but could easily become fish bait if a major group establishes a satellite office and draws the business of a large employer. The key is to know who your potential competition is and what they are doing. This requires a continual ear to the ground and regular contacts with the local provider community through conferences and professional organizations. Every successful practice we have observed has a well-developed "intelligence network" of contacts within its region—and beyond.

There are a number of variables to explore in assessing the competition. First, you want to get a sense of the maturity of your local practice environment. A mature environment is one in which there are numerous multispecialty practices, each with multiple locations. A less mature locale is one typified by a preponderance of solo practitioners and small, single-location groups. A quick review of the Yellow Pages will give you a sense of the marketplace. Clearly it will be more difficult to establish a start-up with distinctive strengths in a mature market; all other things being equal, the competition has raised the bar with respect to access and comprehensive coverage. In a less mature market, even a relatively small group practice may place you well ahead of the pack.

Once you have a sense of the proportion of behavioral practice that is accounted for by groups in a region, it is helpful to establish the extent to which your competition is attracting business from MCOs. This can be determined by contacting provider relations representatives from the major managed care firms writing business in your region. Specifically, you want to know (1) whether the MCO is contracting with groups as opposed to individual provider networks only, (2) whether the MCO routes referrals preferentially to groups, (3) which groups are currently under preferential MCO contracts, and (4) the degree to which current contracts involve risk assumption among provider groups. Once you have made the rounds, you will have a sense of the amount of referral business that is being generated by MCOs, the portion of this that is going to groups, and the specific practices that are gaining a lion's share of this business. The latter probably will be among your most significant competition.

Finally, you will want to determine which practices are growing in your region. Sometimes this can be ascertained by comparing older and newer versions of the Yellow Pages. Fast-growing practices will have added staff and locations, may take out larger advertisements, and so on. It is especially worth talking with practitioners affiliated with the various enterprises. Many groups and networks, for instance, engage solo practitioners as independent contractors as a way of adding capacity to their systems without allowing overhead to mushroom. By talking with the independent contractors, you can gain a sense for how business is faring with a competitor. If the contractors are getting a dwindling number of referrals and voicing displeasure with the situation, this would tell a very different story than if the referral flow were booming.

In most larger regions, such an analysis will reveal several strongly positioned, growing competitors. If you are contemplating starting a new collaboration, these will provide benchmarks that you must meet. If you are an individual practitioner looking to join a multispecialty practice, the strong competitors will reveal the types of services and service delivery features that you will need to provide in your marketplace. The key is to create a distinctive competitive advantage for your practice; **the level of competition in your region will play a major role in determining the speed with which you will need to implement many of the ideas within this book.**

DEFINING YOUR PRACTICE STRATEGY AND MISSION

From your own constellation of strengths or those represented within your start-up and the array of opportunities uncovered by your assessment of the national and local environments, you should be able to define a niche for your individual practice or for any new venture you would undertake. The ideal niche plays to your strengths, covers an unmet need in the local environment, and offers distinctive advantages to referral sources. This niche forms the backbone of your practice *mission*: It shapes the identity of your work. You cannot and should not be all things to all people. Your practice should fill an identified need in the marketplace.

Defining a Core Practice Strategy

The range of possible strategic visions is endless, but several common alternatives link sets of strengths with areas of opportunity.

Low-Cost Strategy

These collaborations consist largely of master's-degree clinicians working in con cert with one or more medical professionals. The practice salaries the clinicians at reasonable, but not extravagant, rates or brings on clinicians as independent contractors. Incentives are frequently created for clinicians to see large numbers of clients. The practice openly courts discounted and managed care referrals and lets referral sources know that, within reason, price will not keep someone from receiving help. By doing a high-volume (albeit lower-margin) trade, it generates considerable word-of-mouth action in a relatively short time and is able to attract some higher-paying clientele as well. Such undertakings are tightly managed, with strong administrative skill, and keep overhead to an absolute minimum. This can be especially successful in locales in which high HMO penetration and large numbers of providers place downward pressure on reimbursement rates.

High-Service Strategy

The practice designs its services to be highly accessible and user-friendly for patients. Patients are seen quickly after they call and referral sources are given rapid feedback. Special efforts are made to treat clients to attractive waiting-room areas and pleasant offices. There is a conscious effort made to accommodate clients' work schedules by arranging meetings on evenings and weekends. Offices are wheelchair-accessible and conveniently located, often in multiple locations near clients' homes and worksites. The practice can be reached 24 hours a day, 7 days a week in case of emergency. It follows up with patients even after they've terminated and monitors patient satisfaction. Over time, the collaboration generates high praise from patients and referral sources and becomes a favored site for referrals. This can be an attractive referral option for behavioral MCOs that emphasize quality and service.

Specialty Expertise Strategy

The collaboration consists of professionals who have developed expertise in a particular area of mental health practice. They teach courses and/or offer seminars at local educational institutions and have published articles in professional media. They use the publications to market themselves to referral sources in the area, especially medical practitioners and other mental health professionals. Accordingly, the practice is often used as a consultant for difficult cases and becomes a preferred site for referral sources needing a particular set of services. Examples of specialty expertise niches: a specialty clinic at a medical center for treating depression, a group that specializes in work with clients of color, and an intensive outpatient program for eating disorders. These practices may not be large and often are not the lowest cost in a region. Rather, they rely on patients to come to them because of their reputation.

Geographic Strategy

The practice is located in a variety of areas, many of which are lacking in mental health services. Each service site is small (as small as one practitioner per locale) and the collaboration is held together by a central office that coordinates marketing, communications, contracting, and so on. Medical staff cover several locations when there is not a need for a full-time psychiatrist at each individual site; the practice also coordinates medical care with primary care physicians in each community. There is a central telephone number by which clients can access help and receive a referral to someone in their community. Not infrequently, the providers located in the small communities make special efforts to be integrated into the social services, school systems, and civic organizations of those towns. This can be especially effective in regions with low population density.

Managed Care Strategy

The practice makes a concerted effort to deliver efficient, effective services to patients seen under managed care plans. Presenting problems are routed to brief therapy as treatment of choice unless contraindicated by factors in the patient's history. Routine psychopharmacological needs may be handled by primary care physicians, especially in HMO networks, with close coordination between behavioral clinicians and those physicians. When possible, the practice develops a variety of outpatient alternatives to hospitalization and bundles these at attractive rates. It also expresses a willingness to risk-share with MCOs and becomes desirable as a core group for several MCOs, guaranteeing a referral flow. Strong management skills and substantial investment in information systems allow the practice to track managed care patients effectively and keep a lid on costs.

Data-Driven Quality Strategy

The collaboration includes members with strong assessment, research, and computer skills and makes a commitment to ongoing data collection. As a result, it has detailed information on the quality and efficiency of services provided by all its members, including data on clinical outcomes. The practice, moreover, expresses a willingness to share aggregate data with MCO partners, giving those MCOs a unique and potent marketing tool. This "mutual marketing" approach creates a broader level of collaboration and allows the partners to enhance each other's market share and develop a favorable reputation among employers for accountability. The practice also uses its data to establish best-practices care guidelines, so that patients can be routed to optimal treatments. These guidelines are under continuous revision as part of ongoing quality improvement programs.

Note that these strategies are not mutually exclusive. Most practices will incorporate aspects of several of the strategies to address the unique needs of a region. For example, the managed care and geographic strategies could coalesce into a potent mission for a network practice. The low-cost and high-service strategies might be linked to market the concept of "value." Smaller collaborations will tend to gravitate toward specialty expertise, low-cost, and/or quality-driven niches to offset their liabilities in terms of specialty and geographic coverage. Larger ventures may take advantage of their management expertise and broad coverage to pursue managed care strategies. Groups consisting largely of psychiatrists and doctoral practitioners will have a hard time implementing low-cost strategies and thus might lean toward specialty, quality-oriented niches. **Each strategy is tailor-made for particular mixes of strengths, weaknesses, and environmental demands.**

Figure 2.1 describes what we call the Collaborative Strategy Matrix (CSM). The horizontal dimension on the grid captures the scope of the multidisciplinary collaboration. This is the breadth of services and professional entities included in the practice, as captured in Chapter 1's Collaborative Cube (Figure 1.1). A small-scope venture integrates relatively few mental health specialties; it is a first-order structure. A large-scope practice combines a diverse multispecialty practice with other mental health entities, such as facility providers and/or insurers.

The vertical dimension describes the overhead cost of the collaboration's professional staff and service offerings. By this, we mean the relative mix between (1) high-priced providers of behavioral services (psychiatrists and doctoral

Scope of practice organization

	Small	Large
Overhead *Low*	Traditional single-location group practice cash market niche	Multispecialty care network Managed care/HMO niche
High	Practice boutique Specialty expertise niche	Facility/provider entity Integrated system of care

FIGURE 2.1. Collaborative Strategy Matrix (CSM).

staff) versus lower-paid providers (master's staff) and (2) high-priced behavioral services (longer-term therapies, intensive treatments) versus lower-priced services (short-term and group therapies). A group practice in an academic department of psychiatry, in which the majority of providers are salaried psychiatrists providing individual therapy and inpatient psychiatric services, would tend to have a high overhead structure. Its cost per treatment episode for an index case would be higher than that for, say, an outpatient network in which most practitioners are master's clinicians doing brief, outpatient therapy and intensive group work. This is important because overhead structure is a major determinant of the fee-for-service or capitated reimbursement that provides an acceptable return on investment to the practice's founders.

The CSM thus describes four core strategies:

1. **Small scope, low cost.** This is a common start-up configuration: a multispecialty practice offering cost-effective services to a defined region. Such a strategy can work well in several environments, including areas in which there are many underinsured and uninsured clients and rural areas in which managed care does not dominate the marketplace. This strategy is especially attractive for providers seeking to operate outside third-party, managed care frameworks.

2. **Large scope, low cost.** The large, cost-effective practice strategy is increasingly seen in regions with high HMO enrollments. The HMOs require considerable geographic coverage and, because of the design and pricing of their benefits, require sharp cost containment. This strategy may be implemented in a variety of network-model collaborations, such as IPAs. Indeed, it is not uncommon for such practices to eventually link with HMOs and/or multispecialty medical groups as part of their strategic vision.

3. **Small scope, high cost.** This is our specialty expertise niche. The practice may be small and cover a quite limited geographic region. The practitioners are apt to have considerable specialty training. They do not at-

tempt to be all things to all referral sources but do one or two things very well. Because of their boutique status and reputation, they can attract clients willing to pay a premium for their services, either through POS insurance plans or pure cash reimbursement. In the best of all worlds, they have such a strong reputation that insurers are forced to court *them*.

4. **Large scope, high cost.** This is what might be called a "system of care" strategy. Many times, the anchor for this strategy is a facility: a hospital, medical center, or chemical dependency rehabilitation program. By their nature, these facilities have high fixed overhead in terms of physical plant and specialty mental health staff. They seek to broaden their exposure to the outpatient arena and develop integrated systems of care. Most provider–hospital organizations and other facility–practitioner entities would fit into this category.

The CSM indirectly suggests two fundamentally flawed strategies: low-overhead collaborations that cannot document their cost-effectiveness and high-overhead collaborations that cannot document their quality. The low-overhead practice that does not collect data regarding utilization and cost loses a major source of potential strategic advantage. It will be vulnerable to competition from provider affiliations documenting high quality. Similarly, high overhead practices need quality data to justify higher reimbursement rates, lest they become vulnerable to competition from lower-cost providers. **Clinicians looking to affiliate with a collaboration are best served, therefore, if they identify the degree to which the practice under consideration is truly accountable for its core strategy.** Your practice's success might be as a Honda, Cadillac, or Porsche. What is important is that your strategy fit your strengths and address the needs of your marketplace.

Developing the Mission Statement

A key component of any business is what it is about and what it stands for. The purpose of a mission statement is to capture, in a relatively concise manner, the essence of your practice's values and directions. Alice's interaction with the Cheshire Cat in *Through the Looking Glass* addresses the value of having a mission statement:

> "Would you please tell me where to go from here?"
> "That depends a good deal on where you to get to," said the Cat.
> "I don't care much where," said Alice.
> "Then it doesn't matter which way you go," said the Cat.

Without a sense of goals and mission, your venture is much like Alice's, lacking knowledge and purpose about its direction.

Mission statements are frequently misused and misunderstood by organizations. At one extreme are ventures without any sort of mission or mission statement. They pursue all business, with little sense of priority or focus. Their employees respond to the challenges of the moment and lack a big-picture sense of purpose. Such businesses often become bogged down in nonessentials, preventing them from positioning themselves for the truly valuable opportunities. They also lack a clear identity in the public eye, which they try to address—in vain— through ever-greater advertising and promotion.

At the other extreme are organizations that become mired in overly detailed strategic plans and mission statements. Endless meetings focus on minute wording changes, political wranglings, and turf battles. Once the massive documents are assembled, the parties breathe a sigh of relief—and promptly retire the volumes to a dusty shelf. Instead of promoting singularity of purpose, the plans and statements paper over the fact that none exists.

Properly conceived and constructed, mission statements capture the essence of an organization's animating values and strategic visions. In considering a mission statement, you need to ask yourself, "What are the core values and purposes of this organization?" "What are the things that we really want other people to remember about us?" "What should be the overarching priorities of our employees?" A good mission statement captures the soul of a practice.

There are two advantages to constructing mission statements. First, the process promotes an aligning of priorities within organizations. The ideal mission statement is neither vague and platitudinous ("We will provide the best quality at the best price") nor mired in detail. It is sufficiently elaborated to highlight the means and ends of an organization, the priorities that should be evident in each business transaction. In fashioning such a statement, it is inevitable that disagreements will arise within the practice leadership. This is helpful. Such disagreements expose important differences in perspective that need to be worked through if the collaboration is to function as a cohesive unit. In requiring leaders to articulate their assumptions, values, and priorities, mission statements can facilitate communication and consensus building—powerful preventive medicine for future conflicts.

The second great advantage of mission statements is the impact they can have on clients and referral sources. A well-constructed mission statement declares to the world that the practice takes its business seriously and *stands for something important*. It conveys a measure of professionalism and commitment. Most important, it helps the public form an image of the enterprise that will create top-of-the-mind awareness when it is time for referrals. When Dr. Steenbarger's university medical center-based group, PrimeCare, was organized, it sought to capitalize on the center's image as a site of research and training. An important part of the group's mission was the concept of "quality, research-based care." This image quickly stuck in the minds of referral sources and greatly facilitated the group's acceptance in the community.

If you are starting your own practice collaboration, a helpful exercise is to assemble the principals and/or the senior staff and simply ask each individual to construct his or her own mission statement for the venture. The statement should capture the basic strategy of the practice and the priorities underlying that strategy. Each participant's statement should then be copied and distributed to every other participant, allowing for comparisons, contrasts, and plenty of discussion. The goal is to reach some basic consensus regarding "Who We Are." One network-style practice that went through a version of this exercise became embroiled in heated discussion when a statement constructed by a leader emphasized the integration of science and practice and the utilization of "empirically based treatments." Several members objected violently, viewing this as a hidden endorsement of of cognitive-behavioral and psychopharmacological approaches over other psychotherapies. They also expressed concern that this would lead to a preferential routing of incoming cases to certain clinicians over others, rather than an even distribution of cases. The theme of the debate became, "Who are we doing this for: patients or ourselves?"

We were present throughout this discussion, and we can tell you that it was not always pleasant. Nonetheless, the exercise was tremendously helpful. It led to the assignment of a committee to develop and recommend practice guidelines that synthesized the diversity of approaches represented by the group and the body of literature supporting particular modalities. It also sensitized leaders to points of view within the practice, allowing them to avoid land mines in the future.

We cannot overemphasize the importance of uncovering and resolving conflicts early in a collaboration. We have consulted to numerous practices that have buried important issues only to have them blow up during the middle of a contract negotiation or during a critical episode of care. This gravely wounds the reputation of a practice. Dana (1996) offers a wonderful exercise for team leaders in which they are required to estimate the cost of such a conflict to their organization. When you take into account the number of people embroiled in the issue, multiply that by their total compensation for that period (salaries plus benefits), and then add in the costs of lost productivity and absenteeism, it becomes clear that a major conflict can cost any business many thousands of dollars. That is money saved if a mission statement exercise can resolve basic disagreements **before the new practice ever opens its doors.**

A Model Mission Statement

Below we've included an example of a mission statement that was assembled by Dr. Budman and his colleagues at a consulting company he founded. The mission statement for Innovative Training Systems (ITS), a behavioral health care consulting, training, and new-product company in Newton, Massachusetts, has been an important centering instrument during a period of rapid growth. It projects a consistent image to staff and customers, serving as both a motivational and a marketing tool. Note that it succinctly integrates a description of the major activities of the organization and its core values and priorities.

☞ LOOKING AHEAD

A mission statement is your organization's face to the world.

　　Innovative Training Systems' mission statement at the end of this chapter (Reader's Resource 2.5) offers one possible model for your practice.

At ITS, all employees have the mission statement in their offices and use it as the basis for the various projects they undertake. ITS came to this statement through an iterative process that took many months of writing and rewriting. Input from employees, colleagues, and potential clients helped to sharpen the statement's focus and impact and address remaining areas of vagueness. Such a mission statement is a living, breathing document. It must change to reflect what your practice is doing and how things are changing. A valuable exercise, we believe, is revisiting the mission statement yearly. Is this still our central, core view of things? Are there any major deletions or additions we wish to make? Such a review helps to keep your eye on what is *really* important: the visions and dreams that initially brought you to this field.

☞ LOOKING AHEAD

Interested in joining a collaborative group practice? How can you ensure that its mission fits with your own?

　　Our personal mission statement exercise at the end of this chapter (Reader's Resource 2.6) might help you identify what is truly important to your own practice.

CONCLUSION

In this chapter, we have seen that there is much more to joining and forming a collaborative group practice than simply signing some agreements and hanging up a shingle. The successful practice synthesizes the strengths of practitioners with the opportunities in the environment to offer distinctive advantages to clients and referral sources.

　　Clearly, there is no single strategy best for all clinicians and markets. In general, those wishing to form or join small, intimate practices will tend to locate in relatively low-population-density areas and/or create specialty expertise and high-service niches that insulate them from high degrees of price competition.

✔ SUMMARY

- Those who succeed in forming collaborative group practices combine a high degree of risk tolerance with a strong desire to coach and mentor others.
- Those who succeed in joining collaborative group practices combine a strong desire for teamwork with an intrapreneurial mind-set.
- The ideal start-up group combines solid financing, managerial, and technological expertise with multispecialty clinical talent.
- There is no single strategy or mission that is right for all groups and markets. Smaller collaborations can establish specialty niches and thrive in more rural markets; larger collaborations are needed for low-cost/high-volume/high-access strategies in more urban, managed markets.

Those seeking to maximize referral flows will tend to offer price-competitive services with wide geographic accessibility, especially in urban regions. The key to success is to (1) identify what you will be doing that is truly distinctive and (2) figure out how you will demonstrate to referral sources that you are truly achieving your distinctive advantage. The groups worth forming and joining are those that have dedicated themselves to a mission and accepted the responsibility of being accountable for its implementation.

READER'S RESOURCE 2.1
Conversation with Greg Alter, PhD

"What everybody's most pleased about is the sense of professional autonomy."

Greg Alter, PhD, is a founder and principal, along with Neil Dickman, PhD, of Pacific Applied Psychological Associates (PAPA), one of the largest behavioral group practices in the country. The group has approximately 11 practice sites, employing more than 55 staff clinicians and contracting with a network of more than 300 providers. A frequent presenter at national conferences and a well-known behavioral health consultant, Dr. Alter has an enduring passion for the integration of medical and mental health care and the use of technology in assisting group practices. He is currently creating a consulting practice, AlterMedX, which assists behavioral group practices with strategies for medical integration and online information system development. He recently spent some time with Brett Steenbarger talking about behavioral health care and the competitive California marketplace.

STEENBARGER: Tell me about your work with PAPA.

ALTER: My jobs . . . have varied from doing everything, from intake, therapy, business planning, business development, et cetera. to, at the end of my job life with the organization, only doing business development. . . . I currently am not even employed by my own business any more. I'm currently back in private practice, as far as my own salary goes, and I am only acting as a principal in the company. I still have my ownership stake. We're so intent on saving cash flow that it made more sense to pull my salary out and let me go solo again.

STEENBARGER: You make it sound as though the margins are pretty tight.

ALTER: The margins are tight. We're talking California. I try to keep in mind that California is not the rest of America. But we look forward to a time when we can be confident of 3% margins. . . . We go between losing a little and making a very little on any given year. Even though we see mechanisms by which we could achieve 8 to 15% margins, every time we start to approach that, there will be another round of cost cuts from the HMOs that get passed on down to us or something occurs that knocks the legs out from under our profit margins.

STEENBARGER: What kind of capitations are you looking at in the California market these days?

(cont.)

ALTER: Capitations for all professional services—hospital, CD [chemical dependency], outpatient, inpatient—consistently under a buck[1]. . .

STEENBARGER: Oh, my goodness!

ALTER: . . . with a low I would say for all professional services with no CD— as low I've heard as 25–30 cents—and high, you still see people with $4 capitations for certain types of contracts. But don't ask me to name any of them, because I don't know any currently!

STEENBARGER: I can see why the margins are very, very tight.

ALTER: The big thing now is to reduce northern California professional services to southern California rates. The competition in southern California has been much more extreme over a much longer period of time, because the volume of patients enrolled in the HMOs has been much higher.

STEENBARGER: Do you find your size gives you meaningful economies of scale?

ALTER: Just starting to. . . . We're all over the northern part of the state. Now we have 11 offices all over the northern part of the state, so there are some obvious administrative economies of scale. I think we're just at the beginning of seeing any possibility that affects our bottom line in a happy sort of way, because at the same time as we are benefiting from some of these economies of scale, we have to make additional infrastructure investments in phone systems, computers, software, and all sorts of stuff like that.

STEENBARGER: Perhaps you can give me some idea of your group's size. You mentioned that you have offices across northern California.

ALTER: Well, our fully capitated business covers over 300,000 lives. Then there's a whole fee-for-service business and business that's not capitated—case-rated—for the managed care companies. That's another 20% of the business. We're about 90% managed care in one way or the other. And we were, say, in 1994, a 3¾ million dollar business and we've grown about 30% each year.

[Note how practice volume has grown faster than profits. This is not unusual in a tightly managed market. By linking a variety of providers across a wide area, PAPA has successfully marketed itself to HMOs but is finding it difficult to turn a sufficient profit to reinvest in information and communication systems.]

---

[1]This compares with a more typical capitation rate of about $2 per member per month in other parts of the country.

(cont.)

READER'S RESOURCE 2.1 (*cont.*)

STEENBARGER: Maybe you can tell me how you're organized.

ALTER: Our philosophy of how we wanted to provide the services from the very beginning was to take what we thought were the best aspects of the community mental health model and see what was good in that and attempt to apply that in a managed care context. So extrapolating from that, the kind of things that we've done have been to maintain as much as possible a staff model. I think it's been one of our major differentiating features from our competition both in general health care and in behavioral care. . . . Most of the staff model medical groups—with the exception of Kaiser—have gone under. The PPO or IPA model has done much better in general medical care in the past couple of years. In behavioral health care, almost all the large MCOs—maybe with the exception of Biodyne in its early years—gave up very quickly on trying to provide services in a staff-model. . . . We are just bound and determined to keep pushing to more integration of our staff model and see it as an ongoing struggle to keep the quality of services up by having as many people maximally involved in the whole culture of the organization.

STEENBARGER: And how do you accomplish that involvement?

ALTER: Everybody gets—and again this harkens to the halcyon days of community mental health—at least an hour of professional supervision a week: individual professional supervision. People who have been on staff more than a couple of years may go into a peer group supervision model and make less use of individual supervision, but individual supervision and consultation are a big part of the glue that holds people together. Especially in the first couple of years, there's an active mentoring program for people so that they get a sense of how we operate, what our philosophy of care is, down to the level of specific treatment protocols.

[This commitment to staff development, even in the face of extraordinary financial pressures, is truly remarkable and distinguishes PAPA as a collaborative practice.]

STEENBARGER: And how do clinicians like that?

ALTER: Well, clinicians now—everybody—would say that the thing they like the best about working for us is the sense of autonomy that they have. They don't brag about their salary, they don't brag about their other working conditions. What everybody's most pleased about is the sense of professional autonomy. I think it proves that professional consultation and supervision aren't necessarily in contradiction with a sense of professional autonomy.

(*cont.*)

STEENBARGER: That's interesting. A staff model is not usually thought of as the model that maximizes autonomy.

ALTER: Right. They're contrasting it in California with the prospect of working with a dozen different managed care companies and dealing with case managers from all of those different managed care companies and filling out the paperwork with no help for all those managed care companies. As opposed to working with us, where we try to minimize the amount of stuff that they have to do that they don't get some central office support for. Eighty percent or more of our services to these HMO customers are where we're in charge of it because we're capitated and we have one set of standards for all those patients.

[This is an excellent example of a trend we believe will become increasingly common: multispecialty group practices accepting the financial risk for care and performing many of the functions previously reserved for managed care organizations].

STEENBARGER: So it's freeing the clinician to do their work.

ALTER: Right. And we don't dictate to them—except in a collegial discussion—what we think the therapeutic plan ought to be.

STEENBARGER: With so many sites—11—and so many clinicians, the communications alone and the computer system. . . .

ALTER: Yeah, it's been inadequate to the job. . . . And yet with the rates we're getting paid, there's not anywhere near the opportunity we would like to upgrade systems to keep up with the level of complexity. So it's an unresolved issue.

STEENBARGER: How are you trying to resolve that?

ALTER: Trying to find more cost-effective mechanisms. . . . We will initially do our appointment scheduling through an Intranet . . . but within a few years we expect we'll have it set up so that all the clinicians will be able to log into our Internet Web site and do their scheduling directly. . . . And it's very cost-effective. . . . These are the sorts of things that, as this computer business gets more sophisticated, it shouldn't get more expensive. It should get more cost-effective . . . And I don't think we've really benefited from the cost efficiencies. By "we" I mean everybody in behavioral health care. It's just gotten bloody complicated and expensive so far. . . . We have hope that it's going to get more cost-efficient.

READER'S RESOURCE 2.2
The Practice Temperament Assessment

The Practice Temperament Assessment (PTA) can help you assess your own temperament and whether it might be best suited for the work of forming versus joining a collaborative group. Simply respond true or false to the following items to indicate your dominant preference.

It is very important to me . . .

1. To have a job that offers a secure salary and little chance of layoff.
2. To do my work in my own way without outside interference.
3. To have work that allows me to be competitive and strive for victory.
4. To teach and learn from my colleagues.
5. To have a stable, harmonious work environment.
6. To figure out my own problems, away from distracting influences.
7. To maximize my income, even if that means taking risks.
8. To have daily contact with peer professionals, socially and professionally.
9. To work in a setting that is not pressured and competitive.
10. To have ultimate control over my practice.
11. To work in a setting that undergoes continual innovation and challenge.
12. To work in a setting that allows open participation and consensus building.
13. To have considerable time for my friends, family, and personal pursuits.
14. To work in a setting where I have full responsibility for decision making.
15. To work long and hard and achieve all I can.
16. To not make difficult clinical decisions before getting the full input of colleagues.

SCORING

Note that the PTA defines two primary dimensions: Risk Taking and Affiliation. Risk takers tend to be achievement oriented and competitively driven and, thus, may be well suited to the development of large practice ventures. Affiliative professionals crave interpersonal contact and sharing of decision making and thus gravitate to group—rather than solo—practice settings.

Scale 1 (Security seeking): Add the number of "yes" scores on items 1, 5, 9, 13

(cont.)

Scale 2 (Autonomy seeking): Add the number of "yes" scores on items 2, 6, 10, 14

Scale 3 (Achievement seeking): Add the number of "yes" scores on items 3, 7, 11, 15

Scale 4 (Affiliation seeking): Add the number of "yes" scores on items 4, 8, 12, 16

Risk-taking index: (Scale 3 – Scale 1)
Affiliation index: (Scale 4 – Scale 2)

The intersection of these dimensions (high/low risk, high/low affiliation) creates four temperaments that can be matched to collaborative formats:

- **Quadrant I (High Risk/Low Affiliation)** describes the classic entrepreneurial "owner-operator," building his or her own practice and retaining significant control over ownership and leadership. Such a professional might be drawn to the development of traditional group practices, where staff conduct a large part of their practice through the group (high integration) and where the owner can exercise hands-on control of the business (vertical governance).
- **Quadrant II (High Risk/High Affiliation)** captures the "empire builder," an enterprising systems builder who is apt to seek out large-scope projects such as networks, joint ventures, and mergers. The desire for affiliation manifests itself as a tendency to delegate and share authority, creating more horizontal governance structures. Inclusion, rather than control, is a management priority.
- **Quadrant III (Low Risk/Low Affiliation)** describes the classic "solo practitioner," a lone wolf who enjoys a high degree of autonomy and a small, stable practice. The desire for independence attracts these professionals to low-integration networks. Often, they do not wish to be burdened with management tasks and prefer delegating such work to MSOs and other vertically governed entities.
- **Quadrant IV (Low Risk, High Affiliation)** categorizes the typical "group practitioner," who seeks stable employment in a collegial setting. These clinicians enjoy participation in horizontal governance structures such as committees and are willing to trade the independence of solo practice for the advantages of ongoing teamwork in a staff-model group.

These are idealized types. Mental health professionals often embody various mixtures of practice traits. Nonetheless, it is instructive to administer the PTA to yourself and gauge your own practice temperament. High scores on any of the dimensions probably indicate a strong set of personal needs that must be addressed in your career planning.

READER'S RESOURCE 2.3
The Practice Assessment Checklist

Your assessment of a practice to join or form will require you to evaluate the groups already in existence in your region. The Practice Assessment Checklist (PAC) will help you to focus on the characteristics of practices that are most worthy of your consideration.

Instructions: Check the following items for each practice entity that you are considering joining or forming.

CAPITALIZATION

1. Does the practice have sufficient cash on hand to weather an initial period of slow referrals or the unanticipated loss of a key referral source?
2. Has the practice sufficiently invested in computer and communication systems that support the goals of accountability for cost and quality?
3. Does the practice generate sufficient free cash flow to fund needed growth and the associated expenses for marketing and specialty (legal, information systems, accounting) consultation?
4. Do the founders of the practice bring a large and stable referral flow and a strong investment of time and money?
5. How much do affiliated clinicians give up to support the overhead of the practice and is this made up for by a stable flow of referrals and an easing of paperwork/administrative burdens?

PERSONNEL AND MANAGEMENT

1. Does the practice consist of a diverse set of all-star clinicians with solid ethical reputations, strong experience, and low turnover?
2. Is the management and staff of the practice committed to quality and cost-efficiency?
3. Are the relationships among management and staff constructive, with an overarching sense of teamwork?
4. Does the management of the practice have sizable experience with marketing, contracting, financial management, and human resource development?
5. If any functions within the practice are outsourced (billing, marketing/contracting), what is the track record and stability of the hired company?

(cont.)

INFORMATION SYSTEMS

1. Does the practice have a reliable, flexible, and user-friendly computer network and software for efficient claims filing, financial management, and authorizations?
2. Is the practice able to capture data from practitioners regarding the types of treatments being offered, patients being seen, number and types of visits offered, etc.?
3. Is the practice able to capture data concerning client satisfaction and clinical outcomes?
4. Does the practice have a phone/reception system to efficiently schedule clients, handle referrals, and triage urgent and emergent calls?
5. Does the practice have adequate communications systems (fax, phone, e-mail, electronic billing) to handle intrapractice communication needs and communications with referral sources?

CLINICAL SERVICES

1. Does the practice offer a broad array of child, adolescent, adult, and family psychotherapeutic, substance abuse, and psychopharmacological services?
2. Does the practice offer a range of individual, group, and intensive outpatient clinical services?
3. If the practice does not cover a broad range of services, has it developed a specialty niche and distinctive expertise in a particular area of behavioral health?
4. Does the practice utilize written practice guidelines to assure a standardized level of care for all clients?
5. Does the practice coordinate specialty services, including psychotherapy, psychopharmacology, and substance abuse work?

READER'S RESOURCE 2.4
Conversation with Paul Curtin

"We're going to live or die as a unit. . . ."

Paul Curtin is the owner and operating head of Alcohol Services, Inc., a Syracuse, New York, outpatient clinic specializing in the treatment of alcoholism. From an inauspicious start as a solo practitioner, Mr. Curtin has built a practice that now extends to three sites and employs approximately 20 full-time practitioners. Most recently, he has taken a significant step by leasing space in a satellite medical practice for a large academic health center. Over the past 10 years, Alcohol Services has made several major transitions, including the shift toward managed care and away from an exclusively public-sector clientele. Recently, Mr. Curtin took the time to talk with Brett Steenbarger about the development of his group.

STEENBARGER: Tell me about the history of Alcohol Services, how you've evolved to this point.

CURTIN: We started in June of 1983. I had worked with the Council on Alcoholism doing programs for adolescent alcoholics and their parents. . . . It worked so well that we got a large group of parents that were really grateful that their children found appropriate help. They wanted to pursue their own health, [because] many turned out to be alcoholic, married to alcoholics, or from alcoholic families themselves. I started Alcohol Services in June of '83. We decided we would focus mainly on family members. Most of the other places focused on just the alcoholic, but we wanted to focus on family members. . . .

We got free office space from the Catholic Diocese in exchange for 6 hours a week of counseling that they never used. Next the Episcopalians gave us free office space. We became licensed by the state as an Alcoholism Counseling Program, but that category disappeared and was upgraded to what was called an Alcoholism Outpatient Clinic. We were struggling along and then the big change came in '84. New York State mandated that group health insurance sold in the state, with relatively few exceptions, give 60 outpatient visits/year for alcoholism. That's when we really started to take off. After a year and a half, we were able to make enough money to rent office space, so that's when we moved. . . . It grew rapidly. This is also the same time when the ACOA (Adult Children of Alcoholics) movement took off and so it was the land of milk and honey. We were really growing.

(cont.)

[Again and again, we see the same formula for success: minimize overhead and detect and capitalize on opportunities.]

STEENBARGER: Were you incorporated?

CURTIN: Yes. A regular business corporation. For the first year, it was a d/b/a [doing business as], but then in September of '84 we were incorporated. This meant that not only were we licensed as a facility, but we were an incorporated one as well. . . . There's a real difference in terms of philosophy between mental health practitioners and alcoholism agencies. Most mental health organizations view themselves as a collection of individuals. Alcoholism clinics are structured to be a single entity. In Syracuse, there's an interesting split. A lot of the other private alcoholism clinics really are compilations of mental health individual practitioners operating under an alcoholism clinic banner. We really believe in doing it as a multidisciplinary team. That's why we have full-time people rather than part-time. We won't contract as individuals with managed care companies. We contract as "Alcohol Services" or not at all. So that's a difference in philosophy that we're finding . . . we're going to live or die as a unit, as a facility, rather than as a compilation of individuals.

[Note here the concern that successful practice heads exhibit regarding the culture of their organization. While minimizing overhead is important, creating staff cohesion and teamwork is an even greater priority.]

STEENBARGER: Maybe you could give me a sense of your growth in numbers.

CURTIN: Right now we have about 170 [patients] in Cortland and 240 in Syracuse. We grew from just the three of us to bringing on more counselors as the years went by. We had a bit of constriction about 3 years ago and we had to redo some things, but now it's starting to pick up again.

STEENBARGER: How many total staff do you have?

CURTIN: Around 20.

STEENBARGER: All your staff are employees rather than independent contractors. What's your thinking behind that?

CURTIN: We think we work best as a team. We are all in the same boat. That includes clerical people as well. We figure the best way to do that is to have everybody salaried and go from there.

STEENBARGER: Which means you have some overhead.

CURTIN: Yes! High overhead and a low forehead!

STEENBARGER: You said there was a constriction a few years ago. What was that all about and how did you weather it?

(cont.)

READER'S RESOURCE 2.4 (*cont.*)

CURTIN: We were really pushing the boundaries of what could be defined as alcoholism counseling. We were long on lengths of stays; there were advanced sobriety issues that we were dealing with. And then right on the day the Gulf War started, Blue Cross—which made up maybe 60% [of the group's income]—said they're going to review all of our cases. They were going to limit their view of what alcoholism counseling addresses. The alcoholism benefit is better than the mental health benefit, so they wanted to make sure only alcoholism counseling was being performed. Right away we had 60% of our revenue threatened on 3 weeks notice.

STEENBARGER: Wow!

CURTIN: And in addition to reviewing all the current cases, they were going to preauthorize all treatment and only do so in 10-visit increments.

STEENBARGER: How did you respond to that?

CURTIN: Well, by losing around 12 pounds and experiencing a lot of anxiety. Until then, like I said before, it was the land of milk and honey, with unlimited availability. Treatment could go on and on. Under the category of alcohol counseling, we were able to provide some pretty advanced care. What was missing was the notion that patients would have to pay for the treatment if insurance didn't reimburse us. Our counselors weren't prepared to ask patients to pay for their care.

You see, the alcoholism field, in my mind, tended to have an inferiority complex in terms of the notion of asking people to pay cash for services. When people weren't going to be covered by insurance, the counselors weren't confident enough in themselves to sell it. If you want advanced, ongoing care, it's going to have to come from your own pocket. There was a dropoff in terms of the people coming; there was a great deal of anxiety on the part of the staff. At the time, I thought it was the worst period we could have gone through. Now my perceptions have changed. I was talking with the head of Central New York Blue Cross telling him that he did us the biggest favor possible. Five years ago, we were going through what the alcoholism field is going through today. So it allowed us to prepare and learn from our mistakes and position ourselves nicely.

[Successful practices have a knack for turning adversity and challenge into opportunity. Alcohol Services used the changes in financing of services to rethink its mission and core business.]

STEENBARGER: How much was your business down during the worst of the crunch?

(*cont.*)

CURTIN: There were cash flow problems. They would hold up the cash while they reviewed the cases. I made sure the staff got paid, but I went through periods of time where I wasn't getting paid. At that time, I had to really shuffle things around.

STEENBARGER: So it really forced you to work in a managed care-friendly way.

CURTIN: Definitely. As a result of that, we asked ourselves: What does alcoholism treatment mean? What do we want people to come away from here with and how can we give it to them in the best possible way? That allowed us to develop the structured program that we have right now, which is very effective.

But also you realize you're never going to win in an adversarial relationship with these giants. . . . After getting kicked around an awful lot, it finally dawned on us that the best thing we could do is not view insurance companies—or, later, managed care companies—as the enemy. But to actually view them as partners. And that is a huge difference. . . . The big dawning for us is that we have some mutual interests with these guys. If we go out and actually begin to talk and develop relationships, things usually go pretty well. In any field, there are some bad guys, but what we've been finding is that by developing relationships, it makes a difference.

I'm on the Governor's Alcoholism Advisory Council. . . . One of the other members is the head of Blue Cross of Rochester, one of the first to get into the HMO business for the Blues upstate. Around 2 years ago, everyone was moaning and groaning about how managed care was going to destroy the alcoholism field and all that. Finally he became fed up and admonished us: "You're sticking your heads in the sand! You're all moaning and groaning! You should view this as an opportunity!" All the people around the table looked at him as if he were speaking Greek. But to me it was a turning point.

A couple of months ago, we continued the conversation and he said to me, "The first thing you have to realize is that we don't want to put you out of business. Because if we did, we'd have to reinvent you." And I said, "Oh!" As a result, I started to do research in terms of what alcoholism costs the medical field. It's astounding. The alcoholism field unfortunately has viewed itself as part of the criminal justice and social services system. We give lip service to the fact that alcoholism is an illness or a disease, but we stay completely away from medicine. So what we're trying to do is hook up with the medical field. What we're finding is that the people who are most receptive to it are the business managers of practices, managed care firms, and the bean counters. We find the most resistance from physicians.

(cont.)

READER'S RESOURCE 2.4 (*cont.*)

[In our experience, this is one of the major differences between quality MCOs and ones that are narrowly opportunistic. The quality companies are in the business for the long run and have to develop ongoing relationships with provider organizations. Their goal isn't simply to quickly win and milk contracts; they want to establish themselves as a partner.]

Everyone is scared about capitation and yet we're tremendously excited by it. Right now physicians have a financial interest in not treating alcoholism and continuing to rack up billings for cirrhosis, pancreatitis, and all the rest of it. . . . But if you have capitation and a limited amount of money in the pool, that $1 you spend in treatment could save $7 in medical costs. Now they have a financial interest in it. Unless they identify and refer alcohol-related patients, the financial drain to practices under capitation will be difficult to sustain.

READER'S RESOURCE 2.5
Innovative Training Systems' Mission Statement

Innovative Training Systems is a company of behavioral health care researchers, consultants and clinical trainers all of whom employ time- and cost-effective concepts to our work, ever remaining sensitive to the varying needs of society in light of the changing healthcare environment. With each other, we strive for mutual respect and collaboration, the sharing of responsibility, and effective resource management. We take these core values to our consulting clients so that they, in turn, will bring them back to their workplaces. These values also permeate our research and new product development efforts.

As researchers and developers of innovative behavioral health care tools we have a responsibility to maintain the highest ethical standards in carrying out our studies and to develop products that will be useful and beneficial to the diverse populations in our society. As trainers and consultants, our first mission is to educate health care organizations, corporations, and providers in high-quality, time- and cost-effective methods for their members, subscribers, and clients. Here too, we value diversity and are committed to the highest quality treatment of all populations.

We recognize the difficulties and challenges inherent in the changing healthcare environment, and we hope that from these changes new possibilities and exceptional opportunities will emerge. Through our new product development and applied research we seek to help significantly improve the delivery of health care services both nationally and internationally. Through our consultation and training, we seek to enable those we serve to identify and refine their existing skills while providing them with options for new approaches to optimize those skills. Our new product development, training, and consultation are continuously evolving, based on the ongoing integration of current knowledge, information, experience, and research.

Revised September 17, 1995

READER'S RESOURCE 2.6
Personal Mission Statement

The purpose of a mission statement is to focus attention on essential values and goals. This aids in internal planning, keeping a practice on track, and makes a powerful statement to referral sources and other external constituencies. The following is a form for a personal mission statement that can help individual practitioners align their priorities with those of a group that they might join or form.

[My Practice Name] was founded on [date] in [location] as a type of practice organization/structure]. It was originally established to provide types of services to targeted clientele in a manner consistent with core practice values. Unlike other practices, I sought to establish a service that offered [key benefits to clients] and [key benefits to referral sources]. Accordingly, [My Practice Name] drew upon my training in the field of [mental health specialty] and my extensive experience with [prior experience and postgraduate training].

Since its foundation, [My Practice Name] has evolved to offer [new services] to [new targeted clientele]. These services have maintained [core practice standards] while offering [distinctive benefits] to clients. [My Practice Name] has been especially responsive to the changing needs of referral sources by offering [new and distinctive services]. This reflects our ongoing commitment to [single most important core practice value].

In the future, [My Practice Name] is committed to delivering services at the highest levels of [core practice priorities] in a setting that facilitates [professional values] among peer professionals and [core service values] with clients and referral sources. [My Practice Name] is prepared to demonstrate these commitments through [specific steps pertaining to accountability].

CHAPTER THREE

Legal Structures for Group Practices: Fitting Form to Function

There is one very important principle . . . you never have to work in accordance with your force, but always beyond your force. This is a permanent principle . . . you always have to do more than you can; only then can you change. If you do only what is possible, you will remain where you are.

—P. D. Ouspensky, *The Fourth Way*

INTRODUCTION

Establishing a strategic mission is only the beginning of your planning process. Once an overall vision is achieved, a host of smaller but crucial choices lies ahead. Your practice will need a name, a location, a business plan, an incorporation, a marketing program: a seemingly endless list of features that make it come to life. Of these features, perhaps none is as important as organizational structure. It is as true in behavioral health as in architecture: Form follows function. In this chapter, we review the various collaborative practice structures and their strengths and weaknesses in carrying out strategic functions.

Note: In this chapter, we will be touching on a range of legal and organizational issues. This will be helpful to those starting a collaborative practice, as well as to those evaluating practices for possible affiliation. No textbook presentation, however, can substitute for the capable advice of legal and accounting specialists, who can address your specific questions and concerns. Our presentation will greatly aid you in making optimal use of these specialists, **but it cannot replace expert consultation.**

☆ IN THIS CHAPTER

- Partnerships, corporations, and other organizational forms: Which are right for your practice?
- Matching the legal structure of a practice to its core strategy
- The governance of group practices and its importance to *your* practice
- Developing a name and site for your group
- What to look for in employment and independent contractor agreements

---

STRUCTURING THE GROUP PRACTICE

Although all practice organizations have certain features in common, there is a multitude of available business structures and legal forms. Each of these arrangements exists because people found that it met their needs. Your challenge is to decide on the format that will best accommodate your mission. How you structure the collaboration depends entirely on what you want it to accomplish.

Unincorporated Structures

Your first decision is whether you wish to formalize the practice entity as a legally recognized corporation or company. The simplest structural alternatives to incorporation are (1) sole proprietorships and (2) partnerships. Both of these are relatively easy to establish and are often found among small group practices. Both also have distinctive drawbacks. (See Table 3.1.)

A *sole proprietorship* is simply a business in which you are the sole owner. The business may operate under its own name (in which case you register it locally as d/b/a, indicating that you are "doing business as" the company), but there is no separate tax filing as a company. Rather, you as an individual simply include the income and expenses of the enterprise on the appropriate schedule of your federal income tax and pay taxes on the income at your personal rate. If you were a psychologist owning a professional practice doing business as "The Growth Center" with one secretary and a part-time marriage and family therapist as employees, you would have a sole proprietorship.

A *partnership* is a legally constituted form of business organization in which ownership is shared among two or more individuals. The partnership is established through documentation outlining the terms of partnership and the roles and responsibilities of the partners. In a general partnership, all partners participate in the running of the enterprise and all share liability for debts incurred by

TABLE 3.1. Summary of Practice Structures

Structure	Typical examples	Typical advantages	Typical disadvantages
Sole proprietorship	Solo practice	Ease of formation and administration	No limits on liability; few tax advantages for benefits
Partnership	Small group practice	Ease of formation; liability limits for limited partners	No limits on liability for general partners; few tax advantages for benefits; inflexibility (cannot survive changes in general partners)
Limited liability company	Staff-model practice or practice network; MSOs	Limited liability; taxation passed through at personal rates	Modest tax advantages for benefits; inflexibility (difficulty surviving changes in ownership)
Professional corporation or general business corporation	Staff-model practice or practice network; MSOs	Limited liability; tax advantages for benefits; flexibility (ownership is fully transferable)	Double taxation of income; limited to single specialty in some states

the company. All partners in a general partnership have an equal stake in the venture unless specifically provided otherwise and all partners have the ability to bind the company. This means that all general partners are empowered to act on behalf of the partnership.

A limited partnership, alternatively, allows for a class of partners that remain relatively silent (e.g., uninvolved in the running of the firm) and whose liability is limited to their initial investment. Specific guidelines ("safe harbors") exist that outline the management activities permissible to limited partners. As long as these are followed, the limited partners will enjoy limited liability. The general partner assumes responsibility for the day-to-day management of the partnership and thus assumes most liability. Note that general partners can be corporations, ensuring their liability protection.

Unless stipulated otherwise, partnerships are dissolved on the loss of a general partner, so that partnerships do not have the same continuity of life as corporations. There are ways in which partnerships can be maintained in such an event, through the concerted action of remaining partners, but this can be a weakness of the partnership form. A limited partnership may completely dissolve, for example, if the general partner decides to end all involvement, dies, or declares bankruptcy. Income from partnerships is divided among partners, declared on each partner's federal income tax, and taxed at the partner's personal rate. Partnerships thus avoid the double taxation incurred by corporations, which can be an advantage.

Younger et al. (1996) note that at least 19 states have enacted legislation enabling the creation of registered *limited liability partnerships (LLPs)*. These are similar to general partnerships but limit the liability of individual partners for acts of malfeasance, negligence, or incompetence on the part of other partners. The LLP would, for instance, shield the personal assets of one partner from malpractice claims against another. Younger et al. (1996) observe that most states protect the partners in an LLP from tort claims but not contract claims. This suggests that partners would retain personal liability for claims arising from normal business debts. The advantage of the LLP is that it allows partners day-to-day involvement in the running of the practice while shielding them from major sources of liability. The American Psychological Association Practice Directorate (1996a) notes that the LLP is permissible as a multidisciplinary structure in many states, including Connecticut, Delaware, District of Columbia, Indiana, Iowa, Kansas, Louisiana, Maryland, Missouri, Montana, Nevada, New York, North Dakota, Ohio, Oregon, Pennsylvania, Tennessee, Texas, and Virginia.

Although sole proprietorships and partnerships are easy and inexpensive to establish and relatively free of government scrutiny and regulation, they have three major disadvantages:

1. **Unincorporated businesses do not protect owners from financial liabilities incurred by the firm**. If the business owes $100,000 to creditors but only has $30,000 in assets, the creditors can attempt to recover the remaining $70,000 from the *personal* assets of the owners. In other words, all debts of the practice become the liabilities of the owners. In a general partnership or an LLP, each partner can be fully liable for the business debts of the partnership. Although this liability can be minimized in a limited partnership arrangement, the limitation comes at a cost: The limited partners cannot actively participate in running the business.

2. **Unincorporated businesses do not share in the tax advantages of corporations**. Corporations can establish employee benefit plans and, in most cases, deduct the costs of these—as well as certain other employee-related costs—as legitimate business expenses. There are far fewer tax benefits available to sole proprietorships and partnerships. For example, a corporation can deduct 100% of owners' health insurance premiums for the purpose of taxation; sole proprietorships and partnerships cannot.

3. **Partnerships are restricted to their original structure**. If a general partner wishes to exit the arrangement or a new general partner is sought, the entire structure may have to be dissolved and a new partnership created. Corporations, conversely, can change ownership freely, through transfer of stock. This can mean that limited partners are at the mercy of general partners and may have little say in the dissolution of the enterprise.

Most practice organizations desire some form of limited liability to protect against the financial risks of doing business. When we have seen practices operating as sole proprietorships and general partnerships, these are usually "groups of convenience." That is, the participants have entered into a cooperative arrangement to share expenses but do not really want to function as employees of an integrated group. This can be a dangerous situation. If the practitioners hold themselves out to the public as a group, by selecting a group name or promoting themselves as a group entity, courts will treat them as though they are a group. The cooperative would thus become exposed to all of the financial liability and malpractice risks of a formal group, but without any of the protections. Younger et al. (1996), for example, observe that a general partnership will be deemed to exist even if no formal papers have been drawn. Courts will view the intent to do business jointly as sufficient evidence that a partnership exists. In such an event, practitioners would incur all the liabilities of general partners, including liability for acts of negligence and malfeasance on the part of another partner.

Limited Liability Companies

As a viable means for providing liability protection, most states allow for the formation of limited liability companies (LLCs), which blend the ownership structure of partnerships with the limited liability of corporations. The "members" of an LLC enjoy the status of limited partners: Their liability is limited to their investment in the firm. The members may share in management responsibilities ("member-managed LLC") or delegate management responsibilities to a specific party ("manager-managed LLC") (Younger et al., 1996). Income derived from the company passes through to members and is taxed at their personal rates, thus allowing the LLC to avoid the double taxation of corporations. The ability of the LLC to involve members in day-to-day management, shield them from business liabilities, and avoid double taxation has made the LLC a popular form of organization. As with partnerships, the LLC must be dissolved once new ownership is established, although the IRS allows for continuity of existence as long as those holding a majority of interest in the LLC so choose.

Many states do not allow members of licensed professions to establish traditional business entities such as LLCs. In such cases, the state oversees the creation of professional limited liability companies (PLLCs), which enjoy the basic advantages of LLCs. Our experience is that most collaborative practices organized as LLCs/PLLCs are structured in a manner akin to limited partnerships, blending vertical (the "general" partner, who holds majority interest and control) and horizontal ("limited partners") governance.

We have observed an increasing number of practice collaborations organized as LLCs in recent years. The LLC structure is relatively easy to establish and serves as a flexible mechanism for the pass-through of clinical income to practitioners. This arrangement can be ideal for low-integration collaborations that allow clinical staff to maintain their own offices and practices in a network. The clinical staff member can join the network practice as a LLC member without being salaried as a practice employee. The advantages of self-employment (Keogh plans, tax deductions for business expenses) are thus blended with the benefits of collaborative affiliation.

The LLC also possesses some distinctive tax advantages and disadvantages (Corporate Agents, 1995). The LLC avoids the double taxation of profits levied on corporations and avoids double taxation of distributions on dissolution. The LLC also enjoys considerable flexibility in allocating profits and losses for taxation. The LLC, however, does not enjoy the same tax deductibility of benefits as corporations (25% vs. 100% of health insurance premiums are deductible, for example) and the marginal tax rate of LLCs (like partnerships) is higher than that for general corporations. This means that, in a year of relatively small profits, the LLC's income tax rate—levied at the personal rates of the members—could be higher than the graduated general corporate rate.

Although LLC and corporate structures have broad protective benefits, they do *not* protect owners from all liabilities. Providers are always individually responsible for their professional practice and remain liable for acts of malpractice. The practice structure also will not allow owners to evade taxes. Earnings retained by the company and not distributed to members/shareholders are subject to taxation, which become the personal responsibility of the owners should the business fail.

It is also important to note that liabilities may be imposed by lending institutions, as well as by state and federal governments. If you are starting a company with a limited track record, your creditors are aware that this is a risky undertaking. Frequently, they will ask that a loan be collateralized *personally* by the principals of the new firm. That is, you may need to use your home or other assets to guarantee the repayment of your loan or credit line. Once your company has a track record, this personal collateral may be replaced by assets pledged by the firm. In the event of a bankruptcy, the practice's limited liability will not protect the collateralized assets of the principals.

The American Psychological Association Practice Directorate (1996a) notes that a number of states permit multidisciplinary ownership of LLCs or PLLCs, including Alaska, Arizona, Arkansas, Delaware, District of Columbia, Florida, Georgia, Idaho, Indiana, Iowa, Kansas, Kentucky, Louisiana, Maryland, Mississippi, Missouri, Montana, Nebraska, Nevada, New Hampshire, New Mexico, New York, North Carolina, Oregon, Pennsylvania, South Carolina, and Virginia. Most other states allow LLCs, but there may be ambiguity regarding their potential for multidisciplinary integration. Legal consultation is therefore strongly suggested if an LLC is contemplated as a collaborative structure.

Incorporation

A corporation is a legally recognized business entity that has the following four characteristics:

- **Limited liability**. Owners of a corporation are shielded from tort and contract claims arising against the firm.

- **Continuity of existence.** The existence of the corporation does not depend on its ownership. Changes in ownership do not necessitate the dissolution of the firm.

- **Transferability of ownership.** Ownership in the corporation is facilitated by the issuance of shares of stock to owners. These shares are easily transferred from one party to another in the event of an owner's retirement, death, bankruptcy, and so on.

- **Centralized management.** Corporations have a designated board of directors empowered to run the firm.

Any business possessing these features qualifies as a corporation. To avoid some of the disadvantages of corporations, such as the double taxation of profits, other structures (such as partnerships and LLCs) must demonstrate that at least two of the above four features are absent.

Generally, when we think of corporations, we refer to general business or C corporations. In a general business corporation, there are no limitations on the number of shareholders and all profits are taxed at a graduated rate. If those profits are distributed to owners as dividends, they are taxed a second time at the owner's personal rate. This double taxation can be a major impediment to C corporations and provides professional practices with a major incentive to distribute revenues as salaries and bonuses, not dividends. An S corporation, on the other hand, is limited to 35 shareholders and allows profits to pass through to owners for taxation at their personal rates, much in the manner of partnerships. S corporations, however, are more limited than LLCs in their ability to pass losses through to owners to offset active income. Such losses are limited to the amount of the owner's investment in the corporation (his or her "basis") and can only be deducted if the owners materially participate in the running of the firm. S corporations are also more limited than C corporations in their ability to deduct fringe benefits of owners as business expenses. Our experience is that when multispecialty practices want the advantages of a corporate form, they generally opt for a C structure or the professional corporation (PC) arrangement described next.

Laws concerning incorporation vary on a state-by-state basis, so you will need to consult an attorney regarding the regulations applicable in your locale. In many states, members of professions such as medicine, social work, and psychology cannot form traditional for-profit corporations as practice structures. Rather, state departments of education (or their equivalents) regulate the creation of *professional service corporations* (also called professional corporations or professional associations) within each discipline or across groups of related disciplines. Just as the state government approves the licensure of an individual practitioner, it must approve the formation of a professional corporation.

In most respects, PCs look and act like any corporation. They are governed by articles of incorporation and bylaws, issue stock representing ownership, elect board members, and hold meetings. If the PC is small, as in the case of a solo practitioner incorporating a practice, the governance of the company and structuring of the ownership is quite straightforward. Larger PCs may have more elaborate structures of governance, with officers, a board of directors, committees, and so on. In such practices, ownership may be divided among multiple parties.

One important difference between PCs and traditional for-profit corporations lies in their tax treatment. PCs are taxed at the maximum corporate rate regardless of their income, whereas general business corporations have graduated rates of taxation. This creates an even greater disincentive to the retention of large amounts of money in the PC, because the income would be doubly taxed: once at the end of the year at the maximum corporate rate and again at the owner's individual rate when it is distributed as dividends. For this reason, PCs with superior tax planning will show little excess revenue on their statements, reimbursing owners with salaries and bonuses and plowing profits back into the firm rather than distributing them as dividends.

In the eyes of the law, the PC, like any corporation, is an entity separate from its owners. The PC has its own name, taxpayer identification number, expenses, and liabilities. With some notable exceptions (state and federal taxes, wages owed to employees, fraudulent transactions), the liabilities incurred by the corporation stay with the corporation. A declaration of bankruptcy by the corporation hence need not wipe out the assets of its owners. As a separate entity, the PC is structured to survive its present ownership. A document known as the *articles of incorporation* establishes the name, location, and purpose of the business, whereas a set of *bylaws* establishes policies and procedures for the governance of the firm. These relatively brief and simple documents provide for the continuation of the practice even if there are substantial changes in leadership and/or ownership.

We have alluded to the distinctive benefits of the corporate form, including the ability to deduct expenses associated with fringe benefits and pension and profit-sharing plans, limited liability, and ease of ownership transfer. We also mentioned the double taxation drawback of corporations: Income from operations and from the dissolution of the enterprise will be taxed twice, once at the corporate rate and again at the personal rate of the shareholders. Note also that losses do not pass through to shareholders in C corporations, as they would in partnerships, LLCs, and S corporations. For these reasons, we highly recommend consulting with a qualified tax accountant when choosing an organizational form.

In addition to the previously mentioned concerns, PCs have one major shortcoming in some states. Where they are formed and regulated on a discipline-by-discipline basis, PCs can only be owned by members of the relevant discipline. That can severely limit the founders' ability to establish a multidisciplinary practice. If a psychiatric nurse and a social worker wish to jointly own a group practice, they may need to resort to other structures to accomplish their ends. This issue is especially acute in the state of New York. Note that the limitation of PCs to a single discipline is not a problem if one professional is considered an employee and the other an owner. A psychiatrist could, for example, own a practice that employs a staff of licensed professional counselors and social workers. Only multidisciplinary *ownership* is prohibited.

That having been said, you may find that attorneys automatically assume that it is impossible to create a desired practice structure in a given state because of the various laws. This is not necessarily the case; state laws vary considerably in their flexibility with respect to multidisciplinary practice. There is also considerable ambiguity in state laws and their enforcement. We highly recommend the American Psychological Association Practice Directorate (1996a) text, *Models for Multidisciplinary Arrangements: A State-by-State Review of Options*, which reviews rules on a state-by-state basis. We have summarized some state-by-state guidelines in Table 3.2. Note, however, that such laws are subject to change. Careful consultation with a well-informed attorney is necessary to ensure that the structure you are creating is legal in your state.

Overall, a number of states do permit general business corporations to engage in multispecialty practice (American Psychological Association Practice Directorate, 1996a), including Alabama, Florida, Kentucky, Louisiana, New Hampshire, New Mexico, Oklahoma, South Dakota, Utah, Virginia, and West Virginia. Many other states allow the corporate form as a multidisciplinary vehicle through the PC structure.

A Note about Not-for-Profit Corporations

One important corporate variant is the not-for-profit corporation. In some situations the not-for-profit corporation may be tax-exempt; otherwise, it is a taxable, not-for-profit corporation. Not-for-profit corporations do not issue stock and thus do not have owners in the traditional sense. Rather, they are membership organizations and are capitalized through the contributions ("dues") of members. A major limitation of not-for-profit corporations is that they may not distribute profits (excess revenues) to members and that, on their dissolution, they may not be sold for members' gain. Rather, when a not-for-profit corporation is dissolved, its assets are generally dedicated to another nonprofit entity. This clearly will not be appealing to practice founders wishing to cash in on their businesses. Not-for-profit institutions, such as academic health centers and hospitals, may wish to organize practices in a not-for-profit manner, however, if they seek the collegiality of a membership structure and do not envision selling the practice.

Federal laws also allow for the creation of tax-exempt, not-for-profit corporations. These are sometimes referred to as 501(c)(3) corporations, in recognition of the Internal Revenue Service statute allowing for their creation. In most instances, behavioral health practices would not qualify for tax-exempt status because they are not primarily organized for the purpose of public benefit. Federal law stipulates that a 501(c)(3) company be organized and operated for charitable, educational, religious, literary, or scientific purposes (Mancuso, 1994).

In limited circumstances, however, a practice entity may qualify for tax ex-

TABLE 3.2. Multidisciplinary Arrangements by State

States in which multidisciplinary ownership of business corporations, PCs, or (P)LLCs appears to be permissible

Alabama	Montana
Alaska	Nebraska
Arizona	Nevada
Arkansas	New Hampshire
Delaware	New Jersey
District of Columbia	New Mexico
Florida	North Carolina
Georgia	North Dakota
Hawaii	Oklahoma
Idaho	Oregon
Indiana	Pennsylvania
Iowa	Rhode Island
Kansas	South Dakota
Kentucky	Utah
Louisiana	Virginia
Maryland	West Virginia
Massachusetts	Wisconsin
Mississippi	
Missouri	

States with significant restrictions on multidisciplinary ownership

California: PCs may have multidisciplinary ownership, but must be primarily organized and owned by a single specialty.

Colorado: Limited to general partnerships; multidisciplinary ownership of LLCs is unclear.

Illinois: PPO networks are registered with the state and may have multidisciplinary composition.

Maine: Multidisciplinary partnerships are allowed.

Michigan: Taxable nonprofit corporations and general partnerships may have multidisciplinary ownership.

Minnesota: General partnerships may have multidisciplinary ownership.

New York: LLPs and PLLCs may have multidisciplinary ownership. Networks (IPAs) may contract with single HMOs only.

Ohio: LLPs may have multidisciplinary ownership.

Tennessee: LLPs and general partnerships may have multidisciplinary ownership.

Texas: LLPs may have multidisciplinary ownership.

Vermont: General partnerships may have multidisciplinary ownership.

Washington: Multidisciplinary PCs may only contract with HMOs.

Wyoming: Multidisciplinary ownership of LLCs is uncertain; general partnerships may be multidisciplinary.

With the exception of New York State and the state of Washington, all states permit multidisciplinary organization of mental health professionals in networks. Individual states may impose particular registration requirements upon these networks. In New York, networks must be organized as IPAs and can contract with single HMOs only. Hence, providers may need to form a separate IPA for each HMO contract entered into. In Washington, multidisciplinary networks can contract with MCOs on a fee-for-service basis but may need to obtain separate licensure as a "health care service contractor" to enter into at-risk arrangements.

Note. This information is paraphrased from American Psychological Association Practice Directorate (1996a). We strongly recommend that readers consult this text and a qualified attorney before choosing a multidisciplinary structure.

emption if it operates with a religious mission (e.g., pastoral counseling) and if it is willing to service all clients, regardless of ability to pay (charitable mission). Such agencies can enjoy the benefits of the 501(c)(3) structure, including tax exemption, eligibility for public grant funds, and reduced rates for postage. A tax-exempt group, for instance, might be able to qualify for state or federal social services grants, whereas a for-profit group would be ineligible. Tax-exempt organizations are also eligible to receive charitable contributions, opening a source of funding (Whitman, 1994).

It is also conceivable that a behavioral practice could operate under tax exemption as part of a medical foundation. A medical foundation is a tax-exempt, nonprofit corporation that acts as a provider of care through contracts with medical/practice groups (for a thorough discussion, see Younger et al., 1996). In some cases, the foundation may be established by a hospital as a way of creating an integrated delivery system (Korenchuk, 1994). The foundation, like other tax-exempt entities, is required to engage in such activities as research and charity. It may, for example, be required to provide care for indigent populations. Foundations also have at their disposal financing through tax-exempt bonds, which can be more attractive to investors (and less costly to the organization) than traditional debt or equity financing.

There are many disadvantages of the tax-exempt, nonprofit status for independent practices. Their requirements may prevent them from actively seeking large-scale contracts with managed care organizations because since these could jeopardize the charitable mission. Too, if the practice is largely composed of pastoral counselors, it may be ineligible for managed care contracts, due to the absence of licensure for such providers in many states.

The IRS also expects that tax-exempt entities will be responsive to their communities. Hence, control of the collaboration's board of directors must be vested in community members—not its professional leadership. This could create management and governance difficulties in large practices, reducing the leadership's ability to maneuver.

In short, the tax-exempt structure imposes important commercial limitations but may fill particular community needs. If tax exemption is to be sought, it is probably best found in the context of a medical foundation, where a hospital organization can meet many of the research, educational, and charitable service mandates. Once again, legal consultation is essential if you wish to operate under 501(c)(3) status.

ESTABLISHING NETWORK PRACTICES

Even in states permitting a variety of forms of multidisciplinary ownership, professionals may opt to retain their self-employed status and affiliate through networks rather than staff-model practices. In such a situation, the members do not want to become employees of a practice because that would jeopardize their

Keogh plans (retirement plans for self-employed individuals) and threaten their autonomy. They also might not want to assume the risks and responsibilities of becoming an owner of a large practice organization. Accordingly, the individual providers will practice in solo or small group structures and the network will assume an organizational form that will not threaten the members' self-employment. As Table 3.2 suggests, most states do not place significant restrictions on the development of multidisciplinary networks.

Independent Contractor Model

There are several mechanisms by which networks can be structured. In one variant, the overarching network practice can organize as a PC or LLC and establish *independent contractor* relationships with each of the professional members. Status as an independent contractor is established via a contract that clearly outlines that the professional:

- Assumes all risk for work to be performed.

- Is solely responsible for control of the work performed.

- Is not an employee or agent of the practice.

- Is not entitled to any benefits provided to employees.

- Is free to contract with other firms for the provision of similar services.

- Is responsible for his or her own liability insurance, tools, and equipment.

The independent contractor model has several advantages and disadvantages. One advantage is related to overhead: Independent contractors are not employees and hence are not paid the fringe benefits (health and life insurance, social security contributions, vacation days, etc.) that are associated with employment. This means that the compensation structure of the network starts with a 20+% advantage over staff models that use salaried clinical personnel. The contractor model is also quite explicit in its emphasis on independence, which will be perceived as an advantage by clinicians who don't want to be tied to a particular network.

A major disadvantage of the independent contractor model is that it *prevents* networks from hiring clinical staff as employees. This is because the IRS forbids independent contractors from performing work that is substantially identical to the tasks performed by salaried individuals. In such an event, the IRS will view the contractor arrangement as a vehicle for tax avoidance (e.g., avoidance of withholding and employer-mandated social security contributions) and can seek payment of back taxes and penalties. We have encountered groups that freely mix salaried staff and independent contractors. Although this is an attractive way of cheaply adding clinical capacity, it could place the practice at jeopardy by triggering costly audits.

A second shortcoming of the independent contractor model is that it is very unintegrated and may provide practice management with little control over the practice patterns of clinical staff. Indeed, one of the crucial stipulations of the independent contractor contract is that contractors must maintain control over the performance of their work. Groups that attempt to dictate practice patterns to contractors, therefore, may find that they have few means at their disposal to enforce their mandates. Because of the independence inherent in the contractor relationship, there may be little perceived loyalty between network and practitioner, making it difficult to assemble a cohesive and truly collaborative staff.

Relationship Enrichment Center (RFC), LLC, profiled in Chapter 7, is an excellent example of a network-style practice that makes use of independent contractors. As Bret Smith, one of the founders, notes, the group has addressed some of the potential shortcomings of a contractor model by making every clinician a partner in the LLC and by blending "facility" providers (those who acquire practice space and full administrative support from the group) and "satellite" providers (those providing their own space in separate locations). Such an innovation allows REC to blend the cohesiveness of a traditional group practice with the advantages of a contractor-based network.

Membership Models

In a membership model, the individual practitioners establish their own network entity (practitioner organization), which they own and control. This could take the form of a management services organization (MSO) or an independent practice association (IPA). A membership MSO would be structured as a taxable not-for-profit business corporation, not a PC. This is because the MSO is a business organization—a lay entity—and not entitled to deliver clinical services in states regulating the formation of PCs. It only provides business and administrative support for clinicians. The MSO becomes the contracting body, linking the individually incorporated practices of the clinicians to managed care organizations (MCOs) and other referral sources. If the MSO is organized as a for-profit corporation, its founders own stock to signify their shares of ownership. When the MSO is organized as a not-for-profit association, membership replaces stock ownership. The money contributed by founders for purchase of the stock constitutes the start-up capital of for-profit MSOs; the dues and initial assessments levied on members are the primary vehicles of capitalization among not-for-profit MSOs.

The IPA also may be structured as a for-profit or not-for-profit entity, with a similar distinction between stock ownership and membership. The IPA, however, is often established as a general business corporation or PC and is not viewed strictly as a business entity. This distinction may make the IPA and not the unintegrated MSO the vehicle of preference in contracting with HMOs and other managed care organizations. As Table 3.2 indicates, this is a requirement in New York State.

The practice organization Dr. Steenbarger helped to found, PrimeCare, is established as a membership model MSO/IPA. It links a core group of faculty within an academic department of psychiatry to clinical faculty and community practitioners across Central New York. The network is empowered to negotiate contracts on behalf of members, which they can accept or reject. If a member rejects a contract, he or she cannot independently contract with that insurer. This gives the network teeth in representing the interests of a large number of practitioners.

Any network has an identity distinct from that of its constituent professionals and hence must be assured of limited liability either through an LLC, an LLP, or a corporate organization. Should lawsuits arise, the network as well as its members could be named. Hence, networks, like group practices, must obtain their own liability coverage and other necessary forms of business insurance. An informal network with no legally recognized form guaranteeing limited liability and without separate professional liability coverage could place all its members at financial jeopardy and hence is quite risky.

Independent MSO Network

Akin to a membership-model network is a network established through an independent MSO. The defining feature of the *independent MSO network* is that the collaborative structure is not established by members. Rather, it is a separate business corporation that contracts with self-employed practitioners to provide business services and represent their interests in contracting and marketing. In this model, the providers are removed from the collaboration itself because they have delegated most collaborative functions to the MSO. The MSO, which is reimbursed either through a set fee or a percentage of clinical revenues, often serves as a supplement to the independent private practices of the clinicians. Accordingly, the MSO represents the providers in MCO negotiations but may not provide services for cases that come to providers through other referral sources.

The independent MSO network may exist in an unintegrated form in which the participants are self-employed and can freely accept or reject contracts signed by the MSO. This amounts to a network practice with an outsourced set of business services. Alternatively, the MSO network can be highly integrated, with the MSO purchasing the assets of the practices and employing the practitioners. The advantage to the latter arrangement is that clinicians still operate out of their own offices but have the security of affiliation with a larger organization. This is a common mechanism when hospital organizations wish to create outpatient networks to cover a full spectrum of clinical services (PHO, or provider–hospital organization). The asset purchase provides a one-time cash infusion to practice owners and, for a reasonably modest investment, allows facilities to move toward the ideal of an integrated delivery system.

Advantages of Network Organization

At first blush, networks look too good to be true. They offer many advantages that aren't found in traditional group practices, including the following:

- **Access.** A network can consist of individual practitioners from multiple neighborhoods and counties, covering all major ZIP codes within a region.

- **Breadth of service.** A network can embrace professionals with a variety of specializations, creating a "one-stop shopping" option for referral sources.

- **Choice.** Large networks offer patients a wider choice of providers and thus are likely to accommodate a range of needs.

- **Availability.** The network can be large enough so that practice openings are assured in any of the specialization areas.

- **Cost efficiency.** Because network members maintain their own offices, the cost of practice expansion is reduced.

- **Attractiveness to providers.** Solo providers who do not want to feel like employees of a traditional group practice may find participation in a network an ideal combination of group affiliation and independence.

- **Increased marketing power.** The network can pool resources and become competitive for large-scale managed care contracts unavailable to solo providers.

- **Access to resources.** The network, if sufficiently capitalized, can offer providers access to financial and administrative resources that would be beyond the means of the solo providers, including sophisticated information systems.

It is not unusual for solo practitioners to first turn to networks as options when considering collaborations. They view the network as a way to maintain their autonomy in the face of managed health care trends. The horizontal governance of most membership models and the appeal of retaining self-employed status offers networks a collegiality and flexibility that many professionals appreciate.

Shortcomings of Networks

Indeed, networks often prove to be too good to be true, succumbing under several constraints:

- **Lack of coordination.** Unless the network members are connected electronically (an expensive proposition; see Chapter 5), it is extremely cumbersome to coordinate central billing, record keeping, and quality control among members.

- **Loss of control**. When clinical staff are employees, it is easier for management to monitor their performance and change practice patterns if necessary. Within a network, practice managers may have reduced control, especially if much of members' practice is conducted outside the network.

- **Lack of funds**. Although networks avoid many costs associated with bricks and mortar, they can be expensive to establish and maintain, with added legal and consultative costs and significant expenses associated with practice management and coordination. Networks may have difficulty raising needed start-up capital and are often chronically undercapitalized.

- **Legal challenges**. Large networks may be viewed as anticompetitive by regulatory authorities, especially if the networks include more than 20–30% of professionals within a discipline in a given region. Because the network members are considered competitors, their efforts to join forces and obtain favorable fee-for-service reimbursements can be considered price fixing and a violation of antitrust laws (DeMuro, 1994).

Our experience is that the latter problem is unappreciated by many of those contemplating joining or forming networks. Large networks have been prosecuted for violations of antitrust law, especially when it has been clear that the effect of the affiliation has been to forestall managed care penetration or raise provider reimbursements (Younger et al., 1996). This problem can be addressed in one of two ways. First, the network can engage in substantial financial risk sharing in MCO contracts (capitation, case rates, or withholds of 20% or more) to prove a level of financial integration and cost-effectiveness. Often, in this case, the network will take the form of an IPA. Second, the network can refrain from negotiating fees, relying instead on a third party to collect fee data (market levels of reimbursement) from practitioners and convey offers from MCOs ("messenger model"). Neither solution is perfect: The former imposes a level of risk that is unacceptable to many providers; the latter greatly limits the network's negotiating clout. As the federal government relaxes antitrust constraints upon provider networks, we may see a much more heated battle for benefit dollars between provider care organizations (PCOs) and MCOs. At present, however, legal consultation is essential if one is forming a large network that will contract on a fee-for-service basis.

Networks are often viewed by practitioners as ways of enjoying the benefits of group affiliation without experiencing the drawbacks. They are also viewed as potential refuges from the competitive pressures of managed care. As a result, providers are often more invested in their individual practices than in the network, using the collaboration as a supplemental referral source only. This generally means that the members are not truly committed to the network's success and are unwilling to adequately capitalize it. For this reason, some refer to these organizations as "group practices without money"! Networks are most likely to thrive when they are central to the practices of owners/members, who are actively involved in the group's formation, management, and governance.

Unique and Complex Collaborative Structures

A significant challenge for practice leaders is to combine the advantages of integration with the appeal of practitioner autonomy. Most organizational forms arise out of the desire to harmonize these elements in a manner that provides a rich array of services across a wide area. These include the following:

- **Satellite group practice**. Here the group practice is organized as a PC, business corporation, LLC, or LLP. It establishes satellite locations at various sites and hires all clinicians as employees, thus combining geographic diversification with a tightly integrated staff model.

- **Centralized network practice**. Here the group practice is organized as a PC, an IPA, a business corporation, a not-for-profit corporation, an LLC, or an LLP. It has a central location from which providers offer services, but the providers are self-employed and affiliate with the network as independent contractors or as members of a not-for-profit corporation. The network group thus combines elements of central location and management with wide access and low overhead.

- **Integrated group practice without walls**. The GPWW is established as a traditional group practice, utilizing the PC, business corporation, LLC, or LLP forms. Clinicians affiliate with the group as employees but keep their own offices and locations. This combines high integration with geographic diversity. The group entity may take the form of an integrated MSO that purchases the assets of clinicians and provides an array of administrative and business services.

- **Provider–hospital organization**. The PHO is a structure created by the melding of a provider organization with a hospital. This can be accomplished in many ways but often involves the creation of a third entity (which can be an MSO) to purchase the assets of the providers and coordinate business functions among the providers and between the providers and the hospital.

The latter forms of organization are *much* more complicated to assemble than simple group practices or networks (see Table 3.3). This is because GPWWs and PHOs usually entail the purchase of individual practices by the integrated entity. As a result, a significant number of issues come into play that are beyond the scope of this book, including the proper valuation of practices and the legal

TABLE 3.3. Complex Forms of Collaboration

Collaborative structure	How it is established	Practice advantages	Practice disadvantages
Unintegrated network practice	Solo practitioners networked through MSO	Geographic coverage; autonomy for practitioners	Complex governance; reduced managerial control
Integrated network; GPWW	MSO purchases solo and group practices	Geographic coverage; tighter managerial control	Reduced practitioner control and autonomy
IPA	Practitioners form and own a multispecialty practice	Geographic coverage; autonomy for practitioners	Complex governance; reduced managerial control
PHO	Hospital forms or purchases an outpatient network	Referral flow to hospital and providers multiple levels of care	Legally complex; may be viewed as a feeder

ramifications of integration. PHOs, for example, can consist of the merger of a not-for-profit, tax-exempt entity (the hospital) with a for-profit practitioner organization. Care must be exercised to ensure that the transactions do not jeopardize the facility's tax-exempt status. Issues with respect to prohibition of self-referrals (Stark laws) also tend to arise in large integrations. For instance, a hospital may be prohibited from paying a premium for the goodwill of a group practice because this could be construed as a buying of referrals—a violation of Medicare fraud and abuse laws. As one moves from first-order collaborations to collaborations of greater scope and integration, the start-up process and associated financial and legal issues become considerably more complex.

Matching Structure to Strategy

If there is anything certain about practice management, it is that you will make many mistakes and explore numerous dead ends. Flexibility is important. You may pursue one structure or strategy, only to find out that another is more favorable. In the words of W. C. Fields, "If at first you don't succeed, try, try again. Then quit. No use being a damn fool about it."

We've been surprised at the frequency with which groups reorganize at some point in their lives. They may begin as unincorporated entities, then restructure as PCs. Recently, we have seen a few PCs reorganize as LLCs, taking advantage of the latter's blend of partnership and corporate advantages. Networks may form more tightly integrated organizations over time, with principals becoming employees of the new entity (integrated GPWWs, PHOs). Clearly, strategic planning is an ongoing process, allowing groups to respond to changes in the marketplace and the law. As internal and external factors shift, groups can reinvent themselves, matching their structure to their strategy.

In general, network models are best suited to groups that need wide geographic coverage and broad multidisciplinary composition. They can add members or independent contractors with little additional overhead and thus enter new markets at relatively low cost—a distinct advantage in a highly managed market. The low-cost strategy is especially well suited to entities employing clinical staff as independent contractors. Because networks of contractors do not lend themselves to managerial control, they are more challenged in implementing specialty niche or data-driven quality strategies.

Staff-model groups, in which clinicians are salaried by the group and/or conduct all their practice within the group, find it easier to establish, monitor, and control practice patterns and assess clinical outcomes and service quality. Generally, though not always, these staff-model practices are smaller and more compact than networks. Staff models more easily implement ongoing case consultations and in-service training and thus can be valued for their perceived level of teamwork and collegiality. This can work very well with specialty niche strategies, as well as tightly knit practices within small communities.

☞ LOOKING AHEAD

If you are looking to join a group, how do you find the right structure for your market and objectives?

Our Strategy–Structure Matrix at the end of this chapter (Reader's Resource 3.1) might be of help!

Though it is a gross generalization, we would say that, on balance, networks tend to have the edge on cost (because of their contractor/member structure) and integrated groups have the edge on quality (because of their ability to control practice patterns and coordinate programs of care). Practices attempting to blend group and network forms are clearly seeking a synthesis of the advantages of each.

ESTABLISHING THE PRACTICE

Before the structuring of a collaboration can proceed, the founders need to establish a few basics that will be reflected in legal documentation. Specifically, the practice will need a *name*, a *governance structure*, and a *location*. The practice will also need specific mechanisms for formalizing the linkages between practitioners and their practice organization.

The Name of the Practice

The practice name is a critical part of its identity. The name should be one that is easily recognized, informative, and distinctive. It never fails to surprise us that practice organizers select names that sound almost identical to those of competitors in their regions. If you call your group "Psychological Services" and there is already a group called "Psychological Associates," it is quite likely that referral sources will be confused. Be creative! A large HMO with which we are familiar chose, for various reasons, to change its name. In a process that took 3 months and cost about $80,000, the HMO hired a firm whose only reason for being is helping large corporations rename themselves. We didn't think much of the name the firm came up with, but then again, no one is paying us thousands to come up with names. Be thoughtful and think about what you want to communicate to anyone who reads or hears the name. This is a very important decision.

Your practice's name must be approved in the state in which you are incorporating to guarantee that it does not conflict with an existing business name. Your attorney can assist you in conducting an appropriate name search. Should your desired name be taken, you might be able to modify it slightly to gain approval. For example, "Behavioral Care, PC" may be unavailable, but you might successfully modify the name to "Behavioral Care of Northeastern Ohio, PC" or "Quality Behavioral Care, PC." The idea is to avoid confusion in the minds of consumers.

In selecting a name, keep in mind that the name will probably be seen on stationery, signs, and business cards. That is a strong incentive to keep it short. The ideal name captures the identity and strategy of the practice and meshes well with a logo that appears in public displays and correspondence. Dr. Steenbarger's academic department, for example, selected a name (PrimeCare) that connotes both quality and a connection to primary medical care. It is easily remembered and lends itself to visual display, which are strong marketing advantages.

The Governance of the Practice

Before papers are filed, organizers need to establish the leadership structure of the practice. This usually consists of a set of director/owners but may include other positions as well. In a small group practice with a corporate structure, the founders may be the officers, directors, and stockholders and share in nearly all aspects of the group's maintenance. Larger groups are apt to have differentiated structures that place directors and members/shareholders in defined roles of authority (see Table 3.4).

Two documents are central to establishing a corporation: the *certificate of incorporation* (sometimes referred to as the articles of incorporation) and the *bylaws*. The certificate of incorporation is a relatively brief form that sets forth the name of the corporation, its purposes, its indemnification of directors, its num-

TABLE 3.4. Governance: Characteristics, Strengths, and Weaknesses

Governance structure	Characteristics
Vertical	Majority of ownership and decision making vested in a single party or a limited number of shareholders
	Limited incentive options for staff (equity sharing, bonuses)
	Strategic planning limited to a core group of officers
	Strengths: ability to make decisions and act quickly, simplicity of governance processes, increased control for group owner/founders
	Weaknesses: limited input from clinical staff and possible reduced emotional investment in the practice; potential conflicts with the autonomy needs of professionals
Horizontal	Ownership and decision making shared broadly through organization
	Broad incentive options for clinical staff (equity sharing, bonuses)
	Strategic planning broadly delegated to teams and committees
	Strengths: high degree of professional staff input and potential high emotional investment in the practice.
	Weaknesses: consensus building can reduce decision-making efficiency and bog down the organization

ber of shares authorized for issue, its address, and the name(s) of the incorporator(s). The bylaws establish the corporation's governance structure and are somewhat lengthier. At a minimum, the bylaws set forth the name and address of the corporation, the date of its annual shareholders' meeting, the number or percentage of shareholders needed to call special meetings and the advance notice required for such meetings, the number of authorized directors and means for their election, the number of directors required to call a special meeting of the board of directors and the advance notice required for such a meeting, the mechanisms and time frame for filling vacant board positions, the number of officer positions and their terms, and the time frame in which vacant officer positions must be filled (Mancuso, 1992). The bylaws in a sizable entity, such as an IPA, may also define a number of positions, including:

- **Board of directors.** This is the central decision-making body of the practice. The bylaws define who serves on the board and how those individuals are to be chosen. The bylaws also define the responsibilities of board members and stipulate their terms of office and procedures for removal.

- **Officers.** Although a board may meet only periodically to consider large issues of strategy, the day-to-day affairs of the enterprise are managed by its officers, including a president, vice president, secretary, and treasurer. Frequently, officers are major shareholders in the group; the bylaws outline how they are elected, their terms of office, and their duties. Generally, officers are elected/hired by the board and comprise a subset of the board.

- **Practice manager.** In a large practice, a full or part-time position might be defined for a practice manager who attends to administrative tasks such as billing, marketing, and data collection. When the practice manager is not one of the principals of the practice, he or she is typically an employee and might hold an ex officio role on governance bodies, such as the board or committees.

- **Medical director.** The medical director is the clinical leader of the practice, as distinguished from the practice manager, who is the business and administrative head. The medical director helps to set clinical policies and procedures and will frequently oversee such provider-related committees as credentialing and utilization review. Generally if a dispute arises concerning the care of a patient, it will be adjudicated by the medical director.

- **Committees.** When the tasks of running a practice exceed the span of control of the officers, committees might be established as a means of delegating responsibility. The committees are often chaired by an officer or senior staff member and might consist of owners and employed staff. Committees typically have defined areas of responsibility, such as quality improvement, and serve in an advisory capacity to the group's leadership. When the officers form the day-to-day leadership of a practice, they may constitute an executive committee. Committees are often found among staff-model groups and membership-model practices.

Although all of the leadership positions are important, the positions of secretary and treasurer bear specific mention. The secretary is responsible for all record keeping regarding meetings of the board and executive committee. Minutes of board meetings are used to document the transactions of the leadership, much as a therapist's session notes document clinical work. In the event of a lawsuit, the minutes may become very important in establishing the actions and intent of the leadership. Minutes also aid in establishing continuity between meetings, especially helpful for absent members.

The treasurer typically handles the financial affairs of the practice, including payment of salaries, oversight of billing systems, and purchasing. It is extremely important that the treasurer keep meticulous records of financial transactions. This will greatly speed the work of the accountant and protect the practice in the event of an IRS audit or lawsuit. The treasurer should be conversant with accounting principles and software and should be able to provide ongoing financial reports to the management team.

In addition to defining leadership positions, the bylaws dictate that the corporation hold an annual meeting in which business is transacted and officers and board members are elected. Large practices may have detailed position descriptions for the officers and directors, clearly outlining duties and expectations. In a small group practice, this meeting may be little more than a formality. Large practices, however, may use this meeting to bring staff together, establish and update committees, and review strategic plans. This is especially important in networks, where clinical staff may have little face-to-face time with practice managers and colleagues.

Documentation Needed to Form LLCs and Partnerships

There are some differences in the documentation needed to establish LLCs and partnerships, as compared to corporations. The LLC's equivalent of a certificate of incorporation is known as the *articles of organization*. It also is a relatively brief document, summarizing the name of the company, its duration of existence (often 30 years), purpose, address, the contributions of founding members and stipulations for additional contributions, the conditions under which new members may be added, the contingencies for continuation of the business in the event a member leaves the company, the manager of the company, and arrangements for the election of managers (Corporate Agents, 1995). The *operating agreement* is the LLC's version of bylaws, setting forth the governance of the company. Such an agreement typically includes the name and address of the company; its duration of existence; provisions for the continuance of the company in the event of a member's loss; the names, addresses, and contributions of members; mechanisms for the distribution of profits and losses to members; the names, addresses, powers, and means of election of managers; conditions of indemnification of members and managers; compensation of managers; bookkeeping requirements; and terms by which interest in the company may be transferred (Corporate Agents, 1995). It is important that these documents reflect the limits of continuation of life and limits on transferability of interest that differentiate LLCs from corporations. Failure to do so may result in an IRS challenge and the imposition of an additional layer of taxation (and penalties) on distributed income.

The relevant documentation for establishing a partnership is the *partnership agreement*. This can be a fairly brief form summarizing the name of the partnership; its term; its purpose; the names and addresses of all partners; their initial contributions to the partnership and any mechanisms for future contributions; provisions for the distribution of profits and losses, as well as the retention of profits within the partnership and payment of salaries; the management responsibilities of each partner and ways in which decisions are to be made; accounting arrangements and arrangements for handling money within the partnership; limitations on the outside business activities of partners; division of ownership of assets in the event of the partnership's dissolution; and provisions for the hiring of a managing partner, including the specific responsibilities and salary of the managing partner (Clifford & Warner, 1995). A good partnership agreement is designed to clarify the working relationship and financial arrangements among partners, so as to minimize areas of future disagreement.

A Note about Equity and Profit Sharing

A major challenge to practices is the issue of reimbursing the practice interests of stakeholders who resign or retire. The practice organization's documentation generally provides for the division of equity in the practice and the disposition of equity at the time a co-owner or member leaves the practice. At the time of incorporation, the firm issues stock, which are shares of ownership. The founders divide equity according to mutually agreed on criteria, which might include the money and effort invested by each person in the practice's formation. If and when the group is liquidated or sold, the proceeds—minus outstanding debts—are disbursed according to owners' stock holdings. In an LLC or a partnership, equity is based on the contributions to the company made by member/partners.

Should an owner or member leave the practice, a set of understandings called a buy–sell agreement dictate how the departing individual will be compensated. The agreement may require compensation from remaining owners/partners according to a valuation formula or may make provisions for the sale of the departing professional's interest to a new owner/partner. Note that if remaining owners/partners are required to buy out their colleague, it will be necessary for the practice to establish a timetable for the buyout and a funding mechanism. For example, each partner may be required to contribute regularly to a sinking fund that is held in escrow for the explicit purpose of buying out departing members if and when that eventuality occurs. Accountants can be quite helpful in establishing such mechanisms. The key is to ensure that the practice is not financially hamstrung by the need to buy out retiring owner/partners while still protecting the investments of those individuals. It is important to review such agreements carefully in any venture that involves equity sharing. If buy–sell agreements and mechanisms are not present, any equity that might be obtained during the start-up or offered as compensation may be worthless if you should leave the practice.

Note that the distribution of equity is not the same as profit sharing. Equity reflects the underlying ownership of the practice and guides the distribution of assets upon the sale or liquidation of the business. Profit sharing may be instituted without equity distribution as a means of enhancing compensation; it is also possible to offer shares of ownership as part of a compensation package. Both strategies can be effective in giving staff members a stake in the practice's success and enhancing the collaborative culture of an organization.

Having observed a number of practices in formation and operation, we would counsel prospective leaders to follow Lao-tzu's advice and "manifest plainness, embrace simplicity." Almost all the successful collaborations we've seen have started relatively small and simple and have grown as a result of hard work and distinctive business and clinical skills. Whenever they have developed complex administrative and governance structures, these structures have been responses to rapid growth, not internal politics. We recently received a prospectus from a massive provider network attempting to begin operations as an entity covering multiple major metropolitan areas. Membership in the network required thousands of dollars, no contracts had been obtained, and the governance structure—for political reasons—reflected the vast provider and geographic diversity of the network. The prospectus confidently asserted that the group would do business with managed care organizations, as well as engage in direct risk contracting with purchasers. (Why managed care firms would want to do business with a group that sought to be a competitor was not addressed.) In trying to be all things to all people, the network had developed complexity at the expense of coherence. Generally, it is far better to start simply and allow complexity to emerge with the growth and success of the practice.

Developing a Site for the Group

The practice's location, like its name, should be tailored to its basic strategy. If the founders are attempting to implement a low-cost strategy, keeping overhead down will be a prime consideration in selecting a location. A group offering interventions in behavioral medicine, alternatively, might do well to locate near potential referral sources, such as primary care practices and hospitals.

Hanna and Ritchie (1992) suggest that the location of a practice be determined by four factors: accessibility, visibility, image, and expandability. The ideal practice location is highly accessible to public and private transportation, with easy egress to the road and ample, free parking. It is helpful if the location is visible from the road and highlighted by a sign. Accessibility for patients with disabilities or medical problems should be easy, with a ramped entrance, properly equipped rest rooms, and elevator (if needed). An attorney can alert you to design requirements under the Americans with Disabilities Act (ADA).

A central office's image is conveyed by the manner in which it is decorated and furnished. Bare, painted walls and inexpensive furniture will convey a "public clinic" appearance and possibly turn off clientele. Neutral colors, comfortable and attractive waiting-room furniture, wood accents, and plants often provide a more soothing appearance. We are often surprised by the number of practices located in highly unattractive buildings that lack private entrances. Although these locations may offer the lowest rents, they may cost the practice in referrals. It is not unusual for MCOs to conduct site visits before awarding contracts. A shabby appearance tells the MCO that this is not a location that will be valued by executive employees of the companies purchasing benefits.

Chances are good that the space you find for your start-up will need redesign. If you are leasing space, the costs of redesign can be folded into the lease payments. Your landlord may have relationships with contractors who can assist you with issues regarding heating, ventilation, and air conditioning (HVAC), plumbing, and the allocation of space. Before consulting with one or more contractors, you need to identify your space needs clearly. Generally, you will need at least the following in a central location:

- A waiting area.

- A reception/business/records area.

- An office for each full-time equivalent (FTE) clinical staff member.

- Rest-room facilities.

- A lounge/lunch/meeting room for staff.

- At least one room for group therapy.

- At least one playroom for child work.

- Ample, convenient parking.

- One or more small rooms or closets for supplies, equipment, and other storage.

The space should be designed in such a way as to allow easy entrance from the parking area to the office waiting area. The waiting area should interface with the reception space for business transactions and to announce arrivals, but the two should be sufficiently set apart to preserve patient privacy. Too many practices place their reception areas in close proximity to clients in the waiting room, allowing them to hear conversations over the phone. This invites violations of confidentiality. It is also important that the clinical space be as soundproof as possible. New buildings often have thin walls through which sound can carry and/or ventilation ducts that become public address systems.

The space also needs to be designed with the staff in mind. Patient records should be located in an area that is accessible to both clinical and administrative staff in filing systems that are locked and secure off-hours. If there are multiple staff members performing billing and business functions, it is helpful to create a business suite for the practice, where computers are networked and staff can readily share information and materials. Often the business suite will be located adjacent to the reception area, making it easy for clients to settle their accounts upon entering or leaving.

Clinical staff also have distinctive space needs. Offices should be sufficiently large and well furnished as to comfortably accommodate family therapy sessions. Walls need to be soundproofed to ensure patient privacy; windows greatly enhance the appeal of the offices. It is very important to have an attractive meeting space that can be used for staff meetings, business presentations, and other administrative functions. Often this space will house resources for the clinical staff, such as journals and books. The meeting room may also do double duty as a group therapy area or staff lounge if space is tight.

Clearly, accessibility is enhanced if a practice has multiple locations, covering clientele in different locales. Indeed, this may be part of the group's strategy. The cost of such an approach can be meaningfully reduced by establishing satellite locations. These may be as simple as subleasing one or more offices within an established building or sharing space with a current tenant. Alternatively, the main practice could link with independent contractors at their own sites to create a network at relatively low cost. In such a distributed structure, the satellite office does not need to have the benefit of the spacious reception area and business suite of the main practice but can be linked to the main practice electronically for record keeping and billing. Larger satellite offices may house a receptionist/billing clerk; this person can be linked to the main group in a wide-area computer network. By creating multiple satellites, the practice covers a maximum area with minimum overhead. At a time when fees and capitated reimbursements are under pressure, a single main office per region is usually sufficient; additional site development should be accomplished electronically whenever possible.

LINKING PRACTITIONERS TO THE ORGANIZATION

If you are looking to join a collaborative practice rather than form one, the documentation described in this chapter will be quite useful in learning more about available groups and networks. In addition, you will want to examine the documentation that links you to the practice: the *employment agreement*, the *independent contractor agreement*, or the *membership agreement*.

Staff-Model Practices

An employment agreement is a contract between the practice and a practitioner/employee. It sets forth, among other things, the date on which employment is to start; the salary and other forms of compensation (such as bonuses or equity stakes); the arrangements for salary increases, including mechanisms for performance review; the benefits accorded the employee; and the specific duties required of the employee.

The contract may also include "restrictive covenants," sometimes called noncompetition clauses, which prevent the practitioner from conducting independent practice outside the group and setting up a competing practice if employment is terminated. Such covenants make sense, but they should not be so restrictive as to prevent clinicians from earning a living if they leave the group. Usually, the covenants define a specific time frame and geographic radius in which a competing practice cannot be established. Without such parameters, the covenants could be construed as an illegal restraint of trade.

It is not at all uncommon for the specifics of an employment relationship to be spelled out in an employee handbook, which outlines general personnel policies and procedures within the practice. For example, a full description of job duties, conditions under which termination can result, and a complete menu of benefits will not be outlined in the employment contract. Rather, the contract will make reference to the handbook for these details. For this reason, it is important to obtain a copy of the handbook and read it thoroughly. The presence of a handbook is a sign of a practice that has some sophistication with respect to the management of human resources. Absence of a handbook or its equivalent means that the practice has no formalized policies with respect to performance appraisals, compensation, termination, and employee grievances. This provides little support for staff clinicians and is not helpful to the development of a collaborative culture. We especially advise clinicians to carefully note the practice's policies and procedures regarding performance appraisal, including incentive payments for excellent performance. A practice committed to appraisals and willing to recognize and compensate high-quality performance is apt to be a successful collaboration.

One of the great advantages of employment for the staff clinician is the presence of a benefits package. This generally includes employer-sponsored or supported health insurance, paid vacation and sick time, and the presence of an employer-sponsored or supported retirement plan. Other benefits typically include malpractice coverage and supported continuing education. The cash value of these benefits can be substantial—20% or more of the entire compensation package—so it is necessary to evaluate salary offers in this light. A lower salary with excellent benefits might be worth more to a new clinician than a higher salary without generous benefits.

Network-Model Practices

An employment contract is only relevant to staff-model practices. If the clinician is hired as an independent contractor, this will be a codified in a contract that establishes the independent contractor status and specifies the nature of compensation. As outlined earlier, the independent contractor agreement will specify that the clinician is not an employee of the practice, retains full control of his or her work, and is free to engage in identical work for other parties. Because the contractor is not an employee, no mention will be made of benefits and there will be no handbook outlining work-related policies and procedures. Clearly, the contractor is trading the advantages of benefits and staff-model policies and procedures for the advantages of independence and autonomy.

Compensation for the contractor will generally consist of a fixed rate for each unit of work completed (e.g., an hourly rate for each therapy session). Care should be taken in the structuring of this reimbursement. For instance, the contract should spell out whether the contractor's fee is a function of billed sessions or reimbursed sessions. If the fee is a function of reimbursed sessions, this places the burden of nonpayments by MCOs on the contractor rather than on the practice. Generally, the contract will enumerate the range of clinical services to be provided by the contractor and the specific reimbursement for each. The reimbursement rate is typically a function of the amount billed by the practice minus a percentage for overhead.

The contractor agreement should also spell out all services to be provided for the contractor by the practice. For instance, many MCOs insist that groups and networks bill under a single taxpayer identification number. Hence, the practice may be responsible for all billing for services performed by the contractor. Care must be taken to ensure that the practice does not provide so many services for the contractor that the contractor is no longer independent. For instance, it would be difficult for a network to perform aggressive prospective review/case management work for contractor clinicians because the clinicians would no longer be empowered to carry out treatment in their own manner. This can make it challenging for networks to operate successfully under risk-sharing arrangements and highlights the need of such entities to find clinicians who practice in ways that are compatible with the philosophy of the organization.

The contractor agreement also will include language spelling out the conditions under which the arrangement can be terminated by either party. Generally, a practice will want to be able to terminate a contractual arrangement "without cause"; that is, without having to prove incompetence or malfeasance on the part of the contractor. It is important, however, that sufficient advance notice of termination is provided by either party and that arrangements are made for care in progress. That is, unless the termination is attributable to suspected malpractice or dishonesty, the practice should continue to reimburse the contractor for cases that are under way rather than force a hasty termination or transfer.

☞ LOOKING AHEAD

Joining a practice? What do you look for in a staff- or network-model group?

Our Group Affiliation Checklist at the end of this chapter (Reader's Resource 3.2) can guide your search!

Independent MSO Networks

In the unintegrated independent MSO network, each of the clinicians is self-employed and hence completes his or her own documentation to establish the corporation, PC, LLC, and so on. The linkage between an independent, outsourced MSO and the self-employed clinician is the *MSO contract*, which is really no different from any standard business contract. It sets forth the rights and responsibilities of the respective parties, including their financial arrangements and mechanisms for terminating the business relationship.

A contract with an independent MSO should clearly spell out the services to be provided by the MSO to practitioners and the manner in which these services are to be delivered. The contract should also stipulate the responsibilities of the practitioners in providing the information to be used by the MSO. For example, practitioners will be expected to provide certain billing and treatment information to the MSO, which is then responsible for preparing the billing statements, maintaining appropriate records and databases, and disbursing the funds from the billings. It is important to specify time frames, so that the expectations of each party are clear. Clinicians, for instance, will be expected to submit claims within a certain time frame and the MSO will be expected to file claims with payers within a defined period.

Should either of the parties become disenchanted with the other, clauses in their contract will spell out the mechanisms for dissolving their relationship. Appropriate notice of termination will be expected so that ongoing business can wind down. The contract should clearly identify the grounds by which the MSO can terminate services to a practitioner. Because the MSO may hold contracts that are essential to the financial well-being of the practitioner, the decision to terminate services can have a significant impact. The contract will state whether terminations are for "cause" (e.g., malpractice or felony conviction) or "without cause." Clearly, if termination without cause is allowed, the MSO offers much less protection to a provider than if cause must be demonstrated through defined mechanisms of due process (review, grievance, etc.).

The MSO agreement will also outline the means by which providers reimburse the MSO for its services. This will either be on a membership basis (fixed annual or monthly fee), a fee-for-service basis (percentage of clinical revenues), or a combination of the two. Overall, it is wise for clinicians to pay the MSO a predetermined percentage of clinical revenues for a defined menu of services. This ensures that the MSO has a vested interest in obtaining referrals for the clinicians. MSOs funded through membership fees alone may lack this incentive.

Membership-Model Practices

In the membership-model practice, as with the unintegrated MSO, the clinicians are self-employed and link to the collaborative entity through a contract. The contract in this case is known as a *membership agreement* and outlines the rights and responsibilities of the providers and the practice organization. Such agreements generally arise if the practice is structured as a not-for-profit corporation. In this case, the bylaws of the practice will reflect its governance arrangements, including the role of members in electing members of a board of directors, participation in committees, and so on. In addition, the membership agreement will outline the services to be provided by the practice organization to members and the responsibilities of members to the organization, much in the manner of the MSO agreement outlined above. Indeed, the membership organization may be an MSO or, alternatively, an IPA established by clinician members and funded with an initial purchase of stock (ownership). In the membership agreement of the MSO or IPA, the range of services and charges to clinicians should be clearly identified. Appropriate mechanisms for termination (including due process) also need to be spelled out because the MSO or IPA can become essential to the health and well-being of clinicians' practices.

A major problem encountered by membership organizations is the potential conflict between the individual providers and the practice organization with respect to contracting. In the unintegrated practice, the provider organization

(MSO or IPA) does not control all contracting for members. Members typically have the right to opt in or out of particular contracts. Under certain situations, a conflict can arise when members have the right to contract with an MCO either as an individual panel member or through the provider organization. This can lead to scenarios in which the actions of members may undercut the negotiating power of their collaborative organizations. To deal with this possibility, the membership agreement may specify that members cannot contract individually with an MCO if a contract between that insurer and the group is in force. The membership agreement might also give the practice organization right of first refusal with respect to the representation of members for upcoming contracts, which is important when there are competing networks to which clinicians belong and questions can emerge as to which network is representing the clinician's needs.

OBTAINING ASSISTANCE WITH THE START-UP: THE ROLE OF CONSULTANTS

The foregoing discussion has probably given you a healthy respect for the amount of thought and effort that goes into the making of a collaborative practice. Before the doors are opened and the first patient is seen, months of effort have been poured into strategic planning, legal consultation, and facilities design. This work may tax the time and expertise of even the most motivated practice developer. Fortunately, consulting assistance is available.

Selecting a Consultant

Numerous consultants have entered the business of behavioral health care, offering guidance on everything from clinical training to computerization and marketing. Many of these individuals have worked in managed care or group practice settings and bring hands-on experience to their work. Although consultants do not come cheaply, they can organize the start-up process and save developers both time and money.

That having been said, there are a number of marginal consultants offering their services to naive clinicians. A common joke defines a consultant as a laid-off managed care executive. Such individuals are not terribly difficult to spot. Their advice is generally "canned" and not well tailored to the specific needs of a region or particular structure. Their advice may also be based on a limited set of experiences. A consultant from a business and managed care background may have little background in the delivery of clinical services, for example, and may not be of much help in designing triage protocols. Similarly, a consultant with a strong clinical background may not have particular expertise in the nuances of contracting or information system design. It is important that the group identify its needs specifically and contract with consultants for only those services falling within the range of the consultant's expertise. Including attorneys and accountants, your practice may very well hire several consultants by the time it is finally established.

According to Bohlmann (1991), consultants address a range of health care concerns and group practice needs, including legal, accounting, information systems, marketing, and contracting issues. Consultants can also be quite helpful in guiding clinical training and developing practice guidelines, outcomes assessment, and quality improvement programs. The fee charged by the consultant typically reflects the prestige of the consulting firm (and, hence, demand for its services), the expenses to be incurred in the consulting process, and the time required by the consultation. Practice managers should always feel free to shop around and negotiate, as fees may vary widely for given services.

☛ LOOKING AHEAD

What consulting needs will your group have?

Our Consulting Needs Checklist at the end of this chapter (Reader's Resource 3.3) can help you use your resources wisely.

The process of hiring a consultant varies across organizations. As Bohlmann (1991) notes, some rely on an informal process in which consultants are interviewed by group principals and selected much in the manner of a job interview. Other groups may issue a request for proposal (RFP), requiring the prospective consultant to answer a range of questions and define and cost out a variety of services. In either scenario, the relationship between group and consultant should be clearly defined by a contract that spells out the specific expectations of the consultant and the exact compensation to be rendered. Ideally, the contract will be quite detailed with respect to time lines and expected products of the consultation. Such an agreement can go a long way toward minimizing misunderstandings.

It is not unusual for large consulting firms to employ a range of professionals, including partners, senior consultants, and junior staff. It is wise to determine the precise individual who will be providing each of the contracted services. Generic concerns, such as orienting group members to managed care frameworks or customizing off-the-shelf information system software, may be addressed by junior consultants at a savings to the practice. More specialized needs, such as those involved in costing out complex at-risk contracts, may require the assistance of relatively seasoned staff. In general, start-ups should be careful to avoid paying for more than they need—and should avoid paying for what they can get through personal networking (see our Resource List in the Appendix).

What to Look for in a Consultant

Our experience is that choosing a consultant or consulting firm with which to work should be like choosing an attorney, accountant, or physician for your family. When seeking the ideal consultant:

- Be sure that your core values are compatible with that of the consultant. (If you are working with a consulting firm, ask the firm for *its* mission statement. If the firm doesn't have one, look elsewhere.)

- Understand that if you are looking to a consulting firm to help you begin your practice, you are really considering a relationship of 2 or more years. What will these people be like to work with over that period?

- Recognize that consulting services are generally costly. You need to understand that in the long run, a good consultant will save or make you money. A poor consultant will lose you money.

- Realize that you can test the waters with a consultant by having the individual or firm do a smaller initial project with your start-up venture and see how you work together.

- If you are unhappy with the services you are receiving, talk with other consultants and see what they have to offer.

These are all commonsense suggestions. However, we have seen consultant relationships that work enormously well and some that work very poorly. **Not infrequently, consultations fail because the practice principals didn't ask the right questions.** When it comes to forming a practice, it is not necessary to know everything, but it is very helpful to know what you don't know.

CONCLUSION

Structuring the practice is a complex process that integrates considerable information from the planning process. If you are forming a group, your choice of a staff or network model and a corporate, LLC, or partnership structure and your selection of a name and location should reflect the organization's core mission and business strategy. Similarly, if you are a clinician seeking to affiliate with a group practice, you will want to identify the kind of group that best fits your personal needs and interests, as well as your career objectives. Fortunately, a wide range of collaborative models are available to practice designers, virtually ensuring a fit between the needs of any marketplace and those of practitioners.

Not infrequently, small groups operating within a specialty niche or a rela-

✔ READER'S SUMMARY

- Most groups seek a legal structure that offers limited liability; this is most commonly found in corporations and LLCs or their professional equivalents.
- The practice structure that is ideal for multispecialty collaborations varies on a state-by-state basis.
- The choice of a staff- versus network-model structure is perhaps the most important factor determining the culture and strategic advantages of a group.
- The name, location, and structure of a group must fit with its chosen mission and business strategy.
- The larger and more complex the group start-up, the greater the needs for specialty consultation.

tively rural area with a dearth of clinicians will structure themselves in partnership or LLC staff-model formats. Larger groups operating in highly price-sensitive markets will gravitate to network models and create opportunities for separately incorporated clinicians to affiliate with MSOs that are established as corporations or LLCs. In either case, success is achieved through a fitting of form to function.

READER'S RESOURCE 3.1
Strategy–Structure Matrix

Success in group practice comes from matching your core strategy and practice objectives with the right structural forms. The matrix below can assist this matching process.

Core strategy/objectives	Common structural elements
Low cost (cash market)	Partnership, PC, or LLC organization; independent contractor model; vertical governance; small scope
Managed care (markets with growing MCO presence)	Distributed group or network/IPA organization; vertical governance; broad scope
Specialty expertise or geographic niche	PC or LLC organization; staff model; horizontal governance; small scope
Data-driven quality (diversified markets)	PC, LLC, or integrated MSO/GPWW; staff model; vertical governance; large scope
Cover wide geographic area	Network-model group practice
Tightly control quality	Staff-model group practice
Keep overhead to minimum	Network-model group practice
Maximize integration of services	Staff-model group practice
Maximize provider autonomy	Network-model group practice
Maximize team collaboration	Staff-model group practice
Maximize security of income for providers	Staff-model group practice

READER'S RESOURCE 3.2
Group Affiliation Checklist

If you are looking to join a group practice, what should you look for in an affiliation agreement? The checklist below can help you find exactly what you're looking for.

JOINING A STAFF-MODEL GROUP

How does the salary compare to prevailing norms in the region?

What direct service responsibilities are required as part of the employment arrangement?

What employee benefits are offered and what is their quality? Health insurance? Retirement plan? Vacation? Professional development expenses? Malpractice coverage?

What is the employer contribution to benefits (health insurance, retirement plans)?

Is there a set of written human resources policies and procedures outlining your benefits, evaluations, conditions of employment, etc.?

Are there bonus and/or profit-sharing plans available as incentives to professional employees?

Are professional employees directly involved in aspects of the group's governance?

Are there formal arrangements by which successful professional staff members can become partners/co-owners in the group practice?

Tip: Make sure you compare apples to apples. A lower salary with a more generous benefits package and greater incentives may be preferable to a higher salary with fewer benefits and incentives.

Tip: Don't neglect the long view. An affiliation with a very successful group that has a bright future is generally preferable to an affiliation with an unknown or a shaky practice, even if the latter offers more money. Look for groups that allow you to grow with them.

JOINING A NETWORK-MODEL GROUP

Does the affiliation agreement make it clear that you are an independent contractor and that you are free to control your own practice and accept referrals from elsewhere?

Are the services provided by the group clearly outlined in the agreement?

(cont.)

Are the conditions under which you may be terminated from the network clearly outlined?

How is the network reimbursed for its expenses? If you are assessed a membership fee, are you assured of a referral flow to cover this amount?

If the network is organized on a membership model, what is the formal voice of the participants in the governance of the group practice?

How much is deducted from your billings to cover the network's overhead? Is this commensurate with the services being offered? How does the overhead deduction compare with the cost of obtaining those services on your own?

Does the network place its providers on an at-risk basis through such mechanisms as case rates (i.e., a fixed, lump-sum reimbursement per referral)? If so, can the network guarantee a sufficient flow of referrals to offset adverse selection risk (i.e., the risk of having a few severe cases assigned to you)?

Tip: A network/MSO providing billing and marketing/contracting services only should be viewed with suspicion if it is deducting more than 15% from the gross billings of clinicians. Networks providing computer systems, data collection, office space, and administrative support may plausibly deduct 50% or more from gross billings.

Tip: Two useful yardsticks: (1) Does the network provide you with a steady flow of referrals? and (2) Does the network meaningfully reduce your paperwork and administrative burden? Networks that provide those two factors may be more valuable for affiliation than those that do not, even though their bite out of billings may be higher.

Tip: See if the network will assure you of a degree of exclusivity within a geographic region. You may wish to make a larger commitment to a network that makes a larger commitment to you. You may also wish to structure your practice in a way to make it attractive to such a network.

READER'S RESOURCE 3.3
Consulting Needs Checklist

The larger and more complex your group practice start-up, the greater will be your needs for specialty consultation. The checklist below will be of help in allowing you to identify potential needs.

LEGAL CONSULTATION

- Assistance in selecting and registering a name, developing articles of incorporation/bylaws/membership agreements, and drafting partnership agreements.
- Assistance in identifying the legal structures appropriate to multidisciplinary practice in your state.
- Assistance in avoiding antitrust risks associated with the establishment of large provider networks.
- Assistance in reviewing and modifying initial contracts with managed care.
- Assistance in drafting employment agreements and independent contractor arrangements and avoiding legal concerns.

ACCOUNTING CONSULTATION

- Assistance with tax filings and payments, withholding for employees, and filing of tax statements for employees and independent contractors.
- Advice regarding accounting software and the maintenance of appropriate financial reports and records.
- Advice regarding cash management and the obtaining of loans, leases, and other financing.
- Assistance with adherence to state and federal laws that pertain to employers, such as Civil Rights Acts, Equal Pay Act, and ADA.
- Assistance to large groups with adherence to federal regulations pertaining to employer-sponsored health and retirement plans (e.g., COBRA and ERISA).
- Assistance in structuring compensation and incentive plans for employees.

INFORMATION SYSTEM CONSULTATION

- Assistance in defining software and hardware needs for a practice, including local and wide-area networks.

(cont.)

- Assistance in purchasing software and hardware to meet a group's present and foreseeable needs.
- Assistance in customizing off-the-shelf software to meet a group's needs.
- Assistance with training professionals in the proper use of hardware and software.
- Assistance with upgrading of the information system.
- Assistance in the development of communications systems and the linkage of these systems to other information functions.
- Assistance in the integration of clinical, financial, and quality-related information.

PRACTICE MANAGEMENT CONSULTATION

- Assistance with the development of MSOs and networks.
- Assistance with clinical training and the development of effective clinical programs.
- Assistance with practice guideline development and utilization management policies and procedures.
- Assistance with marketing of the group practice.
- Assistance with contracting, including the pricing of risk contracts.
- Assistance with the formation of alliances, joint ventures, and other strategies for expanding the group.
- Assistance with the development of continuous quality improvement programs, including outcomes assessment.

CHAPTER FOUR

Developing a Business Plan and Financing the Practice

> *Under peaceful conditions, the warlike man turns upon himself.*
> —Friedrich Nietzsche, *Beyond Good and Evil*

INTRODUCTION

Your strategic planning to this point has defined a vision and corresponding structure for the collaborative practice. During this portion of the development process, you have been an architect, designing the form and function of your practice. Now it is time for building: pouring the foundation, laying the pipes, wiring the structure, and raising the walls. Considerable construction effort goes into practices during the start-up phase, before the first patient ever walks through the door.

Just as a builder needs blueprints to translate the architect's vision into reality, a behavioral collaboration needs a road map to guide the achievement of its strategic ends. This is the purpose of the business plan. Many practices never get to the point of developing a business plan. They lack the business training to assemble a credible document. They tell themselves that they won't need it, because they won't be raising money from outside investors. So they begin building without blueprints.

Even if there is no need to secure financing, the creation of a business plan accomplishes an important aim: It forces developers to articulate and examine their assumptions. Now—not when the practice is up and running and losing thousands of dollars—is when you want to find out which of your assumptions is erroneous. "If it ain't broke, don't fix it" is a prescription for mediocrity. **Test your assumptions until they break, then fix their weak spots.**

This chapter will assist you with the builder's work: assembling the practice's business plan and securing its financing. Most important, it will help you translate *strategy* into *plans*. If you are not forming a practice but are looking for one

---

☆ IN THIS CHAPTER

- Strategies for raising money for a start-up group
- How to assemble a credible business plan
- The basics of financial analysis: A crash course for practitioners
- Creating and executing marketing plans

---

to join, this chapter will give you the tools to evaluate your alternatives and their business potential. Knowing what to look for can save your career a costly detour.

FINANCING THE START-UP

The developers of a small venture may have relatively few start-up needs and hence might be able to finance its creation independently. Those building larger enterprises may lack funds and need to turn to external financing sources. As we mentioned earlier, the most common reason for small business failure is undercapitalization. Often, enthusiastic entrepreneurs overemphasize opportunities and do not plan for pitfalls. When problems arise during the first months of operation, they lack the resources to weather the storm and are forced to close shop. It is far better to seek external financing and start with a cushion than begin life on a shoestring, a wing, and a prayer.

Controlling Start-Up Expenses

As we saw in Chapter 2, new practices have a core set of start-up needs, including office space, insurance, consultations, office and computer supplies, starting salaries, and capital reserves for unexpected needs. These can easily run to $100,000 and more, depending on the size of the start-up.

There are major advantages to controlling start-up expenses and financing the collaborative group internally. A group that finances its own start-up has the greatest control over its own destiny. Also, by controlling start-up expenses, the group is able to keep a larger share of its funds in reserve to hedge against periods of slow referral flows, the possibility of lost contracts, or employee/contractor defections.

Earlier, we observed that there are many ways of keeping these expenses to a minimum. We've observed several common strategies among groups:

- **Space.** Group founders can make sure that the costs of office renovation are folded into leases, spreading them out over time. Even better, it is sometimes possible to share office space with medical practices, churches, and social services organizations, greatly lowering initial expenses.

- **Leasing.** Most assets, such as computers, phone systems, and office equipment, can be acquired on a lease basis with favorable financing terms, reducing the need for large initial expenditures.

- **Consultations.** By doing legwork on their own, group leaders can minimize the consulting time of attorneys and accountants and ensure that they get the insurance they need at a competitive price. A number of do-it-yourself business start-up books offer low-cost, helpful advice (see Resource List in the Appendix).

- **Marketing.** With user-friendly but full-featured graphics programs, it is relatively simple to design stationery, logos, and business cards, limiting out-of-pocket costs to duplication. When Dr. Steenbarger led the start-up of a large network, he created all marketing materials (brochures, meeting overheads, display ads) on a personal computer with Harvard Graphics.

- **Information systems.** Off-the-shelf software can be customized for a fraction of the cost of hiring your own programmer. In many cases, local vendors of hardware and software will offer attractive packages that include leasing, setup, and maintenance that are more advantageous to a group than bargain-basement purchases through mail-order houses.

- **Personnel.** It is not unusual for start-up groups to make use of part-time clerical personnel as a way of minimizing the overhead associated with fringe benefits. Similarly, start-ups may keep the cost of clinical personnel down by relying on independent contractors, thereby avoiding the expenses of fringes and social security withholding.

- **Expansion.** Once a group gets off the ground, it may find that it needs to expand to win key contracts. Such expansion may necessitate greater geographic coverage or broadened coverage of behavioral health specialties. Rather than undertake the addition of significant overhead all at once, groups can form strategic alliances with other behavioral organizations and bid jointly on the contract. Such alliances can become the precursors to more formal joint ventures and mergers, as groups gradually move along the Cube toward greater levels of scope and integration.

There is a fine line between keeping overhead to a minimum and being undercapitalized. Remember CFH Health Care, our Collaboration from Hell (see Chapter 1)? There are many undercapitalized CFHs in the practice world. They estimate their initial expenses to be $30,000 and that is exactly what they raise for the start-up. They are then unprepared to meet any budget shortfalls resulting from slower-than-expected referral flows or unexpected expenses. Worse still, our CFH Health Cares lack key capabilities. For example, they cannot afford to allow their practice managers sufficient time to build relationships among referral sources and effectively market the group. They cannot allocate time or resources to collecting data regarding the quality of their services and hence are no more accountable for their work than the average solo practice. They fail to invest in the technology needed for online management of schedules, authorizations, and billings, miring administrative and clinical staff in hours of unreimbursed, unproductive, and frustrating phone delays.

The key is to find the most cost-effective strategies to achieve those needed capabilities. Though start-ups in behavioral health are far more affordable than those in medical care, given the lesser requirements for medical equipment, space, and supplies, they require a significant initial investment. **Practice developers who finance their own investments are in the best position to maintain control over their practices**. Without outside lenders and investors to satisfy, the leaders can chart their own course. Once the founders have to rely on outside capital, they become accountable to these outsiders. We have seen numerous businesses funded through venture capital firms which secure financing for the company in exchange for shares of ownership that are as high as 80%. In each of these situations, the cost of the financing in terms of loss of control was onerous. Most collaborative practice leaders are attracted to their work by the challenge and potential of running their own businesses. If you do not own 51% of the enterprise, however, you do not own your business. **In a very real sense, a practice head with 49% equity is an employee**.

For this reason, it may be better to start smaller and maintain control over the start-up than to cede authority to an entity that may or may not fully appreciate your vision. Keeping overhead down is essential to this process. If you are relentless in finding ways to keep office, computer, and personnel costs to a minimum, you should be able to finance your own start-up or at least maintain control of your venture, even as you secure initial financing. Successful practice managers are ruthless about the bottom line. They treat every dollar as if it's their own. Because it often is.

Starting the Large Collaboration

When founders seek to develop a large practice network, they frequently look to the network membership for start-up funds. Indeed, one of the appeals of the large multispecialty practice is that it can spread its expenses across numerous providers, reducing any one person's total financial risk. Unfortunately, as we have observed, this is sometimes so alluring as an option that networks are assembled primarily for their ability to raise start-up capital, with little thought going into the quality, motivation, specialty skills, and geographic distribution of the members. Such structures are able to raise cash readily, especially in areas in which the fear of managed care is high, but lack the ability to adequately deploy these funds. The founders have chosen the network structure, not as the result of careful strategic planning but as an expedient for fund raising.

Large networks have a different distribution of start-up expenses than single-location group practices. For example, because network members maintain their own offices, the practice should have minimal rent/lease overhead. A great advantage of group practices without walls is that you don't have to pay for walls. On the other hand, a group of, say, 50 practitioners scattered across several counties would require sizable funds for the design, implementation, and maintenance of an adequate communications and information system (see Chapter 5). Large, membership networks also require more legal and accounting work than traditional groups, given the complexity of membership agreements and contracts with MCOs. They may also have greater insurance needs, especially if they have diverse, active boards of directors and are involved in credentialing and utilization management. Because networks are more cumbersome to maintain, they generally require full-time practice management, which adds to personnel overhead. Although networks appeal to many providers as low-cost start-ups, they are not a panacea. They can easily require start-up investments of thousands of dollars from participating members if organized properly. It is critical to scrutinize the business plans of any start-up network to ensure that the money invested has a reasonable likelihood of paying off in enhanced referral flows.

Raising Outside Capital

If the new practice cannot fund its start-up internally, it will need to turn to outside lenders or investors. A lender, such as a banking institution, will loan money to the enterprise at a defined interest rate over a specified period. The lender typically does not hold an equity interest in the business or reap a percentage of its profits.

An investor (or venture capitalist), alternatively, is one who provides money to the new firm in hopes of receiving an ample return. The investor seeks returns above and beyond those found in fixed-rate instruments and hence will want to be compensated in ways that transcend the bank's arrangement. For example, the investor may seek an equity share in the practice, which could be cashed in once the practice is sold. Because behavioral start-ups are too small to interest mainstream venture capital firms, the parties most likely to be interested in participating in the formation of a practice would be local investors seeking high return and hospitals or other health care groups that could directly benefit from the group's formation. For example, a private psychiatric hospital might have an interest in developing an outpatient provider network.

Given that a venture capitalist will insist on returns well in excess of the interest rates charged for a bank loan, one might wonder why any new enterprise would turn to such financing. There are, in fact, many reasons. If the practice is new and without a meaningful track record, it would not qualify for an unsecured bank loan. Instead, the owners would have to pledge personal capital to collateralize the loan. The venture investors, on the other hand, may be willing to risk their investments without such collateral guarantees. Understandably, they would expect a higher return to compensate for their risk.

The other reason it may make sense to do business with private investors is that these individuals may bring particular expertise to the new practice. If, for example, an HMO or private psychiatric hospital is willing to invest in the start-up, its members might bring management savvy and business contacts that could not be offered by a commercial bank. The bank will not attempt to manage your business; it will only require regular reports of revenues, expenses, and profits. Venture capitalists, on the other hand, may very well assume a share of the firm's ownership and participate in its management. It is not unusual, for example, for the board of directors of a start-up company to include outside investors. This can be a hindrance or a blessing, depending on the expertise of the investors and their working relationship with the firm's managers.

Varieties of Bank Loans

When dealing with banks, a variety of loan structures are possible. (For useful discussions, see American Psychological Association Practice Directorate, 1996b, Milling, 1995.) In general, we can identify three major forms of bank financing:

- Short-term single-payment loans;

- Intermediate-term installment loans; and

- Long-term installment loans.

Let's say that a practice experiences a temporary cash crunch due to an unusually high tax liability, combined with late payment on receivables from an insurer. In such an event, the group will consider a short-term loan (i.e., less than 1 year in duration and generally 30–180 days) to weather the shortfall. Such loans are called single-payment loans (Milling, 1995) because they are repaid all at once at a fixed due date. Typically there is no grace period on loan repayment and the loan is secured by readily available assets such as receivables. In our example, the money owed to the group by the insurer could serve as collateral for the short-term loan to pay tax bills that have come due.

It is not uncommon for small businesses to have peaks and valleys in their cash flows resulting from irregularities in the collection of funds from customers. When these cash flow headaches become frequent, or if business is highly seasonal (perhaps your group is located in a resort or college community and experiences seasonal shifts in referrals), there may be an ongoing need for short-term loans to bridge periods of shortfall. In such a case, an arrangement is made with a bank for a *line of credit*, which is an ongoing source of short-term funds. The line of credit is available to be used at any time at the practice's discretion. Typically, the line will be accessed at cash-crunch times and fully repaid when cash flows are stronger. This minimizes interest expense to the group and maintains solid credit status with the bank. If a group finds itself continuously dipping into a line of credit, it probably has ongoing cash flow problems that need to be resolved and/or needs to consider a longer-term loan.

An *installment* loan, unlike a single-payment loan, is one that is paid off in periodic (often monthly) installments. An intermediate-term loan (usually 1–8 years in duration) is typically sought for the purchase of an important capital asset, such as a computer system. Long-term loans are generally reserved for the acquisition of long-lived assets, such as real estate. Often, a grace period covers the repayment of each installment, beyond which the loan is considered "past due." It is unwise to allow any form of loan to become past due because this can jeopardize the group's credit standing and business relationship with the lending institution.

Banks typically seek collateral to secure their loans in the event of default. This might take the form of compensating balances at the lender institution, where the business is required to maintain savings balances of a certain size. Longer-term loans may involve the pledging of separate assets as collateral and/or the creation of a lien on the assets being financed. As a rule, collateral guarantees vary as a function of the borrower's financial track record. All things being equal, groups that have been in business for a long time and have a solid track record of repaying loans will have an easier time obtaining a loan and will have more modest collateral demands than groups without such a history. This poses particular problems for start-up groups, which—almost by definition—lack solid business and lending histories. Not infrequently, this means that banks will require practice founders to pledge their *personal assets* as collateral for their loans. If, say, four group founders decide to borrow $50,000 toward the start-up of their practice, they may be required to secure the loan by allowing the bank to place a lien on their personal cars or homes. In the event of a loan default, those nonbusiness assets would be at risk.

The frequent need for small business start-ups to secure loans through the personal assets of the owners has two very important implications:

First, although the corporate or LLC organizational structures provide limited liability in the event of business losses (i.e., the corporate veil prevents creditors from laying claim to the personal assets of shareholders), this flies out the window in the event of a bank loan that is secured by personal assets. If group founders are truly interested in limiting their risk and liability, they need to find ways to keep their start-up overhead modest and fund their group's inception internally.

Second, when the owners of a group practice do place their personal assets at risk in a start-up, their backsides are on the line in a way that is generally not the case among institutionally affiliated groups and membership organizations. Not infrequently, this means that the management of such groups will put in the extra hours needed to successfully market and manage the group. Savvy clinicians looking to affiliate with a group may pay particular attention to these practices because they often have the entrepreneurial drive to succeed

When the group practice obtains an intermediate- or long-term installment loan, the structure of the repayment plan may vary, with fixed or variable interest rates and payment in equal installments versus deferred payments. Variable interest rates can be adjusted up or down (sometimes within a defined corridor) as a function of prevailing interest rates, whereas fixed interest rates remain constant for the life of the loan. It is common for intermediate-term loans to be made on a fixed basis whereas longer-term loans often have a variable structure to protect the lending institution from interest rate fluctuations. For example, if a group borrows $100,000 to purchase one of its competitors, the loan might be made at a set percentage above the prime rate (which is the prevailing lending rate to the most credit-worthy borrowers).

Many loans are structured for repayment in equal installments, spreading the debt financing evenly over time. At other times, however, it may be advantageous to allow for deferred payments, permitting the borrower to make smaller payments earlier in the loan period, followed by one or more larger "balloon" payments at the back end. A similar advantage can be achieved by setting an artificially low interest rate early in the loan period, followed by steady rate increases. Such creative financing can be especially helpful to start-up groups, reducing payments early in the loan period (when referral flows are apt to be weakest) and allowing for greater payments as cash flows improve. Accountants can be very helpful to practice managers in determining the most advantageous loan structure and terms for a particular group.

In many cases, financing can be secured from vendors as well as banks. Vendors are often willing to extend a line of credit to the practice, eliminating the need for a short-term bank loan to cover a purchase. Most computer vendors extend leasing terms to businesses, in essence covering the financing of the intermediate-term asset. In financing leases, the vendor often allows for the outright purchase of the asset at the end of the specified lease period at a favorable price. Reliance on such leases for furniture, computers, and software can greatly reduce the need to rely on banks and outside investors.

How a Loan Application Is Evaluated

When a practice seeks outside financing, it needs to provide considerable documentation to prospective lenders and investors. (This is true of IPAs and networks as well, because the recruitment of members can also be a recruitment of investors.) This is one important function of the *business plan*. The business plan is a summary of the practice's current status and future plans. It contains a complete set of financial analyses that specify how borrowed funds will be used and repaid and/or how meaningful returns on investment will be achieved.

Because the lenders and investors reading the plan will come from the business community, it is absolutely essential that practice developers follow accepted guidelines in the execution of their plan. Business plans that are poorly organized, incomplete, or slipshod in their financial analyses are immediate tipoffs to badly managed ventures. Not infrequently, a potential investor will scan the initial summary of the plan and the financials to obtain a sense of the project and its potential. If the impression is not favorable, the remainder of the plan will not be read. Often, practice developers hope to snare investors on the strength of their ideals. Investment, however, does not work that way. First and foremost, the investor wants an opportunity at a meaningful return on investment (ROI) that will justify the risks taken. In an important sense, the investor doesn't care any more about your collaboration than you care about Exxon, AT&T, or General Electric when you buy shares of a mutual fund. **Your plan has to demonstrate the *value* of your practice as an investment and can only do that by speaking the investors' language**.

Consummating a loan with a bank can involve several face-to-face meetings, in addition to the preparation of the business plan. The very first meeting may be little more than an introduction, in which the overall business concept is described, application forms are completed, and business cards are exchanged. At that meeting, founders should also be prepared to leave written material concerning the practice, including a copy of the business plan. Overall, lenders will evaluate several items of information in the course of processing an application for a loan:

- **Financial statements** (profit/loss statements, cash flow statements, and balance sheets) covering the group's operations to date (see the discussion of these financial statements below).

- **Pro forma financial statements** projecting the group's financial status at least 1 year into the future on a monthly basis and several years into the future on an annual basis.

- **A business plan**, describing the group's operations, management, and core strategy.

- **The credit history** for the group, as well as the credit histories of the group's owners/founders.

- **Income tax records** from the group, as well as from the group's owners/founders.

Pavlock (1994) notes that banks will evaluate businesses—including practice organizations—on "six C's" when a loan is under consideration:

- **Character.** Is the borrower experienced, with a good track record of fulfilling business obligations?

- **Capital.** Have borrowers invested their own equity in the business, such that they have a vested interest in its success?

- **Capacity.** Does the borrower have the management skill to use the borrowed funds wisely?

- **Collateral.** Can the lender secure the loan with assets?

- **Circumstances.** Does the lender have a strategic position in the marketplace that will help generate the revenue needed to repay the loan?

- **Coverage.** Is there insurance in place to protect against the death or disability of key leaders within the practice?

If at all possible, it can be very helpful to have a current client of the bank arrange the introduction to a bank official and raise interest in your project. This is much more powerful than approaching financiers or a loan officer on an unsolicited basis. As Milling (1995) notes, however, banks do not make money by turning down loan requests. Generally, if a bank is hesitant to make a loan, it has good reasons for its reluctance. Feedback from a loan officer, even when negative, can be very helpful in modifying future loan requests and in adjusting one's financial and strategic assumptions.

☞ LOOKING AHEAD

Whether you approach a bank or outside investors, you will need to present your ideas to the business community.

How do you prepare a killer business presentation? Our presentation guide at the end of this chapter (Reader's Resource 4.1) may help!

Alternatives to Bank Financing

Suppose you do not qualify for bank financing or cannot make the collateral guarantees necessary to secure a bank loan. In larger markets, it may not be possible to reduce start-up overhead to the point where you can finance a group internally. At that point, then, you have several options:

Bring in New Operating Partners

You can elect to share ownership with a greater number of practitioner founders and, in essence, increase the size of your start-up group. This means that you are reducing the ownership stake of the original founders and spreading the group's profits over more individuals. It also means that governance will be shared with a greater number of participants.

Bring in Silent Partners

A silent partner is one who is relatively uninvolved in the daily operations of the business but invests as a co-owner for a share of profits (and a share of capital gains should the firm be sold at a premium). The silent partner may not be a mental health practitioner and thus will not be invested in the group for career furtherance. Silent partners are typically interested in the return on their capital and, as we noted previously, will seek returns above and beyond the interest rates offered by banks to compensate for their risks.

Establish a Membership Structure

If you are forming a network-model group, you may seek start-up financing from the network participants themselves, as in the formation of an IPA or membership-model network. This can spread the burden of financing quite widely but also creates situations in which governance can be complicated. Note also that, as the membership expands, the demands on the network to generate sufficient referrals to cover the initial investment become significantly greater. It takes a meaningful initial referral flow to justify the investment of 50 or more practitioners in a membership network!

Each of these strategies has its advantages. Selectively adding operating partners can be an effective way to gradually expand the scope of the practice, attract new talent, and increase the pool of financial, clinical, and managerial resources. Relying on silent partners and other outside investors can bring significant financial resources into the group, although this may come at a high cost given the ROI needs of such investors. If they are truly silent, outside investors allow the original group founders to maintain operational control over the practice in exchange for a "piece of the action." Nonsilent outside investors can also be assets if they bring distinctive business expertise to the group. The main thing to keep in mind is that risk and reward are inversely proportional. To the extent that founders reduce their start-up risks by spreading investment over a greater number of principals, they reduce their own profit share and ownership stake, as well as a measure of control over governance.

The membership strategy, alternatively, is the most radical of the financing options. It redefines the organization by dramatically expanding the scope of the group while creating a broad and horizontal governance. Although it reduces the financial risk of each party, it also greatly reduces the profit incentives, because excess revenues are generally plowed back into the enterprise. Membership organizations also are often established for the practice security and autonomy of participants, which may eliminate profit incentives attached to the sale of the group. Although the membership option is a means of financing, we do not recommend that it be selected *primarily* for financial reasons. Rather, the broad scope, low integration, and horizontal governance of the membership network must fit with the needs of the marketplace and those of the practice founders.

Cementing the Financial Relationship

The practice's final arrangement with a bank or outside investor will be codified in a contract, spelling out the obligations and rights of each party. Because lenders/investors now have an interest in the success of the practice, they will need to monitor how it is faring and whether or not it will be able to repay its debts and generate the anticipated return. The *covenants* of a loan spell out the practice's responsibilities and financial expectations during the loan period. For instance, contracts with lenders and investors will require the practice to report financial performance on a regular basis, usually quarterly, and maintain set levels of profitability and cash flow. Should these covenants be violated, penalties can ensue, including the complete liquidation of the loan. Outside funding is *not* a single transaction; it opens the new enterprise to an ongoing business relationship that only terminates when the investment is fully repaid.

Among the indicators of financial performance that banks will monitor during a loan period, several stand out. Ratios of assets to liabilities are an important gauge of the overall financial health of the organization. A trend in the direction of increasing liabilities to assets may signal problems in collections, declining referral flows, and/or difficulties in managing overhead. Trends will also be examined with respect to gross billings and gross revenues, as a way of monitoring the volume of business being conducted and the group's success in collecting its receivables. Expenditure levels will be scrutinized for signs of increasing overhead. An increasing ratio of expenditures to revenues—suggesting that a higher percentage of income is going to overhead—can be a sign of decreasing managerial efficiency and may be a cause for concern.

If the investor in a practice has a stake in the health care market, as in the case of a hospital aligning with a group practice, the contractual terms of the arrangement may extend well beyond finances. Such terms may include input concerning how the practice entity will deliver its services. These terms can also include the provision of management services and other institutional benefits from the investor to the outpatient organization. Silent investors banking on the eventual sale of the group at a profit will want assurances that policies will be pursued in the interest of maximizing the group's value to potential purchasers. Competent legal assistance is necessary to execute and review these contracts and preserve the interests of practice owners (for helpful discussions of financing issues among medical practice groups, see Pavlock, 1994; Yen & Goldberg, 1992).

Financing Issues for Those Joining Collaborative Groups

If you are investigating collaborative practices with which you might affiliate, you may feel that you don't need to be intimately familiar with the foregoing discussion regarding financing. Nothing could be further from the truth. Your understanding of financing may be invaluable in selecting a strong group with a bright future.

Your access to financial data regarding group practices that you might join will vary from situation to situation. If you are joining a group as a co-owner and investor, you are entitled to full financial disclosure and should settle for nothing less. That means that you will be able to see income and cash flow statements, as well as balance sheets, going back several years, and pro forma projections. If these have not been independently audited by a qualified accountant (which is often the case with small businesses, given the expense of independent audits), you may also wish to check financial reports against income tax records. The greater your financial investment in the group, the more important it is that you perform a thorough due diligence. We would be wary of any group that solicited investment from a practitioner or investor without offering full financial disclosure and a contract that clearly outlines the rights and responsibilities of equity holders.

If you are contemplating joining a membership organization, you also are in an ownership/equity financing role and deserve a high degree of financial disclosure, including full financial statements. Dr. Steenbarger's organization, Prime-Care of Central New York, Inc., for example, provides an annual report to members at its yearly membership meetings, which summarizes the past and coming year's budgets, details numbers and types of referrals, and highlights anticipated expenditures. Such information is essential if members are to make informed decisions with respect to the network's governance.

Clinicians seeking affiliation with a network as an independent contractor or looking to join a staff-model practice typically receive much less information with respect to the group's finances. Although owners may share basic data regarding financial performance and growth during an interview, it would be unusual for them to provide a detailed disclosure of financial statements and business plans. That means that it can be difficult to identify groups that have a truly strong financial position. Following are several of the indirect indicators of financial strength that you might factor into your decision making:

- **Practice volume.** How many direct service hours per week are being conducted by clinicians in staff-model groups? Generally, a full-time clinical staff member would be expected to provide direct service for at least 25–30 hours per week. Unfilled hours may be a sign of weak referral flows and/or lost contracts.

- **Referral volume.** Talking with network participants will give an idea of the volume of referrals coming to clinicians. Declines in volume over time may signal problems in obtaining contracts and marketing the group.

- **Concentrations of volume.** Volume may be adequate but may be concentrated in one or two referral sources, such as large MCO contracts. Such groups can be quite vulnerable if these contracts are lost.

- **Delays in payments.** Delays in paying salaries in staff-model groups is the kiss of death and a sure sign of financial crisis. Delays in reimbursement to network clinicians may reflect nothing more than problems in obtaining reimbursement from an MCO. If such delays are occurring across numerous insurers and even with nonmanaged business, this could be a sign of cash-crunch problems.

- **Failure to maintain assets.** Most assets, such as furniture, carpeting, office equipment, and computers, need to be replaced and upgraded periodically. Delays in maintaining and replacing assets may reflect a shortage of funds and future financial problems.

- **Growth.** A growing group practice adds locations and staff members. A shrinking practice experiences cutbacks. You may wish to think twice before affiliating with a shrinking group practice. You could be the next cutback!

By maintaining extensive contacts within a community and talking with local referral sources, you can learn a great deal about group practices, their reputations, and their strength. Although you as a staff clinician may not be investing money into the group directly, you are investing the time and energy of your career. That certainly warrants its own due diligence.

☞ LOOKING AHEAD

How does a clinician go about starting a group practice, adjusting to changes in the practice environment, and manage to sell the practice?

Our featured interview with Warren Throckmorton, PhD, at the end of this chapter offers some insights (Reader's Resource 4.2).

THE BUSINESS PLAN

Lenders or investors will judge the soundness of a financing project based on information contained in a business plan and shared in a business presentation. Not uncommonly, new practices will have no formal plan to present, relying on verbal descriptions and fuzzy projections. This situation undermines the credibility of the owners in the eyes of the lender or investor. Writers on the business of professional practice compare the business plan to the x rays that are ordered by physicians. To adequately diagnose the health of your start-up, lenders, investors, and prospective clinical staff members need to run certain tests and scrutinize pictures of the practice.

Uses of the Plan

As mentioned previously, we strongly advise developers to compose a business plan **even if they are able to cover their own start-up financing.** The drafting of a plan requires a hard look at strategic and financial assumptions. Although the developers may have a global sense of what they'll need to do to survive, a break-even analysis derived from financial statements, for example, can tell them the precise patient volume they'll need to stay afloat. Not infrequently, such analyses require managers to go back to the drawing board and restructure aspects of the practice. Similarly, financial projections lend themselves to "what-if" analyses, in which the impact of adverse events can be objectively evaluated. This can be of incalculable value in planning for adversity.

In membership organizations and networks, the business plan also functions as a recruitment tool. To document the value of an MSO for member providers, a business plan is most useful. The plan can document the financial performance of the MSO to date and detail plans for its future. From the plan, interested providers can determine the adequacy of the MSO's capitalization, its business prospects, and the strength of its management. Just as the group leader uses the business plan to sell a bank or investor on his or her group, the membership network uses the plan to attract talented clinicians.

Having observed a number of practices in the course of our work—as well as the research for this book—we have developed a sense of groups that will succeed and groups that will fail. Usually, within minutes of talking with a manager, our impression becomes clear. Accordingly, we have formulated three criteria by which all collaborative practices can be evaluated via a business plan. These criteria are perhaps the most valuable tool we have to offer clinicians who want to affiliate with a practice.

- Our first criterion of success is **the degree to which the group leaders are willing and able to invest time and money into their venture**. We recently observed a practice network in which the owner/leader was investing 1 hour a week of his time in management. Need we say more?

- Our second defining element is **the extent to which the members are dedicated to the information infrastructure of their group**. As we illustrate in the next chapter, collaborative practices that truly want to be accountable for their work make major investments of time, effort, and money in mechanisms for improving accountability.

- Our third benchmark is the **presence of a simple, clearly articulated mission, strategy, and plan**. Successful practices have a direction and are committed to specific actions to achieve this direction.

Please attend to the following sentences carefully and burn them into your brain: The advice they contain will save you far more time and money than you will invest in this book. **Be very careful about doing business with a practice or other health care entity that lacks these three elements. Be hesitant to choose them as a partner, employer, or payer. In fact, do your best to locate your practice in a region where most of the competition lacks these three elements.** Practices that are invested in a vision and develop concrete plans to be accountable for that vision are the ones that will succeed in the future of mental health. They are the practices most worthy of your investment.

Writing the Plan

There are no absolutes for the ideal length and format of a business plan, but a few guidelines hold true across settings. According to Abrams (1993), the plan should be:

- Professionally executed, preferably with laser printer, and bound attractively with a cover.

- No fewer than 10 pages and not more than 30, not including appendices, with the total length of appendices not exceeding the length of the preceding plan.

- Well organized, with sections of the plan clearly delineated, allowing for an easy scanning of the content.

- Free of hype and unsubstantiated claims but not shy about describing the strengths and potential of the venture.

- Unique to your group and not from a canned program.

- Detailed about anticipated financial performance, with month-to-month projections for the first year of operation and quarterly projections for at least the following 2 years.

Pavlock (1994) suggests that a business plan is divided into sections that summarize the following:

- **Objectives and action plan.** The overall aims of the practice.

- **Organization and management.** Overview of the practice's structure and leadership.

- **Market data.** Description of the market sought by the venture and its plan for marketing.

- **Planned services and programs.** Variety of professional services offered by the practice.

- **Financials.** Projected revenues, expenses, profit, and cash flows.

An especially detailed presentation of business plans is offered by Abrams (1993), who breaks the document into the following categories:

- Executive summary

- Company description

- Industry analysis

- Target market

- The competition

- Marketing plan

- Operations

- Management and organization

- Long-term development and exit plan

- Financials

- Appendix

Abrams (1993) stresses that the executive summary and financials are the most important parts of the plan, simply because they are read first. Loan officers swamped by proposals will screen candidates based on the information contained in these two sections. Your task in the plan, then, is to win attention by capturing the essence of your start-up in a few pages and then convincing the reader that it is a superior investment.

Crafting the Plan

Introduction

Your introduction, or executive summary, will be approximately one to three pages in length. It provides the reader with an overview of your practice, emphasizing its distinctive strengths and financial potential and the expertise of the leaders. The introduction should be a summary of the major elements of the plan, highlighting the practice's structure and organization, its market position and marketing strategy, and its present and projected financial performance. Most of all, the introduction should interest the reader in your venture. After scanning those two or three pages, the reader should have a good grasp of what you are going to do, how you're going to do it, and how successful it's likely to be.

Practice Overview

The next portion of the plan must go into detail about the specifics of your practice's purpose, legal structure, ownership, and leadership. A mission statement, capturing the vision behind your start-up, might be followed by a description of the behavioral health services offered, the history of operations, and the practice's legal status and ownership. The overview must also include information pertaining to the organization and governance of the business (including an organizational chart), its management (including qualifications of practice managers), its operations (how services are delivered at each site), and the competitive advantages achieved by the practice. Flow charts are especially helpful in describing processes, such as triage and quality improvement systems. Column charts can be used to highlight a practice's strengths. Pie, bar, and X–Y charts can effectively summarize statistical data, such as utilization trends or historical revenue growth.

Market Overview

In this segment of the plan, you will summarize the regional marketplace, including population estimates and demographics, and its need for mental health and chemical dependency services. You will also highlight recent trends in the market, including relevant managed care trends and population shifts. A summary of the competition might be followed by a description of your marketing plan: Who will need your services, how you will let them know of the services, and how you will monitor the quality of service delivery and clients' satisfaction with the services. The marketing plan must include strategies for *all* referral sources that you will seek, including primary care physicians, managed care organizations, EAPs, educational institutions, and the general public. Upon perusing this section, the reader should be able to clearly identify the niche in your market that your practice will occupy.

Financials

Here is where you emphasize the bottom line. Your business plan should summarize the historical performance of the practice by including income statements, balance sheets, and cash flow statements for the past several years. The plan should also project financial performance for the next several years. Abrams (1993) recommends that the first year's projections be monthly for income and cash flow statements and quarterly for balance sheets. Subsequent years should be quarterly and annual, respectively. If you are raising funds, this section should clearly identify how these funds will be used and how they will be paid off. Of course, your projections of future revenues and profits will be predicated on certain assumptions concerning the future; these should be spelled out clearly in a subsection of your financial presentation.

Appendices

Material that is relevant to your practice but would clutter the main presentation of the plan can be organized in an appendix. This might include curriculum vitae of the founders, copies of any articles written about the practice, and professional references. Information that is critical to an accurate appraisal of operations and performance should *not* be included in an appendix but should appear in the plan's body.

Preparing the Plan's Financials: Preliminaries

For any bank that would assist in the capitalization of a practice, the bottom line is whether or not the owners are likely to be able to pay off the loans. Outside investors will scrutinize the business plan to determine whether the venture can offer a competitive return on their investments. Even when the investors are the practice members themselves, as in some networks, they will want reassurance that the enterprise is financially viable. These needs make the financials section of the business plan critically important.

Few mental health professionals, however, have had experience in accounting. Assembling income statements, budgets, and cash flow projections may be a daunting prospect. In the sections that follow, we run you through a few basics of constructing financial statements. These statements, properly prepared, document for the reader the past and anticipated profitability and viability of your practice. Equally important, they will uncover for you any weaknesses in your planning, enabling you to avoid costly cash crunches.

A set of financial statements are only as reliable as the information from which they are drawn. That is why it is absolutely essential to keep thorough and accurate records of all income and expenses. The processing of financial data is part of the management information system (MIS), which we discuss in the next chapter. Without accurate records, it is impossible to assemble adequate financial statements and your ability to file accurate state and income tax returns will be impaired. Having a complete and organized set of records greatly reduces the time that accountants need for preparing tax forms and can help the practice survive possible IRS audits.

If you are getting a new practice off the ground, you will not be able to give an accounting of historical financial performance. Nonetheless, you will be expected to make reasonable and thorough financial projections. At the very least, you can audit the records of each founding member of the enterprise and determine the number of patients seen per year, average fee-for-service revenue per patient, and gross practice income. Summed across the founding members, this can give a preliminary estimate of group income during the early months.

Once you have estimated income during these months, you will need to project expenses, including rent, utilities, supplies and equipment, salaries, and consulting fees. These will generally be known in advance or can be accurately estimated on the basis of founders' practice experience. During subsequent months and years, you will make certain assumptions regarding the growth in patient volume and revenue, need for new staff and space, and demand for additional equipment and consulting time. These assumptions should mesh reasonably well with founders' own experience and with the current dynamics of the marketplace. For example, if members' practices are currently growing at 10% per year and there are no preferred group contracts being offered in the region, it would be misleading to project higher growth rates on the basis of winning a contract. All assumptions, as mentioned earlier, must be clearly identified for business plan readers—and should undergo your own skeptical scrutiny.

A most helpful exercise—not necessarily part of the business plan proper—is the construction of a break-even analysis. Here the practice estimates its fixed overhead (rent, salaries, etc.) and its average fee-for-service rate of reimbursement. From these figures, it is easy to determine the level of patient volume that would be needed to avoid losing money. Even further, if the practice strives for a certain utilization target—say, an average of six sessions per outpatient—it is possible to estimate the precise number of new patients that the group needs to obtain to break even. Such analyses are essential to capitation contracting, where one must know utilization, population size, and expenses to accurately determine a per-member per-month (PMPM) premium that will adequately cover expenses and yield an acceptable profit.

Two Formats for Accounting

Although most behavioral practices retain the services of a professional accountant, it is important to know a few basics of accounting. Many mental health professionals are intimidated by the numbers and jargon of accounting and lack any formal orientation to the field. As a result, their practices remain information-poor.

The building blocks of accounting are straightforward: income, expenses, assets, and liabilities. How these are computed, however, can be tricky. In general, there are two major reporting formats for financial statements: *cash basis* and *accrual basis*. The difference between these formats can be substantial. Not infrequently, managers construct statements on both bases to arrive at a more well-rounded view of the company.

When financial statements are assembled on a cash basis, it simply means that income and expenses are only logged in once the cash actually enters or leaves the practice. Anticipated future payments and receipts are not included in the analyses. Because income tax statements are constructed on a cash basis, it is common for groups to keep their records in this manner. This, however, may yield a limited perspective of the group's finances.

The difference between cash- and accrual-basis accounting can best be illustrated with an example. Suppose Behavioral Affiliates, PC, has 10 clinicians on staff, each conducting 100 billable hours per month. During the month of December, the group as a whole conducts 1,000 sessions of psychotherapy, each of which is billed at an average rate of $70. The computer system breaks down, however, and the group is late in sending out claims. As a result, during the month of January, the group doesn't bring in the $70,000 that was billed but only receives $50,000. Moreover, in January the group has to pay its insurance for the coming year, which amounts to $15,000.

A cash-basis income statement for Behavioral Affiliates, PC, covering the month of January would simply describe funds coming into the group and expenses that were paid during that month. Thus an item for income would list the $50,000 of reimbursements and an item for expenses would list the $15,000 for insurance. Note, however, that although this would give an accurate picture of cash coming in and cash going out, it would give only a partial picture of the group's financial situation. It would not account for the $20,000 in receivables, much of which is likely to be realized in coming months. It would also charge the yearly $15,000 expense to the single month, when in fact this is an expense covering an entire year's worth of practice. Someone looking solely at January's performance would see an artificially negative picture of the group's health: Income would be understated and expenses overstated.

Accrual-basis accounting for the income statement of Behavioral Affiliates, PC, would enter onto a line item the amount billed for the month (minus some adjustment for bad debts and denials from insurers), not just the amount received. Similarly, a position statement would reflect dollars receivable and payable in the future, not just cash that has been received and disbursed. Accrual-basis accounting would also divide yearly expenses into monthly amounts, deducting an insurance expense of $1,250 for January—and every subsequent month—not the full $15,000. Instead of $50,000 of income and $15,000 of expenses for January, the accrual statement would reflect approximately $70,000 of income and $1,250 in expenses: a sizable difference.

When considering the construction of financial statements, there is no single best basis for accounting. The cash and accrual methods provide different lenses through which a reader can assess the organization. The combination of the two perspectives, however, can yield insights not available in any single format. For example, if Behavioral Affiliates, PC, showed a number of months similar to December–January, the combination of cash and accrual statements would alert the reader to potential collection problems.

If your practice is mostly doing cash business, with patients paying every session or every few sessions, the choice between cash versus accrual accounting will not make a great deal of difference. If you are dealing with income and expenses that tend to arrive in clumps, accrual-basis statements will be necessary to give an accurate picture of your financial health. Once groups begin working under capitated and other risk-sharing arrangements, reimbursement is prepaid, which necessitates accrual-basis accounting (Pavlock, 1994).

Three Financial Statements

Although there are many financial analyses that can be performed to assess a business organization, three statements are expected in a business plan: balance sheets (sometimes called position statements), operating statements (also known as income statements), and cash flow statements. Taken together, these statements summarize the assets, liabilities, income, and expenses of an enterprise, allowing a reader to take the financial pulse of the organization.

The purpose of the position statement is to capture the relative balance between assets and liabilities within the organization. An asset is something of value that is owned, such as furniture, cash, or a building. A liability is something of value that is owed, such as a loan that is outstanding or payroll obligations that have not been met. A typical position statement divides assets into two categories: current (including cash and cash equivalents) and noncurrent or tangible (including equipment and buildings). Liabilities are also divided into current (including accounts payable and payroll withholdings) and noncurrent (including the stock holdings of investors). A high ratio of assets to liabilities connotes a degree of financial strength. Because cash assets are not typically held within the incorporated practice (to avoid double taxation), a group may be financially strong without having a high ratio of assets to liabilities. In fact, young, growing businesses often start with a skewed ratio because they have borrowed start-up and/or expansion funds and have not yet realized their potential. The issue of financial strength is thus not so much one of absolute ratios **but of the practice's ability to meet its liability obligations**.

The operating statement examines the relative balance between income to the organization and expenses that have been incurred. Income is usually a reflection of billings for professional services. Expenses may be divided into categories, such as those for personnel, supplies and equipment, physical plant, and general administration. In addition to expenses, operating statements will reflect any nonsalary distributions of income to providers. The net profit (or loss) for the period in question is a reflection of income minus the sum of expenditures and distributions. Profitability is an important sign of a practice's health because it is a major source of funding for future growth and replacement of assets. It is not unusual, for example, for computer systems to be upgraded every few years. Without profits, there can be no pool of money for such upgrades. Note, per the previous discussion, that profitability estimates for any given reporting period can vary meaningfully depending on whether a cash or accrual accounting basis is employed.

Cash flow statements are simply a summary of all cash that enters and exits the business in a given period. A positive cash flow means that there is an increase in available cash from one point in time to another. A negative cash flow suggests a decrease in available cash. It is quite possible for a company to be financially strong but cash-poor. For example, a group's real estate assets may gain in value over time, contributing to a healthy balance sheet. The increase in value, however, provides no free cash to the group. Similarly, billings can increase and make an accrual-basis operating statement look good but might not contribute to cash flow if the rate of payment denials skyrockets. A group practice with a healthy, positive cash flow is able to meet its financial obligations in a timely fashion. A negative cash flow can lead to "cash crunches" and difficulty paying off bills, creditors, and employees.

Devon Macrae Behavioral Group: An Example

To concretize our presentation of financial statements, let us take a simple group, consisting of four professionals: Devon, Macrae, Marlo, and Naomi. Devon and

Macrae practice on a full-time basis, averaging a combined gross income of approximately $200,000/year. They invest $40,000 in their group's start-up and hire Marlo and Naomi to work for them on a half-time basis for $24,000/year each. They also hire a full-time receptionist and billing clerk for $30,000/year and pay themselves salaries of $75,000 each. In addition, the group pays out $9,000 per quarter to lease its space, $500 per month in utilities and phone, $3,000 a year in malpractice insurance fees, $1,000 a month in health insurance benefits for the full-time staff, $3,000 biannually for life insurance benefits, and $500 a month in supplies and office equipment. The group recently borrowed $10,500 and put down $9,500 to purchase a reconditioned computer system and an integrated software package. Payments on the loan come to $500/month. A $3,000 bonus is divided among employees on a quarterly basis, based on performance reviews.

Drawing on the discussions of Pavlock (1994) and Schafer (1991), we can construct simple versions of the three basic financial statements. (Note that these are simplified versions of financial statements, for the purposes of exposition only. They should not be taken as literal templates for your own practice's statements.) The statement of financial position compares the group's assets to its liabilities and determines its net worth. The operating statement compares income to expenses to ascertain whether money was made or lost in that reporting period. Finally, the cash flow statement looks at the cash transactions during the period and indicates whether there was a net inflow or outflow of cash to the group (see Figures 4.1–4.6).

Note the cash-basis income statement, statement of position, and cash flow statement for the Devon Macrae group. The income statement compares revenues actually collected to operating expenses associated with human resources, services purchased, physical resources, administration, and distributions of income. The statement of financial position compares cash and physical assets to liabilities associated with debt and withholdings to track changes in the net worth of the practice. The cash flow statement summarizes infusions of cash from collections and investment minus payments of cash for expenses, distributions, and reduction of debt, thus tracking changes in the group's cash position. Each of these statements is issued on a monthly basis and summarized at year-end by a set of annual statements.

Now note the same three statements constructed on an accrual basis. Instead of reflecting income and expenses from cash transactions, accrual-based accounting looks at the impact of achieved, but not yet realized, gains and losses. For example, the income statement reflects total billings, not just those collected. The accrual statements also smooth the reporting of periodic expenses. The lease, for instance, is $9,000 on a quarterly basis but shows up on the accrual-basis statements as $3,000 monthly. In situations in which there might be large expenses paid once annually at the end of the year, accrual-basis accounting provides a sense of impact on the monthly statements leading up to the actual expenditure. Were cash-basis accounting to be used only, the group owners might develop a

			Month			
	1	2	3	4	5	6
Revenue						
Collections	20.00	30.00	25.00	30.00	25.00	20.00
Operating Expenses						
Human Resources						
Salaries, prof.	4.00	4.00	4.00	4.00	4.00	4.00
Salaries, admin.	2.50	2.50	2.50	2.50	2.50	2.50
Salaries, owners	12.50	12.50	12.50	12.50	12.50	12.50
Life insurance	3.00	.00	.00	.00	.00	.00
Health insurance	1.00	1.00	1.00	1.00	1.00	1.00
Total human resources	23.00	20.00	20.00	20.00	20.00	20.00
Physical Resources						
Lease	9.00	.00	.00	9.00	.00	.00
Utilities	.50	.50	.50	.50	.50	.50
Supplies purchased	.50	.50	.50	.50	.50	.50
Computer	.35	.35	.35	.35	.40	.40
Depreciation	.25	.25	.25	.25	.25	.25
Total phys. resources	10.60	1.60	1.60	10.60	1.60	1.60
General and Admin.						
Prof. liab. insur.	3.00	.00	.00	.00	.00	.00
Interest expense	.15	.15	.15	.15	.10	.10
Other expense	.20	.20	.25	.25	.20	.25
Total G&A	3.35	.35	.40	.40	.30	.35
Total op. expenses	36.95	21.95	22.00	31.00	21.90	21.95
Income before Distributions	(16.95)	8.05	3.00	(1.00)	3.10	(1.95)
Distributions	.00	.00	3.00	.00	.00	3.00
Net Income (retained earnings)	(16.95)	8.05	.00	(1.00)	3.10	(4.95)

FIGURE 4.1. Income statement: Cash basis. Devon Macrae Group, January–June, this year, in thousands of dollars.

false sense of security in the early months, only to be confronted with the large, unaccounted expense in December.

The degree to which cash- and accrual-basis statements will differ is, in part, a function of the time frame selected. Given discrepancies between when income is billed and when it is realized (and discrepancies between when expenses are incurred and when they are actually felt), short-term (e.g., monthly) statements will usually show wider differences between the two accounting methodologies than do longer-term (e.g., annual) statements. To the extent that your practice has income and/or expenses bunched into a single time frame, accrual-basis ac-counting will be helpful. This is often the case when managed care payers ac-

	Month					
	1	2	3	4	5	6
Assets						
Current Assets						
Cash	21.30	29.10	28.85	27.60	30.45	25.25
Total current assets	21.30	29.10	28.85	27.60	30.45	25.25
Noncurrent Tangible Assets						
Equipment	21.00	21.00	21.00	21.00	21.00	21.00
Less accum. deprec.	(.25)	(.50)	(.75)	(1.00)	(1.25)	(1.50)
Total N.T.A.	20.75	20.50	20.25	20.00	19.75	19.50
Total assets	42.05	49.60	49.10	47.60	50.20	44.75
Liabilities and Owners' Equity						
Current Liabilities						
Payroll w/holding	9.00	9.00	9.00	9.00	9.00	9.00
Notes payable	10.00	9.50	9.00	8.50	8.00	7.50
Total current liabilities	19.00	18.50	18.00	17.50	17.00	16.50
Owners' Equity						
Common stock	40.00	40.00	40.00	40.00	40.00	40.00
Retained earn.	(16.95)	(8.90)	(8.90)	(9.90)	(6.80)	(11.75)
Total equity	23.05	31.10	31.10	30.10	33.20	28.25
Total liabilities and equity	42.05	49.60	49.10	47.60	50.20	44.75

FIGURE 4.2. Statement of position: Cash basis. Devon Macrae Group, January–June, this year, in thousands of dollars.

	Month					
	1	2	3	4	5	6
Cash from Operations						
Collections	20.00	30.00	25.00	30.00	25.00	20.00
Expenses	(27.75)	(21.70)	(21.75)	(30.75)	(21.65)	(21.70)
Distributions	.00	.00	(3.00)	.00	.00	(3.00)
Total cash, ops.	(7.75)	8.30	.25	(.75)	3.35	(4.70)
Cash from Investing						
Downpayment, equip.	(9.50)					
Cash from Financing						
Common stock	40.00					
Retirement of long-term debt	(.50)	(.50)	(.50)	(.50)	(.50)	(.50)
Total cash, fin.	39.50	(.50)	(.50)	(.50)	(.50)	(.50)
Net Increase (Decrease) in Cash	22.25	7.80	(.25)	(1.25)	2.85	(5.20)
Cash Balance at Beginning of Year	.00	22.25	30.05	29.80	28.55	31.40
Cash Balance at End of Year	22.25	30.05	29.80	28.55	31.40	26.20

FIGURE 4.3. Cash flow statement: Cash basis. Devon Macrae Group, January–June, this year, in thousands of dollars.

	Month					
	1	2	3	4	5	6
Revenue						
Billings	25.00	30.00	25.00	30.00	25.00	20.00
Operating Expenses						
Human Resources						
Salaries, prof.	4.00	4.00	4.00	4.00	4.00	4.00
Salaries, admin.	2.50	2.50	2.50	2.50	2.50	2.50
Salaries, owners	12.50	12.50	12.50	12.50	12.50	12.50
Life ins.	.50	.50	.50	.50	.50	.50
Health ins.	1.00	1.00	1.00	1.00	1.00	1.00
Total human resources	20.50	20.50	20.50	20.50	20.50	20.50
Physical Resources						
Lease	3.00	3.00	3.00	3.00	3.00	3.00
Utilities	.50	.50	.50	.50	.50	.50
Supplies used	.40	.40	.50	.60	.40	.40
Computer	.35	.35	.35	.35	.40	.40
Depreciation	.25	.25	.25	.25	.25	.25
Total phys. resources	4.50	4.50	4.60	4.70	4.55	4.55
General and Administrative						
Prof. liab. ins.	.25	.25	.25	.25	.25	.25
Interest expense	.15	.15	.15	.15	.10	.10
Other expense	.20	.20	.25	.25	.20	.25
Total G&A	.60	.60	.65	.65	.55	.60
Total op. expenses	25.60	25.60	25.75	25.85	25.60	25.65
Income before Distributions	(.60)	4.40	9.25	19.15	19.40	14.35
Distributions	1.00	1.00	1.00	1.00	1.00	1.00
Net Income (retained earnings)	(1.60)	3.40	0.25	18.15	18.40	13.35

FIGURE 4.4. Income statement: Accrual basis. Devon Macrae Group, January–June, this year, in thousands of dollars.

count for a sizable portion of revenues, given inevitable delays in reimbursement and needs to adjudicate disputed claims.

Note, as discussed earlier, that the juxtaposition of the two accounting formats gives a more rounded picture than any one format alone. Judging by the cash-basis statements, the Devon Macrae group appears to be reasonably healthy, with no great excess of expenses over revenues and a rising cash flow. When we look at the accrual-basis statements, however, it is clear that the practice is not so healthy. Billings have been increasing steadily but collections have not. The group is working harder but not making any more money. Eventually, some of these patient receivables may become so aged that they have to be written off as bad debts and the income will have been lost. On a smaller scale, note that the group shows a major loss during the first month of operation on a cash basis but

	Month					
	1	2	3	4	5	6
Assets						
Current assets						
Cash	21.30	29.10	28.85	27.60	30.45	25.25
Pt. receivables	5.00	5.00	15.00	30.00	50.00	70.00
Supplies on hand	.10	.20	.20	.10	.20	.30
Prepaid rent	6.00	3.00	.00	6.00	3.00	.00
Total current assets	32.40	37.30	44.05	63.70	83.65	95.55
Noncurrent Tangible Assets						
Equipment	21.00	21.00	21.00	21.00	21.00	21.00
Less accum. deprec.	(.25)	(.50)	(.75)	(1.00)	(1.25)	(1.50)
Total N.T.A.	20.75	20.50	20.25	20.00	19.75	19.50
Total assets	53.15	57.80	64.30	83.70	103.40	115.05
Liabilities and Owners' Equity						
Current Liabilities						
Payroll w/holding	9.00	9.00	9.00	9.00	9.00	9.00
Notes payable	10.00	9.50	9.00	8.50	8.00	7.50
Total current liabilities	19.00	18.50	18.00	17.50	17.00	16.50
Owners' Equity						
Common stock	40.00	40.00	40.00	40.00	40.00	40.00
Retained earnings	(5.85)	(.70)	6.30	26.20	46.40	58.55
Total liabilities and equity	53.15	57.80	64.30	83.70	103.40	115.05

FIGURE 4.5. Statement of position: Accrual basis. Devon Macrae Group, January–June, this year, in thousands of dollars.

	Month					
	1	2	3	4	5	6
Cash from Operations						
Collections	20.00	30.00	25.00	30.00	25.00	20.00
Expenses	(27.75)	(21.70)	(21.75)	(30.75)	(21.65)	(21.70)
Distributions	(0.00)	(0.00)	(3.00)	(0.00)	(0.00)	(3.00)
Total cash, ops.	(7.75)	8.30	.25	(.75)	3.35	(4.70)
Cash from Investing						
Purchase of equip.	(21.00)					
Cash from Financing						
Common stock	40.00					
Increase in long-term debt	11.50					
Reduction in long-term debt	(.50)	(.50)	(.50)	(.50)	(.50)	(.50)
Total cash, fin.	51.00	(.50)	(.50)	(.50)	(.50)	(.50)
Net Increase (Decrease) in Cash	22.25	7.80	(.25)	(1.25)	2.85	(5.20)
Cash Balance at Beginning of Year	.00	22.25	30.05	29.80	28.55	31.40
Cash Balance at End of Year	22.25	30.05	29.80	28.55	31.40	26.20

FIGURE 4.6. Cash flow statement: Accrual basis. Devon Macrae Group, January–June, this year, in thousands of dollars.

near break-even on an accrual basis, reflecting the spreading out of multimonth expenses that are paid in January. By viewing their financial status from different angles, Devon and Macrae can best recognize problems as they arise.

Using the Financials to Appraise a Practice

If you are a clinician seeking to join a membership network or if you are contemplating investing in an expanding practice, the three statements described above will provide a good look at the financial strength of the organization that you are considering. Several guidelines are particularly useful in utilizing this financial information.

Make Sure Statements Are Independently Audited

This is absolutely mandatory if you are thinking of purchasing a practice, merging with one, or forming a joint venture. An unaudited set of statements is only as good as the word of the person compiling the information. Statements reviewed and assembled by a recognized accounting firm indicate that there has been outside scrutiny of the information going into the reports. In the absence of audited statements, you may wish to examine a group's tax filings.

Don't Rely on Statements from a Single Accounting Period

Generally, it is essential to obtain statements from several years back, so that trends in income and expenditures can be observed. A single year's statements tell very little about the ongoing health and performance of the firm.

Beware Nonrecurring Items

A single major financial event can drastically distort one's view of an organization. For example, if a practice sells a major piece of real estate, it may log a healthy profit for that reporting period. That says little, however, about the health of the core business.

Keep an Eye on Depreciation

Most assets lose their value over time as a function of wear and tear. A computer system purchased for $25,000 5 years ago is not worth $25,000 now. Such depreciation should be reflected in the position statements of the firm. The business should also be generating sufficient profits to replace depreciated assets.

Examine Outstanding Leases and Contracts

One of us (B.N.S.) nearly learned about this the hard way when he evaluated a health care organization for possible purchase. The firm was barely profitable despite a seemingly strong patient flow. When he examined its expenses, he found that it was paying far too much for its lease space and certain professional services. Gradually, the reason for this became clear: The owners of the firm were the ones leasing space and providing services to their own company. That gave his organization a strong incentive to acquire the company's assets but not its contracts and obligations.

One of the most helpful tools in assessing the strength of an organization is *profit margin*. A profit margin represents the ratio of profits to total income. In calculating profit margins, it is useful to have accrual-basis statements to smooth out the effects of one-time purchases, lump-sum reimbursements from at-risk contracts, and so on. Also make sure that disbursements of income to practice members and owners beyond usual salary amounts are not treated as expenses. The actual profit of a practice and its retained earnings can be very different things. Finally, eliminate nonrecurring items, such as gains or losses from the sale of major assets.

If the resulting profit margin decreases over time even as revenues are rising, this means that the practice is having greater problems in extracting profit from its business. This could be reflective of poor management, a tightening marketplace, or both. In any event, it is a potential warning sign. Generally, as a business expands, it hopes to take advantage of economies of scale and extract greater profits from each additional dollar of revenue. For instance, a network may spend considerable funds to establish its communications system; each clinician added to the system, however, may represent little additional overhead. Hence, a greater share of the business brought to the network by that clinician should go to the bottom line as profits. When revenue growth outstrips margin growth, it means that the practice is not enjoying economies of scale. It is a red flag.

MARKETING APPLICATIONS OF THE BUSINESS PLAN

Embedded within the business plan, though not necessarily identified as such, is a marketing plan for the behavioral practice. The marketing plan can be conceptualized as a miniature business plan dealing with that portion of the practice concerned with maintaining and increasing market share. How will the business promote itself? How will it take advantage of opportunities in the marketplace? What kind of growth in referral flow is it targeting over the next several years? These are key questions addressed in a marketing plan.

Developing a Marketing Plan

Many professionals equate marketing with advertising. To be sure, advertising is an important means of marketing a company's products and services. Marketing, however, extends far beyond advertising. Marketing begins with the very conceptualization of a product and its "packaging" or presentation to the marketplace. It concerns itself with the identity of a practice and its services and coordinated ways of conveying that identity to clients and referral sources. This is sometimes referred to as an "integrated marketing communications" perspective, a tight synthesis of advertising, sales promotion, public relations, and direct marketing to create and sustain a consistent message to the public (Belch & Belch, 1995).

When Dr. Steenbarger helped to found a membership-model MSO/IPA based in an academic department of psychiatry, he began with scores of interviews with managed care firms, medical practices, and behavioral health providers. He quickly discovered that there was a fundamental disconnect in the community between primary medical care and behavioral health. Each primary care practice had its favorite referral sources for patients requiring mental health services, but these were notoriously unreliable. Sometimes they were filled and no longer accepting referrals. Sometimes they could not provide the specific services required. As a result, physicians were left making call after call trying to connect their patient to a provider. Worse still, once the connection was made, little feedback was provided from therapists to physicians. Clearly, this was an untapped market.

Choosing the name PrimeCare for the organization, Dr. Steenbarger hoped to convey two notions: (1) *prime*, in the sense of high quality, and (2) *primary care*, connoting gatekeeping and cost-effectiveness. The group quickly established a single triage phone line that could be readily accessed by physicians. Drawing on a practice network of more than 80 members, it guaranteed callers that patients would be interviewed over the phone and rapidly connected with an appropriate provider. Moreover, the cost of the initial phone assessment was borne entirely by the practice; there was no charge to the patient or the patient's insurance. Promotional materials to physician practices emphasized the ease of use of the network's central triage number and its guarantees of timely referral placements and rapid feedback to referring doctors. Materials prepared for managed care organizations stressed the primary care theme and the practice's capacity to speedily assess clients and deliver services at an appropriate level of care.

PrimeCare's marketing strategy involved an integration of the group's fundamental niche—a department of psychiatry—and the assessed needs of the marketplace, condensing these into a concept (primary care) that was meaningful to referral sources. This differs in scale only from the marketing efforts of Coca-Cola or Procter & Gamble, which attempt to establish brand identities that tap the needs and desires of a marketplace.

Littlefield and Daily (1992) identify a three-phase process for the ongoing marketing of group practices:

- **Assessment of position.** Evaluating the strengths and weaknesses of the practice, the needs of the community, the steps needed to address community needs.

- **Internal reinforcement.** Working with the providers to develop an organizational culture and sense of teamwork that reinforces the practice's identity and ensures that promised services are delivered.

- **External projection.** Projecting the image and message of the practice to the public, heightening awareness of the group among referral sources and patients.

☞ LOOKING AHEAD

How does a collaborative group develop a marketing plan?

Our market planning guide at the end of this chapter (Reader's Resource 4.3) walks you through the process!

The marketing plan is research-based, built on a thorough assessment of the needs of clients, insurers, and community referral sources. Groups that are sophisticated in their management will make internal reinforcement a continuous process, allowing the marketing plan to merge seamlessly with efforts at quality improvement. Sullivan and Luallin (1992) note, for example, that practices can set targets for levels of service delivery (e.g., patients should be seen for a first appointment within X business days of their initial call to the practice) and monitor the degree to which these targets are hit. When the practice falls short of targets, efforts at remediation can be initiated. Bonuses may be offered to clinical staff for the achievement of service targets. Through such measures, the marketing plan suffuses the organization.

Broader Marketing Applications of the Business Plan

As discussed previously, the primary use of the business plan is to document the practice's strengths for the purpose of raising capital. Even the self-financed collaboration, however, will find it helpful to assemble a plan as a means of marketing. There are three elements among the plan's applications:

- **Recruitment.** The business plan can help recruit quality professional and management staff into a membership-model practice by showing the prospective employee the strategic position, financial strengths, and future prospects of the practice.

- **Referral building.** Sections of the business plan can be shared with managed care organizations and other potential referral sources to establish the credibility of the practice as a long-term player in the market.

- **Expansion.** If the group looks for strategic partners for joint ventures or other collaborative efforts, the plan can quickly orient prospective partners to the group's strengths and establish the practice's credibility.

In sum, the business plan concretizes the start-up's strategy and can be used as a means for touting its strengths. Just as strategy needs to be revised periodically to adjust to changing conditions, the business plan is a flexible document. "It is a bad plan that admits of no modification," the Roman maxim advises. Successful practices view planning as a continuous process, identifying areas of strength, weakness, opportunity, and competition and basing decisions on these.

CONCLUSION

Clinicians traditionally shy away from business and financial matters. In this chapter, we have attempted to take the mystery out of business plans and financial statements and provide practical tools by which you can evaluate your own start-up efforts, as well as the groups in your region with which you might affiliate. Although this information will not substitute for the consultation of a qualified accountant, it certainly can help you make optimal use of the consultant's abilities and expertise.

Until a collaborative group's strategy has been detailed in a business plan, it remains little more than a set of general intentions. The plan is a critical element

---

✔ SUMMARY

- Reducing the overhead of a start-up group is essential to maintaining control over the practice and weathering financial adversity.
- Start-up funds can be raised from bank loans, the investments of clinician owners, or the investments of outside investors.
- The business plan outlines the strategy and financial performance of the group practice and documents how the group will raise, use, and repay capital.
- Three financial statements are essential to evaluating the health of a group practice: income statements, position statements, and cash flow statements.
- The marketing plan of a group practice establishes integrated strategies for attracting and maintaining referral flows.

in translating broad visions into measurable objectives, guiding the management of the practice. It also is essential to attracting the interest of lenders, investors, and potential business partners and serves as a potent marketing tool in its own right. Testing and refining your collaboration on paper can save months of costly experience down the line and truly position your group for the success it deserves.

READER'S RESOURCE 4.1
Guide to a Killer Presentation

Knowing how to make a successful presentation is absolutely essential to starting up a practice. It is not at all unusual for practice managers to have to make several formal presentations per month, whether to lenders, referral sources, or insurers. The presentation is both educational and motivational: It seeks to inform listeners about the practice and interest them in it at the same time. **To no small degree, presentations are the foundations from which business relationships are built.** When approaching a lender or referral source, there are several keys to an effective business presentation:

ENGAGE THE AUDIENCE EARLY

We are amazed at the number of practices that set up meetings with lenders or insurers only to approach these parties as potential adversaries. The successful presentation is successful before the first slide is shown, before the first lines are delivered. In the minutes before the meeting, there is active and friendly engagement of the other parties and a true spirit of collaboration and teamwork.

MAKE USE OF SIGHT, SOUNDS, AND HUMOR

Once you have engaged an audience, keep them engaged! Drop-dead gorgeous slideshows on a computer, perhaps with sound and motion embedded, can be entertaining as well as informative. Concrete examples can be extremely helpful in making your points and creating impressions. Instead of talking about your triage system in the abstract, for example, use a clinical example to illustrate how your practice routes cases to appropriate providers and treatments.

GIVE THEM SOMETHING TO REMEMBER

Handouts are absolutely essential to a good presentation. They serve multiple functions. First, you want your listeners to focus on you and your major points, not frantically taking notes and keeping their noses in a portfolio. A second purpose of handouts is that they provide an ongoing reference for lenders and referral sources. This may be crucial in guiding their future decision making. Finally, well-designed handouts can convey a level of professionalism that reflects favorably on your practice.

(cont.)

SPEAK THEIR LANGUAGE

You must address the needs of your audience in your presentation and demonstrate why it makes sense to do business with you. If you are pitching your group or network to a bank or lender group, a clear and powerful presentation of your financial projections is essential. If you are addressing a provider relations team from an MCO, your talk should display your familiarity with the needs of MCOs and show how your practice will meet them.

To create the perfect presentation, take a few minutes to answer the questions below:

- Who will be your audience? What is their level of sophistication?
- How many people will you be presenting to? What will be your needs for space? Handouts?
- What are the main points you want to convey?
- What practical results do you want to see as a result of the meeting?
- How will your presentation identify the needs of your audience and address these in a straightforward manner?
- What facts and statistics can you present that will have a dramatic impact on the audience?
- What tables, charts, or displays can make a visual impact on them?
- What handout materials can you leave with your audience to make an impression after the meeting?
- What stories or examples can you provide to your audience to illustrate your central points?
- How will your presentation engage the audience in a dialogue and capture their interest and involvement?
- How will you follow up after the presentation to keep the momentum and achieve your goals?

The killer presentation does the following:

1. Actively engages the audience.
2. Highlights a problem.
3. Offers a solution.
4. Uses sight, sound, dialogue, and practical examples to maintain the interest and attention of the audience.
5. Follows through afterward to achieve a specific set of objectives.

From an integrated marketing communications perspective, the tone, format, and content of your presentation must fit with the central theme of the marketing plan.

READER'S RESOURCE 4.2
Featured Interview with Warren Throckmorton, PhD:
Developing a Group Practice

"If you're going to integrate financially, you've got to integrate as a culture."

Warren Throckmorton, PhD, is currently an associate professor of psychology and director of college counseling at Grove City College. He has been active in the American Mental Health Counselors Association (AMHCA) and was recently selected as that organization's president-elect. Previously, Dr. Throckmorton worked in a residential treatment setting for children and adolescents; later, he developed his own practice group in a rural community. He recently took the time to discuss his group practice experience—from the earliest marketing efforts to the eventual sale of the practice—with Brett Steenbarger.

STEENBARGER: Tell me how you began your practice.

THROCKMORTON: Well, I worked on meeting people, going to lunch with psychiatrists and ministers and various referral agents to try to get a leg up on a practice in Portsmouth [Ohio]. Once I was done with my doctoral coursework in '86, my family moved to Portsmouth and I started a practice there. It was a solo practice at first; it was basically myself and a two-room office. I got there with four clients and within a month I had none. So that was a little scary! But within a year, the practice had grown to 20 to 25 clients a week and I took on an associate at that point. . . . He started part-time and came on full-time about a year later. . . . It was piecemeal from there, but I started to add part-time folks who wanted to do 1 or 2—or as many as 10 hours a week of clinical work. They were working other jobs in the community.

STEENBARGER: Were these folks hired by you as independent contractors?

THROCKMORTON: Individuals with licenses allowing independent practice were brought in as contractors. Other individuals requiring supervision were considered employees . . . . Inasmuch as I was directing their work and involved in it intimately, I needed to consider them employees. All, at first, were part-time, paid on a percentage of their work. It was a different percentage depending on their work, intensity of supervision needed, et cetera. Along the way I had two full-time employees, though not at the same time.

(cont.)

READER'S RESOURCE 4.2 (*cont.*)

STEENBARGER: Maybe you could talk a little about your marketing.

THROCKMORTON: I was aware that ministers see a lot of people. Among some of the conservative pastors, there's a bit of distrust of mental health services. These ministers don't refer as much, but they see a lot of people and do a lot of counseling. I had known that from a previous survey I had done as an undergraduate. I surveyed Baptist ministers in three states and knew about how many people they counseled a week.

So I felt, "Here's an area I have some understanding about. I can communicate with those folks and understand their concerns." So I surveyed them for their referral practices. . . . I went to the phone book and all the churches in the area. It turned out that the ministers were seeing a lot of folks, but not referring and, more specific to that area, they weren't feeling comfortable with existing services. I didn't put down the other services, but I let them know, "Well, you see a lot of people! Must be real trying. Is there anything I can do to help you?" . . . That seemed to ease many of their concerns, when they learned that I wasn't going to turn people away from their faith. Some of the ministers had heard this from parishioners who had gone to other counseling services.

Most communities have ministerial associations and denominations have their own regional meetings. . . . I went to the Baptist one, which in southern Ohio is a large one, and then I also went to the pastoral counseling service in town and spoke with their director and communicated my results. He communicated them to the rest of the association and that seemed to be enough. That process generated quite a few referrals.

[This is a great example of the expertise niche strategy. Dr. Throckmorton was able to identify an unmet specialized need in the community, and he positioned himself to address this need.]

STEENBARGER: So that's how you built up the referral base prior to bringing on employees.

THROCKMORTON: Yes, I deliberately looked for underserved groups and for referral sources looking for other options.

STEENBARGER: It sounds like the other market you identified as an area of opportunity was the child market.

THROCKMORTON: I had worked with kids in residential treatment and knew it was hard to get outside clinicians to see our kids. When we needed referrals for various kinds of testing at the time, we just couldn't find peo-

(*cont.*)

ple. So I thought if it's true there, it's probably true in other places. I just began to ask around at day-care centers: To whom do you refer when you have a consultation case? . . . They didn't have anyone! I started going to other day-care centers: "And what do you do when you need to refer clients for counseling?" "Well, we don't. We'd sure like to. Do you do that work?" "Well, yeah, actually I do!"

Then I started approaching the university about teaching some child development courses for day-care workers. They liked that idea. . . . Another thing I did was put together a program . . . to teach Head Start and day-care workers child development courses leading to a credential called the Child Development Associate. . . . There was a need for Head Start workers to get this credential, so I approached the university and we approached the Head Start centers and it all came together. The sidelight of that was that they needed mental health consulting. Every Head Start needs a mental health consultant. They often go to the community mental health center or maybe even a school psychologist, but in my area, they didn't use the existing services and so they contracted with me.

[Every successful practice head we've met has been a motivated marketer. Dr. Throckmorton shows a distinctive knack for getting outside the practice, networking with others, and cultivating referral sources.]

STEENBARGER: So that really built your referral base!

THROCKMORTON: [It] built my referral base and also gave me a good platform . . . for attracting other clinicians of like mind. Many of these part-timers were school people: school counselors, school psychologists. So they would come in and see some of the overflow of kids I couldn't see.

STEENBARGER: You mentioned that your practice had the reputation for being *the* child practice in the region.

THROCKMORTON: That was really deliberate. Once it was clear that the child service agencies didn't use the existing services . . . I deliberately set about to establish that reputation.

A lot of folks going into practice do what they want to do and end up doing what 10 other people in the community are doing. . . . I had the experience in residential treatment . . . and was always interested in childhood development and did take a course in my master's program that was offered on doing therapy with children. . . . But many of my colleagues had that and yet wouldn't have thought of themselves—and I didn't either—as a child specialist. So I took some extra credit work . . . and just learned everything I could to gear the practice in that direction and brought in the part-timers with that reputation.

(cont.)

READER'S RESOURCE 4.2 (*cont.*)

[This is the difference between business planning and flying by the seat of one's pants. Dr. Throckmorton was not content to establish a "me-too" practice.]

STEENBARGER: What led you to the decision and opportunity to sell the practice?

THROCKMORTON: I'd done my doctoral dissertation finally in '91. It was on the criteria that third-party payer use to choose mental health providers. . . . The outcome of that—and getting into all the managed care literature and of course having Ohio Biodyne, Medco/Merit into Ohio—just led me to feel like things were changing and practices were going to be squeezed. A lot of competition with larger entitities would probably be coming . . . eventually managed care companies would not contract with people; they'd just start their own groups. I really saw that might happen, so I started to study up on some options for me. Could I continue doing this? Was private practice about to die?

At the time I was doing all this reflecting, the hospital in town . . . was fixing to upgrade their clinical, outpatient behavioral health care work. . . . The psychiatrist who was the premier psychiatrist in town and who I worked with had sold his practice to the hospital and became the medical director. His burning urge was to develop an integrated delivery system. When I heard they were doing that, it occurred to me that they were going to sink a lot of money into it and be a big competitor. So I approached [the psychiatrist] at the time about how I might be a part of it and he was very receptive. We basically struck a deal so that I could come over and help them develop their group; they'd buy up my tangibles and charts, bring over my office management, and I'd go work for them.

[Small group practices and networks often find themselves drawn toward greater levels of collaboration to maintain their competitive position in a community. This often leads to alliances, joint ventures, and buyouts.]

STEENBARGER: I see. How did the process go, in terms of negotiating a value for your practice?

THROCKMORTON: I put together a prospectus. The psychiatrist had asked me to give him a booklet, giving the history of the practice, both clinically and financially. He asked me to put down billings, receipts, expenses, and profit statements on a graph and also the payer mix . . . from where did my referrals come—where did they live—and who referred them. I put all that in a booklet. What they were doing was valuing the practice based upon the tangibles. Part of this has to do with the fact

(*cont.*)

that it's a nonprofit hospital—it was a Medicare hospital, of course—and they had to go with the Stark rules. They couldn't pay for goodwill. There was no valuation based on goodwill. The valuation was based on an average of the prior 3 years' billings.

[Paying for goodwill—the reputation and strategic position of the practice—could be construed as buying referrals and would be in violation of Medicare fraud and abuse laws.]

STEENBARGER: So they're just valuing it based on that dollar amount, not on a multiple of that amount.

THROCKMORTON: That's right . . .

STEENBARGER: In terms of what they were buying, they weren't just buying the tangibles . . . but you were part of the deal as well.

THROCKMORTON: I came in as a salaried employee and my salary was based on my prior years' billings, a percentage of that.

STEENBARGER: The group practice wouldn't have been worth very much if you weren't part of the deal.

THROCKMORTON: Absolutely.

STEENBARGER: What role did you play in this new integrated delivery system?

THROCKMORTON: I came in with the social worker that the hospital already had on staff. They changed his method of compensation at the same time that they brought me in. He was basically on salary, but they offered him the opportunity to base his income on production, in kind of the same way that they looked at my prior production and based my salary on that. So he came into the group, there was another social worker who was part-time . . . and the psychiatrist. And we just all sat down together and decided what we wanted to call the thing, how we wanted to market it, got the hospital publicity people in to put an ad campaign together. The hospital bought a building in the community and refurbished it nicely. Essentially we put together a marketing plan and a business strategy to achieve a certain percentage of managed care business, a certain percentage of cash pay, and we wanted to keep certain percentages of other payers as well. So it was a joint decision-making process.

STEENBARGER: How much of the business that you were going after was managed care?

THROCKMORTON: Well, just to give some perspective, at the time, the percentage of business that was managed care for me in the practice that I sold was 5.3%. That's all. We were looking for maybe 30–40%. Things had changed so rapidly in the area as far as managed care; 1990 was the

(cont.)

READER'S RESOURCE 4.2 (*cont.*)

first year I had any managed care business. By '93, we were looking at most of our major employers going to managed care.

STEENBARGER: Any pearls of wisdom or advice for people who are in solo practice or small groups and looking to make the next steps in their evolution?

THROCKMORTON: There are just a lot of people-type things that are important in making a group happen. Having banquets, having dinners, having recognition. Even in a small group, I began sending out memos recognizing good work that people had done or exemplary cases. I would put out memos to all the part-timers so that they could feel some ownership of the group. I think the development of recognition among the group members and a feeling of we-ness is really important. If you're going to integrate financially, you've got to integrate as a culture . . . and that's one thing I tried really hard to do with the first group. Even though people had their other jobs, I wanted them to feel a part of— and some ownership of—the work they were doing with me.

I think groups that are coming together, they might come into it thinking, "Well, this will be just work. I'll just know these people at work." I mean, if you're going to integrate your lives financially, you're going to have to think about the culture you're creating and the kind of relationships that you're going to develop.

STEENBARGER: That's a really good point.

THROCKMORTON: I think people who run groups will experience problems if they don't pay attention to the subtleties and nuances of developing a culture.

READER'S RESOURCE 4.3
Developing a Marketing Plan

What goes into a marketing plan? According to several authors (Bangs, 1995; Shouldice, 1987; Solomon, 1991), there are a few key elements to be considered:

- **Objectives.** Your marketing plan should include quantifiable objectives. These can be stated in terms of absolute numbers (10,000 billable visits during the coming year) or in terms of year-over-year increases (increase billable visits by 20% next year), broken down by referral source.
- **Situational assessment.** The plan should describe the target markets for the practice, including demographics, coverage of the population by health plans, benefit levels of plans, competition, and health care trends affecting the market.
- **Image of the practice.** The plan should assess how the practice is perceived by the public and referral sources. This would include its physical plant, community visibility, and presentation to managed care entities and medical practices.
- **Patient relations.** The plan needs to evaluate how the behavioral enterprise services its patients. It is often helpful to determine professional response to calls, promptness of scheduling, helpfulness with billing, and sensitivity with which complaints are handled.
- **Professional relations.** The plan should assess how the practice develops contacts within the professional community, including marketing efforts to other behavioral health providers, medical practices, and other professional referral sources (e.g., schools and social services agencies).
- **Hospital relations.** The plan must look at relationships with psychiatric and chemical dependency facilities, including staff privileges at hospitals, ability to hospitalize patients quickly when necessary, ability to accept outpatient referrals from hospitals, and ability to participate with facilities in intensive outpatient programs.
- **Managed care relations.** The plan should clearly identify managed care trends within the community and how the behavioral practice will benefit from these. A clear picture needs to be presented regarding the needs of area MCOs (access, cost-effectiveness, risk sharing) and the degree to which the group can address these. The plan should identify the panel enrollments of the clinicians and strategies for expanding these.

(cont.)

READER'S RESOURCE 4.3 (*cont.*)

- **Community relations.** The plan needs to determine the degree to which practice leaders and clinical staff are active in community affairs, generating business contacts and referrals. Such activities could include participation on community agency boards and free speaking engagements.
- **Communication pieces.** The plan should evaluate the various means through which the practice communicates with patients and referral sources, including educational brochures, advertising, and professional notices. The look and content of these should support the overall marketing effort.

Bangs (1995) suggests that several questions can guide the creation of a marketing plan:

- **What business am I in?** Are you a "mental health professional"? A member of the "managed behavioral health care" industry? Do you provide a variety of helping services, from EAPs to corporate consultations, or are you in the business of helping individuals?
- **What do I sell?** Are you selling a continuum of behavioral health services? A product with a demonstrated level of quality? A program of cost savings? A level of service?
- **Who are my target markets?** Are you selling to the general public? To physician referral sources? To schools? To insurers? Are you seeking business from the general community, from a specific demographic group, from managed care contracts?
- **What are my marketing goals for next year? My revenue and profit goals?** What kind of growth in referral flow are you targeting and from which sources? What specific income and profit are you targeting from each of my major markets: managed care, indemnity insurance, cash paying?
- **What might keep me from achieving these goals?** What are the major challenges you will face in each of your markets? From competition? From declining reimbursement rates? What specific steps will you take to address these challenges?
- **What is my marketing budget?** What time, personnel, and money have you allocated to marketing? How will you allocate these limited resources to your various markets? How will you take advantage of low-cost marketing opportunities, such as participation in speaker's bureaus, public seminars, and media interviews? How will you allocate limited time to relationship building with key referral sources?

(*cont.*)

Successful collaborations set specific marketing goals based upon targeted markets. They tailor marketing materials and approaches to their preferred referral sources and strive to convey a consistent theme or image. Often, the central marketing message cuts across the various marketing components—advertising, sales promotion, public relations—and involves one or more of the following strategic themes that we have touched upon earlier:

- Low cost
- High service
- Integrated, comprehensive services
- High quality
- Superior access and availability
- Superior responsivity to the needs of referral sources

Management by Information: Integrating Science and Practice in the Collaborative Practice

Anyone who fights for the future lives in it today.
—Ayn Rand, *The Romantic Manifesto*

INTRODUCTION

To this point, our discussion has illustrated the steps involved in forming and evaluating collaborative practices. Now, however, we come to the point at which these practices structure themselves as accountable entities. As we stressed earlier, information is the hub around which all collaboration revolves. The new breed of behavioral practices are neither practitioner- nor insurer-based. They are information-based.

In this chapter, we describe the elements of an effective management information system (MIS) and illustrate its use in managing staff, evaluating strategic directions, and documenting the cost and quality of services. We strongly believe that the transition to management by information is the single most important step practices can make to become competitive in the future.

☆ IN THIS CHAPTER

- Assembling and purchasing an information system
- The information you'll need to practice effectively
- Management by information: Making quality count
- At-risk contracting and what it means for your practice
- Revolutionizing practice through collaborative models of management

PLANNING YOUR PRACTICE'S INFORMATION INFRASTRUCTURE

In Chapter 2 we stressed information as a key element of strategic self assessment. Nonetheless, the behavioral practice's MIS is perhaps the most overlooked aspect of the start-up. Information, as we define it, is any set of data that allows a practice to operate more cost-effectively and/or with greater quality. The information system is a tool for capturing, analyzing, and transmitting these data and aiding in financial and clinical management.

Management Information Systems

The backbone of the MIS is a computer system. In a group practice with a well-developed information infrastructure, this system consists of the following elements:

- A central, "server" computer that houses essential data files and the practice's software.

- "Client" computers in the offices of clinical staff members that allow easy access to the server for easy clinical data collection and submission of billing data.

- "Client" computers at the workstations of administrative staff members (practice manager, billing clerks, appointments secretary, etc.) to facilitate access to the server for management of clinician schedules, billing, and management of accounts payable/receivable.

- Applications software for such functions as scheduling, billing, communications, and record keeping.

- Wiring and/or modem connections that allow the computers to communicate with one another and share applications.

A number of peripheral devices assist the information system, as well, including printers, fax modems, and scanners. Some form of automatic backup of data is critical given the potential for data loss in any system.

With the heavy memory requirements of a server (very large hard-disk capacity of several gigabytes of memory and up to 128 megabytes of RAM [random access memory] are common configurations, depending on the size and usage patterns within the network), the need for client computers in staff offices, and the need to network the computers, the cost of an information system can be substantial. The American Psychological Association Practice Directorate (1996c), drawing on estimates from medical groups, reports that a group of 10 providers would need to invest $43,303 on hardware, $10,927 on system software, and $20,215 on application software to manage the practice.

Because the information system does not bring dollars into the practice immediately, it is generally the first place that leaders turn to reduce start-up costs. Even in the current marketplace, which demands considerable information to engage in risk contracting (see below), most practices are still using pencil-and-paper methods for data collection and phone calls and face-to-face meetings for communications. As a result, these practices are like cars heading down a freeway with only a rearview mirror for guidance. They lack the tools needed to evaluate and modify their practice patterns on a timely basis.

In our experience, the MIS of most practices falls into one of several categories.

Primitive

All notes and records are kept by hand. Billing may be computerized, but there is no software to capture utilization data from billings. Use of computers is primarily limited to word processing and generation of bills to patients and insurers. Apart from telephones, there are no communications systems linking providers to one another and to management; communications with insurers is by mail or phone.

Intermediate

Clinicians keep most data by hand but provide core information to administrative personnel for entry into a computer system. In addition, appointments and billing are computerized, allowing for a capture of basic utilization and demographic data. The practice can use its computer system to generate timely reports concerning income, expenses, and accounts payable and receivable. Computers and online communications systems (e-mail) are limited to the offices of a few key clinical and administrative staff members.

Advanced

Computers are located in most if not all offices and networked to allow for intrapractice communication and document sharing. Key data on patient care is entered directly into the computer system, allowing for ongoing quality assessment and data-based concurrent reviews of utilization. A computerized appointments system allows referrals to access a central triage phone number and receive an appointment on the spot. The computer system can generate up-to-date financial and clinical reports broken down by specific work teams/responsibility centers. Claims can be filed electronically to speed payment; outpatient treatment reports can also be filed by computer to speed authorizations.

Fully Integrated

This system is primarily a vision of the future but useful as an eventual goal for large enterprises. Practices are linked to referral sources, including multispecialty medical groups and managed care organizations, for referrals, communications, and case consultation. The process of eligibility checks, authorizations, claims adjudication, and claims filing is primarily electronic. Computer-based communication systems permit interdisciplinary consultation and facilitate the process of obtaining second opinions. Patient records are electronic, greatly facilitating review of charts.

Those starting a behavioral practice can feel squeezed between the need to minimize overhead and the need to have a competitive information system. Often, the choice is forced by undercapitalization: The group lacks funds and decides to do without technology. As Michael Hurst, founder and CEO of Instream Inc., noted in our interview (see Chapter 6), however, consider the opportunity costs of such a choice. The time it takes a practitioner to pull a chart, make an entry, submit billing data, and return the chart may only amount to 10-15 minutes. **At a provider rate of $60 per hour and up, however, this means that the practice is losing $10 of productivity each time a record is accessed and a session is documented.** Over time, an advanced system can pay for itself by reducing or eliminating the time spent in pulling charts and communicating with external reviewers.

We recently consulted to an MCO on issues concerning the design of clinical services. The MCO set up a series of meetings and conference calls to try to bring all stakeholders—medical providers, behavioral clinicians, managers, and so on—into the process. Inevitably, some individuals could make some of the meetings and not others. Minutes of the meetings and resource materials made it to some members' offices but not others. As a result, there was a continual need to postpone agenda items and reschedule discussions. We estimated at one point that the MCO lost several thousand dollars in inefficient use of staff time by relying on management by meetings rather than document sharing in an online communications system. Had the members invested in the productivity of their organization, the additional overhead would have been more than recouped in efficiency and employee morale.

Defining the MIS Structure

Clearly, there is no single system that is ideal for all practices (for a discussion of needs-assessment issues pertaining to information systems, see American Psychological Association, 1996c). Your choice of a system will be dictated by several factors, including the following:

- **Size of the practice**. A small staff-model group occupying a specialty niche may find it possible to keep records and statistics by hand, minimizing the need for an advanced computer system. Larger-scope entities will find the compilation of statistics by hand to be unwieldy and will need significant computerization to track and integrate services.

- **Managed care penetration of your region**. More competitive markets, in which contracting is already being conducted on a risk-sharing basis, demand advanced information systems that help practices monitor their utilization. Markets in which fee-for-service work dominates require less advanced systems. MCOs demanding the collection of quality data also require a meaningful degree of technological sophistication.

- **Centralization of your practice**. Practices located in a single, central location can more easily review charts and collate information, even when the data are kept in pencil-and-paper format. Networks, conversely, have no centralized physical records and thus need an advanced computer system to coordinate referrals, utilization management, and review of charts.

We view the development of an advanced information system as perhaps the single most important investment that a collaboration can make to enhance its competitive position. A good system will enable a practice to control its costs, document its cost-effectiveness, assess its quality, build its communications, and monitor its service record. Armed with information, practices that are operating on a fee-for-service basis today will be better able to make the transition to prepaid financing later. We cannot stress this enough: By the time a practice needs to engage in risk-bearing contracts, it is too late to assemble an advanced information system. To successfully price services in a risk-based market, a group or network needs to know its practice patterns and the utilization characteristics of its populations. Without at least a full year's worth of data, practice managers will be in the dark when contract opportunities arise.

We have a simple rule for defining the minimum MIS for a collaborative practice. Managers and practitioners need to have a system that allows them to keep current on their income and expenditures, cost of providing care, utilization patterns, and quality of services provided. The test of this capacity is to address several basic questions:

- Can you generate up-to-date reports on the number of clients seen and the utilization of various treatments?

- Can you generate up-to-date cash flow and income statements and reports on accounts payable and receivable?

- Can you generate up-to-date reports on measures of service and clinical quality?

- Are staff members electronically linked for rapid communications?

Note that our MIS is not defined by a type of computer arrangement or by a particular size of capital investment. Rather, it is defined by function. The MIS must enable the practice to capture the data needed to perform ongoing evaluations of the following:

- **Staff performance.** How clinicians are stacking up in terms of the quality and cost efficiency of their work;

- **Financial performance.** How the practice is faring in generating referrals and controlling overhead;

- **Overall clinical performance.** How the practice is faring with respect to the cost and quality of its services.

In addition, the MIS needs to be a communications platform from which practitioners can talk with each other, efficiently schedule their appointments, receive rapid feedback relative to their performance, make suggestions to management, and communicate with insurers.

Jeff Zimmerman, profiled in Chapter 7, tells the story of a staff clinician who received positive client satisfaction ratings from his adult psychotherapy clients but much more negative ones for his child cases. This led the practice managers to sit down with the clinician and investigate the situation. It turned out that the parents (who were filling out the satisfaction questionnaire) were happy with the treatment of their children but not happy with the level of communication between themselves and the therapist. Had the information not been collected and rapidly shared, the situation might have gone unchecked indefinitely, reducing the practice's word-of-mouth referral flow. Hard data in real time enhanced the clinician's practice, and thereby contributed to higher quality for clients.

Successful collaborative practices that we have interviewed have displayed a mentality very similar to that demonstrated by Dr. Zimmerman's group. We call it *management by information.* They are passionately dedicated to knowing how well they are doing: Are clients satisfied with the services provided? Is the group offering convenient, rapid access to treatment? Are clients being routed to appropriate care? Are they really improving as a result of the care being offered? Are clinical services being delivered in a cost-effective manner? **Stellar practices want to know the answers to these questions**. At the hub of their clinical, financial, and administrative operations is the MIS, helping them assess and improve what they do (see Figure 5.1).

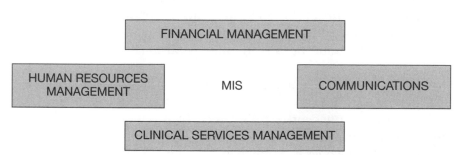

FIGURE 5.1. The management configuration of the collaborative practice.

Unfortunately, it is very common for practices to build their MIS by accretion, adding pieces to the system as they are needed. Typically, the practice begins with billing and accounting software, adds scheduling capabilities, and later purchases packages that can handle outcome data and other quality-related measures. Each software package might be helpful in its own right, but frequently the programs cannot readily share information. As a result, considerable management potential is lost. We know of many practices, for instance, that gather patient data through their billing system (diagnosis, demographics) and outcomes data through another program. The programs cannot readily speak to one another because of incompatibilities in file formats, leaving managers unable to answer such questions as the average satisfaction of clients with different diagnoses. A useful MIS has the flexibility to expand the amounts and types of information collected and relate each piece of data to every other in readily understood reports.

☞ LOOKING AHEAD

What information is essential to collect via the MIS?
    Our Information System Checklist at the end of this chapter (Reader's Resource 5.1) may help you determine your needs!

Networking the Practice

Developing an adequate information system for a small, centralized practice is not especially difficult or expensive. A number of software vendors offer integrated packages that assist with scheduling, billing, and record keeping (see the Resource List in the Appendix). These programs are often priced according to the number of "nodes" in the computer network. If the program is not networkable, it means that information cannot be shared through the practice, imposing severe limitations. This is especially problematic with respect to scheduling because it means that clinicians must continually update triage staff with their calendars, making it difficult to offer immediate appointments. It also adds cumbersome and time-consuming steps to the billing and claims management process because communications with billing staff must occur by fax, mail, and phone.

The network itself can be installed by a reputable local vendor, who will also offer maintenance services. In most small practices, the arrangement of computers will be a local area network (LAN), which connects workstations in a single building. The practice manager, receptionist/appointments coordinator, and billing clerk will be the ones most frequently using a simple system. They should be highly involved in the selection process, testing demonstration copies of the programs and assessing the user-friendliness and capability of each package.

More complex systems will link clinician offices to those of administrative staff, for rapid sharing of schedules, billing data, and clinical information.

Larger practices—and especially networks—require much more extensive computer systems and will probably need outside consultation in designing and shopping for a system. Most likely, this network will link practitioners across a variety of sites in a wide area network (WAN). For example, a network of 50 clinicians may need to access a central server numerous times each day. The system would be connected to multiple phone lines to allow for ready access, have sufficient memory to allow multiple users to access applications simultaneously, offer a high level of user-friendliness and data security, and enjoy extensive maintenance support so that downtime is minimized. Considerable time and effort would also need to be spent in training providers to use the system appropriately.

Maintaining a computer network is a major commitment for the behavioral practice. Bret Smith of REC Management, Inc., profiled in Chapter 7, notes that it is one of his most time- and money-consuming areas of business. Server downtime can grind the practice to a halt, interfering with billing, scheduling, and data collection. There are continual needs for software expansions and upgrades, as well as upgrades of hardware. This means that, as the practice expands, either a significant portion of a staff member's time must be allocated to MIS needs or the MIS must be outsourced to a specialty firm.

Outsourcing MIS Needs

Given the cost and expertise required to build and maintain a network, it is not surprising that a number of practice organizations consider outsourcing their MIS needs to MSO specialists. MSOs have the potential to benefit from economies of scale. As John Hill, former chief operating officer of Value Behavioral Health, pointed out to us, an administrative services organization can contract with firms that provide large server farms and set up their own software, creating MIS platforms capable of meeting the needs of multiple provider organizations. This greatly reduces the MIS overhead to each practice. Indeed, he asserts that the majority of administrative services to a practice could be provided for approximately 5% of gross billings, once economies of scale are realized. Greg Alter of Pacific Applied Psychological Associates observes that such an MSO platform could be Internet-based, creating a comprehensive site that could be accessed by multiple practices.

Two sets of information needs are typically addressed by MSOs and other MIS firms. The first pertain to billing, claims management, communications, and authorizations. The vendor/MSO centralizes all billing and related financial and clinical record keeping for the practice. There are many ways for these activities to be organized. In the case of a company such as Michael Hurst's Instream, the vendor does not actually prepare billings and financial reports for clinicians. Rather, it provides an interface for the electronic filing of claims and treatment reports that is accepted by payers and that links to most widely used practice management software. Traditional MSOs, on the other hand, actually do the claims filing and report generation for the practice, providing the hardware and software required for capturing the needed information. The practice may still employ clerical staff to assemble encounter data from clinicians prior to sending it to the MSO, or the MSO may provide such staff itself, relying on clinicians to enter their own data. The latter is an attractive arrangement for practice networks, which otherwise would have to build and maintain WANs to centralize claims filing and communications. Once the MSO provides the central servers and software, it is simply a matter of connecting the clinician to these to expand the MIS. The savings to the network in hardware, software, and system support can be sizable.

A second set of needs addressed by MSOs concerns the collection of data pertaining to clinical quality, such as client satisfaction and treatment outcomes. Firms such as Compass offer validated and normed tools for the assessment of these, as well as mechanisms for their scoring and interpretation, but do not actually administer the questionnaires themselves. Others, such as DeltaMetrics, actually conduct external outcome studies of a practice, contacting clients on their own, administering questionnaires, and interpreting results. The latter, naturally, is much more expensive but completely frees clinical staff and practice managers from the time-consuming process of periodically surveying caseloads.

An unappreciated advantage of external MSOs is their ability to assist practice organizations in evaluating their data. Let's imagine that 20 networks and groups in a region are contracting with an MSO for their billing, communication, and data collection needs. Over time, the MSO will assemble a considerable data warehouse, with a significant amount of information regarding utilization, client satisfaction, and outcomes. From this database, the MSO could begin to establish norms, such as the average satisfaction level among clients with severe presenting complaints. These norms prove invaluable in managing clinical and administrative services, especially with respect to benchmarking for quality improvement. Over time, we predict that MSOs will serve an important consultative role in quality assurance programs, providing databases that could not be assembled by isolated practice organizations.

Providing Information via the Web

Increasingly, we are hearing about practices developing a presence on the World Wide Web as a means for communicating with the outside world and sharing information within the staff. A good example would be the site developed by REC Management, Inc. (http://www.recmgmt.com). The REC site contains useful information about the practice, a variety of tools for clinicians, and opportunities for those accessing the site to communicate with the MSO. It is especially helpful as a tool for marketing REC to referral sources and interested clinicians.

A Web site can be accessed by anyone wanting to learn more about the practice, including prospective clients. Through the creation of links, designers of sites allow Web surfers to access as much information as they like on topics of their choice. An especially attractive aspect of the Web is its ability to combine sound, graphics, and text in interactive presentations. It is thus possible to have sophisticated sales and research presentations to international audiences 24 hours a day, 7 days a week. As the Web has become an increasingly common part of daily life, we are now seeing clients shopping for providers online in ways similar to—but much more comprehensive than—the Yellow Pages. Unlike the Yellow Pages, Web sites can offer detailed and easily updated descriptions of a practice's treatment programs and philosophies, its participation in insurance plans, and choices of providers.

Developing and maintaining a Web site can be very simple or quite involved, depending on the organization's needs. At one end of the continuum, the members of the practice can do all the work themselves and build a site from scratch. This means designing and constructing pages using HyperText Markup Language (HTML), purchasing a server and software to facilitate access to the site, connecting the server to an Internet service provider (ISP), and registering the Web address in Washington, DC, with the InterNIC (http://rs.internic.net). This may sound unusually daunting, but it should be noted that Web authoring tools have become quite user-friendly and are now built into several major word processing programs. Practices assembling WANs already have much of the hardware necessary to maintain a site and can receive help from ISPs with respect to site design and server software.

An alternative to building a site is relying on the hosting capacity of ISPs and online services such as America Online and Prodigy. Practice managers simply tell the ISP what the site should contain and how the information is to be linked; the basic work of constructing pages can be performed by the ISP. Because the site remains resident on the ISP's server, the practice does not need to purchase and maintain its own hardware and can rely on the security features and superior access of the ISP. The major online services also offer user-friendly software for altering pages, adding links, and so on. Web outsourcing is not cheap, amounting to several thousand dollars in start-up costs and ongoing monthly maintenance charges, but it may be ideal for practices with limited high-tech skills. These costs can be reduced meaningfully if the practice has its own "Web Master" who can assemble the site.

Although the Internet has received considerable media attention, the more powerful business trend has been toward Intranets, which are LAN- and WAN-based online systems linking members *within* an organization. Intranets allow members to send messages, share files and documents, hold conferences, and work on documents simultaneously: They are internal Internets. Intranets can incorporate internal Web sites, allowing staff members to readily access information, including graphics and sound files. An Intranet Web site is not meant to be accessed by the public at large and hence has somewhat more relaxed security needs than public sites. It does, however, allow for the broad, interactive sharing of information in a graphics-intensive format and thus may become useful as a means of archiving and sharing medical records. As organizations move toward

☞ LOOKING AHEAD

How are information technologies enhancing the accountability of group practices?
　　Check out our featured interview with Peter Brill, MD,
at the end of this chapter (Reader's Resource 5.2).

integrated systems, it is likely that internal Webs will facilitate online case consultations and quality reviews, allowing consultants to quickly access and inter-
pret medical and mental health data.

The Evolution of the MIS

One theme we heard repeatedly from founders of successful practices is that their
MIS needs always seem one step ahead of them. It is rarely if ever the case that a
computer system meets the information needs of a practice for all time. For example, group practices often develop satellite locations to expand their geographic coverage. Once that occurs, the LAN is no longer sufficient for all information needs. The computer system must expand to permit communications
and data sharing between satellite locations and the central office. Software and
hardware upgrades are also needed in many cases to exploit newer technologies,
such as groupware applications for online conferences and simultaneous document editing.

Many times, start-up groups can expand their MIS without having to jump
to large computer networks. This permits the MIS to evolve gradually and keeps
overhead controllable. We have found two particular technologies to be helpful
in this regard: document scanning and interactive voice response (IVR) systems.

A scanner is a peripheral device that converts any input, such as type or
graphics, into digital form. Once the typed page or image is scanned, it can be
transferred and manipulated in a variety of ways. Optical character recognition
software allows data to be scanned and read into traditional computer applications. It is possible, for instance, to have clients fill out questionnaires on
scannable forms that can be read into the practice's database program. Although
this may not be quite as time-efficient as administering the questionnaire to
clients directly by computer, it is much more time-effective than simple pencil-
and-paper administration, which requires a separate set of operations for manual
data entry. The broad use of scannable forms also reduces overhead by eliminating the need for computers in every clinician's office. If billings, intake data, and
outcomes/satisfaction forms are in scannable form, they can be completed by
hand and quickly delivered to a clerical staff member in charge of data entry.

Another interesting technology that can assist practices in expanding their
MIS capabilities without investing in expensive networks is IVR telephone sys-

tems. The best way to think of IVR is as a customized voice mail system. Callers dial a dedicated number and receive a recorded message with numerous options. The options, for example, could allow clinicians to update their daily schedules or enter basic encounter data concerning a new client. The IVR program structures the options for the caller, always providing a menu of choices via touch-tone telephone. Thus, if a therapist is updating a schedule, the first menu choice might be for month of the year ("press 1 for January, 2 for February"), followed by day of the month ("terminate your entry by pressing the pound key"), and time of day ("press 1 for A.M., 2 for P.M."). The information entered by phone is captured by the practice's central computer and stored as a separate file. The file can include voice recordings as well as the data entered by keypad. A clerical staff member can then access the file, transcribe voice data, and ensure that the numeric data are transferred to the appropriate software application without clerical reentry.

A very powerful application of IVR is the capture of satisfaction and quality data from clients. Instead of requiring clients to complete questionnaires by paper or on scannable forms, they can be asked to dial a dedicated number for the IVR system. The system then reads the questionnaire items to the client over the phone, allowing for an entry of responses by touch-tone keypad. All data are stored in a text file (in the generic ASCII format) for easy transfer to analytic software. Such a methodology has two distinctive advantages: (1) It requires no reading skill on the part of clients and thus is quite appropriate for clients with educational or visual deficits; and (2) it allows for timely capture of information without necessitating a computer in every clinician's office.

In sum, it is important to think flexibly about MIS needs. Often it is possible to keep overhead down, even as the ability to capture up-to-date data and achieve rapid communications is implemented. The current mergers of technologies, blurring the distinctions among computer companies, regional and long-distance telephone carriers, and ISPs, promise expanding options for growing practices. We find it quite likely that the collaborative practice of the future will be linked to a variety of insurers and health care organizations through an electronic web of applications and communication media, facilitating online audits of cost and quality and consultative services.

Shopping for an MIS

When large health care organizations, such as hospitals, shop for an information system, they typically issue a request for proposal (RFP) to qualified firms and retain a consultant to help them evaluate proposals. This can be a very expensive and time-consuming process, something all but the largest behavioral groups will want to avoid (for complete discussions of RFPs and vendor selection, see American Psychological Association, 1996c; Beebe, 1992; Milner, 1994). Ciotti, Seiter, and Pagnotta (1994) point out that the RFP process can run over $50,000 in consulting fees alone, generating far more detail than the average decision maker requires. They recommend interviewing other health care organizations, conducting site visits, and talking with vendors so as to limit the field to four or five suppliers. They further suggest that the lengthy RFP be condensed into a request for information that assesses the vendor's experience in the field, its client base, and its financial strength (especially important if you need them to be around to service the system). Obtaining copies of user manuals and conducting site visits to representative practices utilizing the systems can help practice leaders adequately evaluate the various options. The goal is to save your money for the computer system, not overly elaborate consultations.

Should you elect to assemble a MIS through a consultant, there are several factors to keep in mind (Doyle, 1990):

- Consultants should have a broad knowledge of the major systems available on the market.

- The consultant should be aware of your budget and needs and should not attempt to sell you systems that are not needed.

- The consultant should be free of any financial ties to particular vendors.

- The consultant should be willing and able to assist you in negotiations with vendors, especially if you are making a major purchase.

Some consultants will try to convince you to build rather than buy an information system. Off-the-shelf software, they will argue, cannot be flexible enough to meet your needs. Although there can be merit to this argument, building a system from scratch is a dangerous proposition. It can be extremely time-consuming and expensive. "Bugs" in the system may not show up for months after the system is first used, creating major headaches. Worst of all, your programmer may not be available later, so that when you must upgrade your system, it will take a long time for a new programmer to learn the system and make the changes. For these reasons, it generally makes sense to stick with a system and companies that have been around for a while.

Knowing Your Information Needs

You can best help a consultant help you (or serve as your own consultant) if you have clearly articulated the information needs of your practice. We have emphasized that the mental health professions are in the midst of a revolution in which the ability to document and deliver quality as well as cost-efficiency will be mandatory. Furthermore, we believe that this will create broad collaborations among insurers, practice organizations, and purchasers of benefits in which providers assume financial risk for their services. Before shopping for a system, it is important to identify the specific information that you will need for cost and quality accountability. Our checklist at the end of this chapter should be of some help in gauging your needs. Recognize, of course, that your demand for information should flow naturally from your strategy. If you are marketing a high-quality service, your MIS should have a well-developed capacity to capture data and generate useful summary reports pertaining to service and clinical quality. If your strategy calls for a high level of cost-effectiveness, you will need the MIS to carefully track utilization as a function of patient diagnosis and treatment modality.

Of the data to be captured by a practice, two elements stand out in our minds: average quality and average cost per treatment episode. Average quality will give a snapshot of the general level of administrative and clinical service effectiveness within the practice. It is very helpful (and impressive) to know, for example, that 95% of all clients were satisfied or very satisfied with the services received, that 90% of all clients were seen for a first appointment within 5 business days of their initial call, and that 85% of all clients reported significant improvements in their functioning over the course of care. Such information is crucial to ongoing quality assurance efforts and will greatly aid in marketing the practice and developing effective compensation systems.

The average cost per treatment episode is important because it prepares the collaborative practice for risk-bearing contracts. To compute average cost in a staff-model practice in which clinicians are salaried, it is necessary to divide the overhead of the practice (rent/leases, equipment/MIS expenses, salaries, utilities, etc.) by the number of patients being seen during that unit of time. This represents the amount of money that the practice needs to obtain from each case to break even.

In a network/contractor model, the overhead would not include clinical salaries. The best way to compute cost would be to divide overhead by the number of sessions offered during that unit of time and then add to that figure the average per-session reimbursement per clinician. If that figure is multiplied by the average number of sessions per case, a total cost of treatment episode will be obtained.

Knowing cost of treatment allows practices to estimate the case rates (lump-sum reimbursement per case) they would need to make an adequate profit. Once case rates are derived, it is only a matter of estimating utilization within a population to arrive at a capitation amount for outpatient services (for a useful discussion of capitation contracting, see Zieman, 1995). If you are a clinician contemplating an affiliation with a staff-model group, network, or an IPA operating in a highly competitive market, determining whether organizations know their average cost and average quality is a quick and straightforward means of assessment. It will help you identify the capabilities of the group's MIS and will tell you

☞ LOOKING AHEAD

What is at-risk contracting and how does it affect your practice and its information needs?

Our Capitation Crash Course at the end of this chapter (Reader's Resource 5.3) may shed some light!

whether the practice managers have the mind-set and commitment needed for success in such a marketplace.

A Note to Those Joining Group Practices

There is an understandable tendency to view MIS-related topics as part of "management," not particularly relevant to the work of the clinician. Nothing could be further from the truth. If you are a solo clinician looking to affiliate with a group either in a network (to maintain your individual practice) or as an employee (to integrate with a collaborative venture), your professional future will hinge crucially on your ability to deliver time-effective services (see Chapter 6). The presence of a sophisticated MIS means that you will have valuable tools in documenting and improving the quality of your work. The MIS, employed properly, is a powerful vehicle for ongoing professional learning and development.

During the latter 1980s and the 1990s, managed care has primarily been something that has been done *to* clinicians. With the burgeoning quality mandates noted in Chapter 1 and the push toward risk assumption in contracting, the need will become intense for clinicians capable of **managing their own services**. Over time, as we see a withering away of external care reviewers and the inefficiencies of time-consuming authorizations, group practices will perform these functions independently, allocating care resources according to research-based guidelines. Your task as a network or staff clinician is not to learn how to work with managed care. It is to learn collaborative strategies for managing your own cost and quality. The MIS is an indispensable part of this evolution. The guidelines contained in this chapter will be helpful in identifying group practices that can truly advance your career.

TOWARD COLLABORATIVE MANAGEMENT

A neglected issue in practice management is the organization of the work units producing the information contained in an MIS. It is often assumed in clinical practice, for example, that the individual clinician is the primary unit of organization. Increasingly, however, the field of management is recognizing the value of *work teams* as organizational units (Katzenbach & Smith, 1993). This has profound implications for MIS development within collaborative practices.

The Construction of Work Teams

In a typical practice, professionals carry out their work in relative isolation, with only occasional coordination in staff meetings and clinical conferences. This creates a need for managers to fill a linking function, ensuring that staff do not work at cross-purposes. In a team-based organization, groups of individuals form integrated work units and coordinate their own efforts. To a large degree, therefore, team-based practices are self-managing. The responsibilities of management are driven down the organizational chart.

An example illustrates the profound differences that team-based organization can make. Let's imagine that Integrated Behavioral Services, PC, undergoes a reorganization. Instead of allowing individual clinicians to pick up cases as they come in, every clinical service is now to be delivered programmatically (see Chapter 6). The practice now will be composed of identified programs for every major type of referral: an eating disorders program, a mood disorders program, an intensive outpatient treatment program, and so on. Each program is staffed by a multidisciplinary group of professionals and led by a senior clinician. The programs are empowered by practice management to develop their own treatment guidelines, policies and procedures, and measures of cost and quality. To ensure that these do not conflict, the heads of each program meet on a regular basis as part of a "clinical management team." When referrals come to the practice, they are assigned to a program, not to an individual clinician. The program clinicians, linked electronically, are then responsible for subsequent triage, treatment planning, and data collection.

In addition, the administrative staff of Integrated Behavioral Services, PC, are reorganized into teams. One team, for example, deals with billing, claims management, accounting, and financial reporting. Another is dedicated to coordination of appointments, triage, and communications with patients and referral sources. Once again, each of these teams has a leader and is charged with specific responsibilities regarding the organization of workflows and collection of data. When policies and procedures need to be changed to improve service to clients or referral sources, administrative team members have the support of the organization in designing and implementing the modifications.

As the practice develops new services, additional teams are created to structure and manage these. These teams cut across the practice, allowing clinicians and administrators to coordinate their efforts. For instance, if Integrated Behavioral Services wants to develop EAP services for local companies, the EAP team might consist of clerical staff, clinicians, and managers, so that issues of accounting, reimbursement, scheduling, quality assessment, and clinical services are not tackled in isolation. Instead of designing the service from above and imposing it upon staff members, the staff members most familiar with their own work are empowered to participate in the design and maintenance of the service.

A key element of team-based management is that **each team becomes a responsibility center**. That is, each team is responsible for developing the following:

- **Goals and objectives in accordance with the overall strategic plan of the practice**. Each team engages in its own planning processes.

- **Criteria by which the achievement of these goals and objectives can be measured.** Each team is self-managing, monitoring, and adjusting its performance.

- **A sub-MIS, supporting team assessments and communications.** The team helps determine how information will be woven into its work flows.

- **The organization and delivery of its own services.** The team is empowered to utilize information to change its services and ways of delivering these.

Each team thus becomes a mini-organization, engaging in its own planning, self-assessment, and quality improvement. Coordination of the teams through a central mechanism (a team of teams) ensures that each team is aligned with the overall mission and goals of the practice, even as it exercises considerable latitude in achieving its pieces of this mission. It is especially powerful when incentive plans for compensation are team- as well as individually based, rewarding the successful collaborations of clinical and administrative staff.

Note that team-based management is not the same thing as management by committees. Committees are advisory bodies to central management; as such, they can be quite useful. Committees, however, rarely represent formal work units and rarely possess an identity outside their occasional meetings. Team-based management formally reorganizes the practice. It is the expression of a systems perspective in which the overall system (the practice) is supported by the interdependent functioning of relatively autonomous subsystems (teams). Committees create collaborations for an hour a week. Team-based management embeds collaboration within the organizational chart.

The Critical Assumptions of Collaborative Management

Table 5.1 summarizes the important differences in underlying assumptions between traditionally managed and collaboratively managed organizations. Traditional management vests decision making in the hands of central planners, who are deemed to possess superior skills and knowledge. Collaborative management is predicated on the notion of *local expertise*: Those closest to the consumer and most immersed in their work flows are likely to have the understandings needed to address consumer needs.

A second crucial assumption of collaborative management is that clusters of affiliated individuals produce synergies that could not be achieved if those same individuals were working in isolation. Traditional practice management assigns a case to an individual clinician and has little input into the subsequent handling of that case, except perhaps through occasional staff conferences or outcome assessments. When the case is assigned to a team, however, there is active, ongoing interdisciplinary treatment planning and coordination. The team takes responsibility for the success of its cases.

TABLE 5.1. Traditional versus Collaborative Management

	Traditional management	Collaborative management
Locus of decision making and responsibility	Managers	Multispecialty teams
Unit of service delivery	Individual provider	Team-based programs
Organizational structure	Hierarchical managers and staff	Decentralized interdependent teams
Priorities	Staff autonomy and management control	Integration of staff and management roles

Finally, traditional management tends to polarize the work of managers and staff, with managers occupying the highest rungs of the organizational ladder. This creates an untenable situation in which ambitious, talented clinicians either have to remain at relatively modest levels of recognition, authority, and compensation if they wish to continue their clinical work or abandon their craft to become full-time administrators. We firmly believe that this subtle devaluation of clinical talent is a major drag on practice organizations. Collaborative management allows individuals to be managers *and* clinicians because it encourages teams of professionals to become self-managing. It thus lends itself to compensation systems in which overall contribution to the practice can be recognized and rewarded. It also prepares the group for at-risk contracting, when it is crucial that clinicians learn how to manage their own care.

Perhaps most important of all, collaborative management places organizational culture at the heart of the practice. Unlike some industrial and service organizations, a behavioral practice consists largely of professionals who have trained to achieve a measure of recognition and expertise in their fields. To ignore this fact and treat clinical staff members as assembly-line workers robs the organization of its lifeblood. Many times practitioners have not developed innovations in their work because these have been neither rewarded nor sought. Clinicians are often expected to put in a maximum of clinical hours and not "waste time" on unreimbursed activity. If an idea for a new clinical service strikes a clinician, there is a powerful disincentive to pursue the thread because the clinician's own revenue will be adversely affected by the time needed to bring it to life. Team-based management creates explicit structures for encouraging and recognizing innovation and drawing on the expertise of staff. This recognition, based on the support and acclaim of one's peers, often means as much to the professional staff person as salary raises and bonuses.

Aligning Individuals into Teams

Our experience is that team development is not easy. Clinicians, by and large, have been trained to work in isolation. Managers have been taught to manage, not to empower others to manage. It is difficult for clinicians to give up perceived autonomy, just as it is challenging for managers to yield perceived control. Nonetheless, collaborations have an uncanny way of tapping into the best that professionals have to offer. Katzenbach and Smith (1993), summarizing years of work with team-based organizations, explain,

> Strong interpersonal commitments drive a number of aspects that distinguish high-performance teams. Fueled by interpersonal commitments, team purposes become even nobler, team performance goals more urgent, and team approach more powerful. The notion, for example, that "if one of us fails, we all fail" pervades high performance teams. (p. 66)

Similarly, Senge (1990) describes the interpersonal environment within team-based learning organizations:

> The fundamental characteristic of the relatively unaligned team is wasted energy. Individuals may work extraordinarily hard, but their efforts do not efficiently translate to team effort. By contrast, when a team becomes more aligned, a commonality of direction emerges, and individuals' energies harmonize. There is less wasted energy. In fact, a resonance or synergy develops, like the "coherent" light of a laser rather than the incoherent and scattered light of a light bulb. There is commonality of purpose, a shared vision, and understanding of how to complement one another's efforts. Individuals do not sacrifice their personal interests to the larger team vision; rather, the shared vision becomes an extension of their personal visions. (pp. 234–235)

These have been characteristics of every successful practice organization we have interviewed. The practice is not simply collaborative because it coordinates work efforts. The members truly care about one another. They are devoted to each other's success and development. There is an esprit de corps that transcends the function of normal working relationships.

A dramatic example has been the extraordinary resources that organizations such as Pacific Applied Psychological Associates (PAPA), Relationship Enrichment Center, and CPG Behavioral Health Resources devote to ongoing staff training. As Jeff Zimmerman of CPG noted, this investment amounts to hiring a clinical staff member and telling that individual to sit there and not generate revenue. Nonetheless, it is a valued expenditure, contributing to the cohesion, as well as education, of member professionals. We recently heard a secondhand report that one of the principals of PAPA remarked that if managed care fees ever became so low that he would have to abandon PAPA's supportive staff model, he would opt to leave the business. This says a lot. Excellent practices begin with extraordinary personal and professional commitments.

A Model for Team Alignment

How does one move from being a traditionally managed practice to a collaborative enterprise? It is not as simple as shifting boxes on an organizational chart or holding more meetings. In many respects, collaboration remakes the practice.

Jamieson (1996) offers a model of team alignment that is a most useful tool in making the transition (see Figure 5.2). At the center of the Alignment Model is "culture," the set of values and expectations that permeate the organization. Jamieson (1996) notes that team management replaces an ethic of within-organization competition with the notion that "sharing expertise and information helps our performance" (p. 308). Surrounding culture are the building blocks of the enterprise:

- **Strategy.** The mission, plans, and goals of the firm.

- **Structure.** The ways in which jobs, teams, and work flows are designed.

- **Systems.** The ongoing policies and procedures of a firm.

- **Practices.** The day-to-day behaviors and interactions exhibited within the organization.

Linking culture to strategy and practices is what Jamieson (1996) calls *vision*, the organization's verbalized depiction of its desired end state: what it strives to be and become. In a successful business organization, strategy is the guiding light for the other components: structure, culture, systems, and practices must reflect the underlying strategy of the firm.

Jamieson's (1996) tool is especially helpful to clinicians attempting to conceptualize what we called the Index of Quality (IQ) of a practice. In a truly collaborative organization, there are clear and tight links among the components of the model. **Moreover, these links and components exist at team levels, as well as organizationally.** That is, each team has its own strategy, driving its culture, systems, and practices. The strategy of a team developing a new clinical ser-

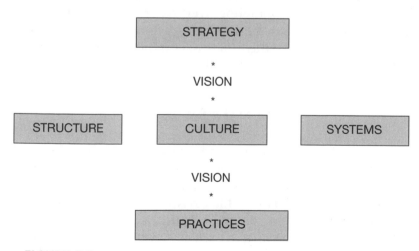

FIGURE 5.2 Jamieson's (1996) Alignment Model of organizations.

vice will be quite different from that of a team engaging in quality assessment, necessitating a different structuring of work flows and responsibilities.

This can be most readily observed in the forms of alignment among collaborative practices with differing strategies and structures. The small group practice implementing a specialty niche strategy may have a closely knit, horizontal governance, with few structured policies and procedures, informal patterns of communication, but highly formalized protocols for assessing quality. Very large networks implementing a low-cost, geographically diversified strategy may not be closely knit, given the spread of providers, and may require more vertical governance, more formalized policies and procedures, and tight utilization protocols. Similarly, the specific capabilities of the MIS will be reflective of the underlying organizational missions. The small group may have relatively few MIS needs with respect to communications but may need ways of accessing clients even after treatment ends to assess outcomes and feed results back to clinicians. The larger network group will have extensive communications needs in order to maintain cohesion.

At its best, alignment within teams and organizations creates an entrepreneurial spirit and a cohesive culture. In a very real sense, team leaders are empowered as "intrapreneurs," innovators within their own organizations, with responsibilities for their own ventures. This creates a culture in which mutual support is blended with a strong achievement and work ethic.

INTEGRATING THE MIS INTO COLLABORATIVE MANAGEMENT

An old saying defines a camel as a horse designed by a committee. Nothing can be more draining than attending team meetings in which members lack the information necessary for effective decision making. Discussion quickly bogs down into turf battles and endless wrangling over matters of opinion. There is much more to collaborative management than being warm and fuzzy and holding endless meetings. A central role of the MIS is to empower teams by giving them the data they need to evaluate and continually improve their efforts.

The Need for Tools

Let us take a look at two of the outstanding organizations interviewed for this book. Each, in its own way, is fueling the creation of collaborative practices through the development of information tools.

Compass Information Services, Inc., has created a database of more than 15,000 cases, capturing the utilization and clinical outcome patterns of clients with a variety of presenting concerns and intensity of needs. Drawing on research and theory concerning the relationship between "dosages" of psychotherapy and clinical outcomes (Howard et al., 1986; Steenbarger, 1994) and the patterning of change over time (Howard, Lueger, Maling, & Martinovitch, 1993), Compass is able to create profiles of anticipated progress for new patients. These provide objective benchmarks for clinicians to determine whether their clients are on track in their therapeutic work or whether changes in treatment plans might be indicated. The Compass tools also allow clinicians to determine, over large caseloads, the efficiency and effectiveness of their work with different types of patients, aiding efforts at professional development.

Particular synergies can be obtained, however, if such tools are utilized in a collaboratively managed organization. Teams are able to structure their clinical services in programmatic ways, developing their own triage criteria, practice guidelines, and care review mechanisms and criteria. With the addition of reliable and valid outcome tools and a large database, the clinical programs now can assess the degree to which their guidelines and case management are actually contributing to cost-effective, quality care. If, for instance, much more negative outcomes are obtained for clients with borderline personality disorder than for similar clients in the database, the team could examine its clinical practices and the elements of its programs to address needs that might be unmet. The Compass database, for example, breaks down outcomes into categories, including client well-being, functional status, and symptomatology. If the program discovers that well-being is being enhanced for clients with severe problems but not functional status, it could develop or link to psychosocial programs addressing social and vocational needs as a way of improving functioning.

As Peter Brill, founder and CEO of Compass notes, a large database allows for the risk adjustment of outcomes data, permitting a tailoring of expectations to the client's presenting diagnosis, problem severity, quality of social support, and so on. Over time, as an increasing number of cases are added to the database, more sophisticated analyses of contributory variables become possible. Instead of working from a simplistic model that says, "All treatment must be conducted briefly, within 10 sessions," teams can define parameters of cost and quality for each client group, delivering *appropriate* care.

In a different way, Value Behavioral Health, Inc., profiled in Chapter 7, is empowering provider organizations by delegating care management to the practices themselves and providing extensive feedback on utilization and quality. Here the team concept is extended beyond the individual organization to encompass the relationship between a practice and an MCO. Each practice is encouraged to manage its own care by conducting internal utilization reviews. Each also agrees to utilize a set of reliable and valid measures, assessing everything from client satisfaction and access to clinical outcomes and number of sessions delivered. VBH compiles the data in a central database and, each month, allows each practice to compare itself to others. Once again, the database creates a set of norms or benchmarks by which the practice can identify whether or not it is doing a good job. The clinical practices can then use this information for their own strategic planning purposes, modifying the structure and content of services accordingly.

An exciting aspect of the VBH program is that it creates incentives for the delivery of efficient and effective care. Practices that meet high standards on the measures are paid bonuses for their work and recognized for their efforts. This truly creates a situation in which insurers and providers act as a collaborative, quality-driven system. The same teamwork that is apparent within collaboratively managed practices can be achieved in the relationship between MCOs and networks/groups.

None of this is possible, however, without information-based tools. **Management by collaboration requires management by information**. If you are identifying practices with which to affiliate, your task is to determine which of the alternatives has the potential to create information-driven, quality-minded, collaborative efforts. We predict such organizations will be winners in the emerging mental health marketplace.

The Role of Communications in Collaboration

The MIS is not just a collection of information tools. It is also a platform from which data derived from these tools can be archived, manipulated, and shared within the organization. Essential to the management of the practice is the timely distribution of information throughout the organization. If teams are to be self-managing, they desperately need data in real time. They also need the ability to merge and manipulate data in their own ways, to achieve their unique ends.

Two of the innovative organizations interviewed as part of our research, U.S. Behavioral Health, Inc. (USBH), and Instream, Inc., have been collaborating to enhance the communications capabilities of practices and insurers. USBH has linked a number of its preferred group practices through Instream's communications platform, permitting rapid interchange of data within the practice and between the practice and insurer. For instance, claims can be electronically submitted in bulk, allowing for rapid processing and payment. Outpatient treatment reports can also be completed and filed electronically, speeding authorizations. These time efficiencies greatly aid the practice in its cash flow management, overall productivity, and staff satisfaction. Who wouldn't want to work for a practice that eliminated phone calls for authorizations and claims disputes?

As Michael Hurst of Instream, notes, however, the benefits of a communication system go far deeper. Once providers and care managers are online, they can talk with each other in an ongoing e-mail-style conversation to consult on matters of treatment planning and referrals. It would be simple, for example, for a group contracting with USBH to talk with a USBH care manager about local resources for a client in need, construct an intervention plan that could be coordinated locally, and provide ongoing feedback about the success of the plan. Although this is technically possible by telephone, it rarely occurs in such a coordinated, ongoing fashion because of the time eaten up playing "phone tag." With the online communications system, clinicians with expertise can be drawn into the conversation, creating virtual multidisciplinary consulting teams.

A communication system also links providers within the organization, allowing for ongoing collaboration without the time and hassle of scheduling and conducting face-to-face meetings. Let's imagine, for instance, that a practice establishes an anxiety disorders program and assigns a team to develop and manage the program. The team will need to agree on basic practice guidelines for the program to determine, say, when clients will be referred for psychiatric consultations, when they will be referred to coping skills groups, and so on. An Intranet-based communication system allows the team to draft the guidelines, share feedback, and make changes as needed, with participants doing the work at their chosen time. It is no longer necessary to synchronize schedules to conduct face-to-face meetings. Teams can include members from satellite locations and maintain their cohesiveness even when they are not in the same room.

As an illustration, the book you are reading is a collaboration between us and The Guilford Press, but we have held only one face-to-face meeting to discuss our work. Most of the writing, rewriting, and discussion has occurred via America Online, through e-mails and file transfers linking the participants. It's eye-opening to recognize that not too many years ago, such a project would have required the manual typing and retyping of numerous drafts and countless phone calls and meetings. Communications technology has reshaped the nature of collaboration, opening the doors to new modes of working.

CONCLUSION

This chapter has made clear that collaboration is much more than throwing your hat into the ring with other clinicians. It entails a fundamental reconceptualization of what a practice is all about and how its services are to be organized and delivered. Our research convinces us that the future lies with data-driven, team-

✔ SUMMARY

- An MIS, linking financial, clinical, and administrative data, lies at the heart of the collaborative practice.
- The ideal MIS depends on the size and structure of the group practice, with larger groups and network-model practices requiring more extensive systems.
- As group practices move toward at-risk contracting, they experience greater demands to engage in management by information and learn how to manage their own cost and quality.
- Team-based organization within the group practice infuses the organization with a collaborative culture and allows clinicians to shape their own information and management systems.

based organizations that are committed to their own learning and development. This is a very new kind of science–practice collaboration, in which the scientists and practitioners are one and the same (Steenbarger et al., 1996).

The planning of your practice should not simply be a mechanism for coping in a difficult competitive environment. It deserves to be a tool for defining the kind of working environment that will nurture your growth, success, and fulfillment as a professional. The move toward collaboration promises a new wave of quality-driven practice organizations that offer distinctive benefits to clinicians, insurers, and clients. For some practitioners, this may be a threat. In our eyes, it is an exciting opportunity to create a professional culture that is equally committed to doing things right and doing the right things.

READER'S RESOURCE 5.1
Information System Checklist

Your information system might be large or small, simple or sophisticated, but it should be *all* of the following:

- **User-friendly.** Systems that are easy to navigate will be used more often and will contribute to productivity. Communications routines should make it simple to send messages to groups of people simultaneously, archive communications, and share files and documents.
- **Powerful.** Memory (RAM) and video memory should be sufficient to allow rapid movement from program to program and function to function. The system should not crawl at a speed that keeps users staring at an hourglass symbol.
- **Secure.** Patient records must be kept confidential, requiring encryption of sensitive data and passwords to protect access to records.
- **Reliable.** The hardware and software should have a good track record, with minimum downtime. Software that has been in use for a while will be less likely to be plagued by surprise "bugs" that shut down your system and cause data loss. Vendors that are financially strong and in business for a while are most likely to be in business later.
- **Redundant.** All data should be backed up at least daily, with backups occurring automatically or with minimum effort and fuss. In case of a system shut down, there should be a back-up system for accessing and entering patient information. Computer downtime should not lead to practice downtime.
- **Well serviced.** On-site service, provided on short notice, is mandatory, especially with large networks. Many service organizations guarantee response within an hour of a call.
- **Integrated.** If you are using different computers and/or software programs, these should be capable of communicating with one another. Data should be entered in recognized formats, not the proprietary format of a single company. Don't get closed out by a closed architecture.

Practical features to look for in MIS software:

- **Does it ease the work of billing?** Will it satisfy the needs of the insurers I work with? Does it allow for easy data entry? Does it archive patient records in a way that is easy to access? Does it allow clinicians to submit billings electronically?

(cont.)

READER'S RESOURCE 5.1 (*cont.*)

- **Does it ease the authorization process?** Does it allow clinicians to stay on top of the need to file treatment reports? Does it facilitate the completion of reports with clinical information that is easy to access? Does it allow clinicians to submit authorization requests and receive replies electronically?
- **Does it ease scheduling?** Does it allow triage staff to schedule appointments for clinicians at the time of the patient's initial call? Does it allow clinicians to easily access and modify their schedules?
- **Does it ease communications?** Does it allow for online communications among clinical and administrative staff? Between staff members and members of other organizations? Does it allow for easy document sharing and file transfer?
- **Does it generate useful financial reports?** Will it facilitate the generation of financial statements? Does it help managers stay on top of receivables and payables? Does it aid in expense tracking for income tax purposes?
- **Does it generate useful clinical reports?** Does it track number and types of patients seen? Sources of referrals? Demographics? Services offered? Breakdown of patients seen as a function of provider? As a function of referral source?
- **Does it generate useful utilization reports?** Does it track the average length of treatment? Utilization of specific programs and services? Does it break down utilization as a function of patient demographics? Diagnosis? Provider?
- **Does it generate useful quality improvement reports?** Does it track patient satisfaction? Outcome data? Performance on service indicators? Does it break these down as a function of provider? Patient diagnoses? Demographics?

If you are joining a group practice, an MIS with most of the above capabilities will become a powerful learning tool, as you document and improve the quality of your work. A good MIS, employed properly, will make you more competitive in the job market and contribute to your growth as a professional.

READER'S RESOURCE 5.2
Interview with Peter Brill, MD,
Compass Information Services, Inc.

"Do they get better? That's probably the only absolute we have. . . . "

Peter Brill, MD, was trained as a psychiatrist but quickly moved into the business world by studying organizations at the University of Pennsylvania's Wharton School. He is currently a Fellow at Wharton, as well as a member of the clinical faculty at the University of Pennsylvania's Medical School. He is best known, however, as the founder and CEO of Compass Information Services, Inc., a company devoted to helping mental health organizations assess clinical outcomes. Early in the history of Compass, Dr. Brill teamed up with Kenneth Howard, PhD, from Northwestern University, a well-known researcher in the field of psychotherapy outcomes. The result has been a set of tools that assess phases of clinical change and the improvement achieved over varying "dosages" of psychotherapy. By collecting thousands of questionnaires, Compass has been able to create risk-adjusted norms for the progress of patients, enabling clinicians to assess the fruits of their efforts.

Dr. Brill kindly spent an hour with Brett Steenbarger talking about the history of Compass and how outcome assessment might be valuable to collaborative group practices.

STEENBARGER: Maybe you could give me a little historical background on how Compass came to be and how you've evolved to the present point.

BRILL: The way I got into it, it's kind of a funny story. My father's a psychiatrist and when I got out of my psychiatric residency, I was headed off to Wharton. I said to my father, "You know, after all this study, I feel like the kid who wakes up on Christmas morning and there's a pile of manure lying on the floor. He comes down and starts digging through the pile of manure and the father says to him, 'What are you doing?' And he says, 'With all this shit, there must be a pony in here somewhere!'" (*Laughs.*)

I came through psychiatry, 1969 through 1972, when we were still at the point where . . . if they were getting better, they really were getting worse, because it was a "transference cure." And if they got worse, they're really getting better because they were immersed in their problems! We had few active medicines at that point and it was pretty confusing to me at times whether you're dealing with a healthy person in an abnormal environment or vice versa. All of that . . . led me into

(cont.)

READER'S RESOURCE 5.2 (cont.)

looking at the person–environment as the issue, but not necessarily assuming the reasonable, expectable environment that we had been taught. . . .

I became very interested in environments and went off and studied organizations—that's how I ended up at Wharton—and went off and studied marriage and families. . . . The problem when you get to that level of analysis is that you never know whether anything is getting better or worse and you never know what level your intervention should have.

That led me to a natural desire to understand outcome. It went way, way back. Later, I got involved in starting a managed care company. . . . As I started to enter the managed care business, my biggest concern was that it was too easy to just say no and that there really was no rational basis for allocating care.

STEENBARGER: Right!

BRILL: . . . We are so much in our infancy as a field. You see, I think we're about where general medicine was in 1910. 1900 was the point at which we had a greater probability of being helped by going to a physician than harmed. We're just past that crossover point. We have about 200 different models of therapy, and we are not able to separate one from the other on any empirical basis. We have a few active medicines . . . but most of the research, you can't differentiate any treatment for anybody. Everything seems to work a little bit and everything seems to get 60–70% better.

[Dr. Brill takes a strong position, but we are inclined to agree. We have reviewed practice guidelines from a variety of sources that attempt to synthesize the current level of research understandings and have found that few practices actually make use of such guidelines.]

When you come down to where you're starting to allocate care to people and you're influencing or choosing providers based on how they're doing, you begin to worry, "Do you have any idea what's going on?" . . . So what you do is enroll a bunch of people on some criteria and then . . . profile people you refer to basically on the number of sessions that they use on the average. Well that's pure cost; there's not a bit of quality in that! If you give out five sessions to patients and I give out six, the presumption is you're doing a better job and they'll refer more cases to you. Well that's nonsense. There's no quality in that at all.

When I got into that business, I was very reluctant to do any kind of case management until I could find a method that I felt at least was

(cont.)

reasonably accurate as a way to determine whether somebody was getting better or not. That's how Compass was born. . . . Compass takes advantage of dose–response and phase theory to take you through the treatment process.

["Dose–response" refers to the work pioneered by Ken Howard, in which curves were drawn to describe the trajectories of improvement of different patient populations over time, thus describing the "effect" of a given "dose" of therapy. Phase theory refers to Dr. Howard's idea that therapeutic change proceeds in three distinct phases: (1) an increase in well-being and hope, (2) a reduction of presenting symptomatology, and (3) an improvement in life functioning. Tools used to assess dose–effect can be used to track clients' progress through these phases to see whether expected changes are truly occurring, to see whether therapists and practices are effective in their work, and so on.]

STEENBARGER: The idea of process modeling is what I see you doing.

BRILL: Absolutely, absolutely. . . . It turns out you can use the first phase, the improvement in subjective well-being, the restoration of hope, to tell you if you're on the right track. So as early as two to four sessions, you can by and large tell whether treatment is heading in the wrong direction. Also, because of the phase interlocking, you can develop actual algorithms to connect the three of them together into a single number . . . so we're able to track whether a person is getting better or worse. The power of that is incredible. For example, if you have a person coming in and they start at a given level and they get worse for the first step to the second step. . . . Let's say they came into the first session at 50% [the 50th percentile with respect to their comparison group]; then they were at 40% at the fourth session and they were at 20% at the eighth session. What percentage will ever get back to 50%, much less get better? Do you know what the answer is?

STEENBARGER: No.

BRILL: Zero.

STEENBARGER: That's amazing.

BRILL: So it looks like an uncorrected course of treatment . . . is a process that doesn't reverse itself. . . . The theory we used to have about that is that people have to get worse to get better. We don't see any evidence of that.

STEENBARGER: That's powerful. My understanding—again in a process modeling vein—is that you can norm that according to various patient and other variables and risk-adjust the norms so that one group of patients may show a certain improvement and that would have one meaning,

(cont.)

READER'S RESOURCE 5.2 (*cont.*)

but another group of patients with a different profile may show the same improvement but with a very different meaning.

BRILL: Well, this is the dialogue I had with Ken [Howard] . . . What I wanted to do was, to use your words "model" or what I call "predict" [negative outcomes] from the moment they walked in the door. Now, why would I want to do that? It's pretty obvious. Why do you use a Pap smear? You use a Pap smear because, if you can grab an illness or decaying process early in its cycle, oftentimes you can cheaply—cheap in both the financial and the human sense—change the direction of the process and correct it. Whereas if you wait longer, you end up with end-stage cancer! I think that's very much what goes on in mental health. I think after a person deteriorates to a certain point, it's irreversible. So I wanted to predict the course of someone's treatment and the path of their care from the day they walked in.

    We are able to find about 20% of people that look to be non-talking therapy responders. From the day they walk in, you could plot their curve. You could put them in talking therapy and they'll stay the same or get worse.

STEENBARGER: Hmmm!

BRILL: So now we're back to the issue of, Can we array dose–response curves from the day they walk in by treatment modality? Medication *A*, medication *B*, group, family, individual therapy? That would then help determine which kinds of treatment you might want to try first.

STEENBARGER: Very interesting. . . . You could base your whole triage system on that.

BRILL: Going back to your group practices, if they set this thing up right, it's very, very possible to do several things. Just by using Compass by itself and not using the provider profiling and the rest of it, they'll discover that about 17% of the people that come in for treatment don't need treatment . . . because they're perfectly well from the moment they walk in. . . . We've done a study: There's no difference in the average number of sessions that a clinic will give to people in the normal range versus people in the 50th percentile or say in the 20th percentile. Because they don't differentiate; they weren't taught to think that way. . . . Those 17% that come in perfectly normal don't need treatment. . . . They tend to get worse on average by being put into treatment.

    The second way you save money is because 30% of cases will not get better without some change in treatment. . . . You can pick them up very quickly and by changing treatment, you can get a lot of them bet-

(*cont.*)

ter, which does one of two things: It greatly shortens the total number of sessions or, if you're one of those places that gives a limited number of sessions to everybody, it increases your quality for the same number of sessions. One of two ways your quality per cost ratio will go way up.

[As an increasing number of practices move toward financial risk sharing with insurers, they will gain an economic interest in monitoring the care that is delivered and making sure that it is achieving its desired ends].

Now you can also go to matching people with providers. Also go to studying those people in your system who, for some reason, are very good with one kind of case and learn from each other. So all of those are ways that Compass immediately could help people who are setting these practices up.

STEENBARGER: One of the themes we have in the book . . . is the multispecialty collaboration as a "learning organization". . . . This strikes me as a mechanism for the learning in the learning organization.

BRILL: Because it gets you out of ideology. The biggest problem I used to have, we'd sit in a group of people [in a case conference], we'd sit and express our thoughts and feelings about the person. Sometimes we'd come to consensus, sometimes we'd have diversity. But the problem was, it was like if you put us back as primitive man and an earthquake happened and we sat around talking about our feelings about what's causing the earthquake without any knowledge of geology!

STEENBARGER: Which of the gods was angered . . .

BRILL: Exactly! (*Laughs.*)

STEENBARGER: . . . and which ones you have to appease . . .

BRILL: See, I think if you use course [of treatment], that's the absolute. Do they get better? That's probably the only absolute we have. . . . That's the only tool we're going to have to slowly go about sorting out fact from fiction.

[Obtaining measures at multiple points in time and examining rates of change—not just pre–post outcomes—allows for a much more sensitive appraisal of quality and helps route clients to treatments that will work efficiently, as well as effectively.]

READER'S RESOURCE 5.3
Capitation Crash Course

Even in this day of highly managed care, most contracts with individual providers and provider groups are on a fee-for-service (FFS) basis. That is, they guarantee the clinician or group a fixed reimbursement for a given behavioral service.

At-risk contracts, on the other hand, make some or all of the provider's reimbursement contingent upon (usually cost-effective) performance. In a *withhold* contract, for example, the insurer may hold back 15% of the traditional fee and return it to the group only if certain efficiency targets are met. A *case rate* goes even further in the risk direction by giving the group a lump-sum reimbursement for each case referred. *Capitation* extends risk contracting to an entire population, as the group is given a per-member per-month (PMPM) fee to manage the behavioral health needs of a defined number of covered lives.

At-risk contracting is attractive to insurers because it places the group practice in a situation in which it is rewarded for cost-efficiency, not for the delivery of increasing service. (This same dynamic makes risk contracting risky because it provides unscrupulous groups with an incentive to deny care.) It would not at all surprise us if we see an increase in risk contracting over the next five years, with bonuses or other incentives tied to the achievement of quality criteria. This would help to address potential abuses of prepaid health care.

It is typical for MCOs to place capitation and other at-risk contracts out to bid, requiring groups to compete for the business. For a group practice to bid for such business, it must be able to calculate its average cost per treatment episode, as well as the demographic and utilization patterns of the covered population, to ensure that it can provide the promised services and still make a profit. It must then be able to monitor the services delivered under the contract *as they are occurring* to guarantee that services are being rendered appropriately and cost-effectively. This means that the MIS under risk contracting must be more extensive than that under FFS.

Here is a simple exercise that illustrates the point. Imagine that your group has just won a contract that will pay a capitation rate of $2 PMPM for all outpatient behavioral health services. The contract covers 5,000 employees working at a local factory and their dependents: a total population of 10,000. This means that every month the group practice will receive $20,000 to cover the population's outpatient needs.

Now let us establish some parameters:

(cont.)

- We will assume that your group needs to retain 10–15% of the contract amount as profit to reward the practice owners, replace aged equipment, finance expansion, and so on. This means that $17,000–$18,000 per month or $204,000–$216,000 for the year will be available to cover the population's needs.
- We will assume that master's-degree clinicians will receive $60/hour for their services, doctoral clinicians will receive $70/hour, and MDs will receive $100/hour.
- We will assume that 50% of referrals will go to master's-degree clinicians, 30% to doctoral clinicians, and 20% to psychiatrists.
- We will assume that the master's and doctoral clinicians average six sessions of therapy per treatment episode per patient. We will assume that psychiatrists average one full-hour evaluation and five full-hour combined therapy/ med management visits (6 total hours) per case.
- We will assume that 5% of the population accesses outpatient behavioral health services during the year.

Based on these parameters, we can conclude:

- 500 patients under the contract will access services. Of these, 250 will see a master's-degree clinician for six sessions at $60 per session for a total of $90,000, 150 will see a doctoral clinician for six sessions at $70 per session for a total of $63,000, 100 will see a psychiatrist for six hours at $100 per hour for a total of $60,000.
- This makes direct treatment costs $213,000 for the year, leaving the group with $27,000 in profit, a roughly 11% margin.
- Given the higher rate of reimbursement for doctoral and psychiatric professionals, the group practice has a built-in incentive to refer as many cases as possible to master's clinicians. An equal referral flow to all professionals would wipe out the profit margin.
- If the utilization of the population is 6% instead of 5%, the practice would either have to (1) reduce the average number of sessions per client from six to roughly five or (2) reduce the reimbursement rates of the clinicians by roughly $10 an hour.

Three important conclusions follow from this exercise:

1. **When contracting at-risk, it is vital that your MIS be able to track utilization as it occurs.** If a few clinicians are averaging 10 sessions per client rather than 6, you need to know that immediately or all profit from the contract will be consumed. Similarly, if a few

(cont.)

READER'S RESOURCE 5.3 (*cont.*)

clinicians are practicing quite efficiently, you will want to refer more cases to them.

2. **When contracting at risk, it is vital that you be aware of the utilization patterns of the population being covered.** A relatively modest increase in the percentage of the population utilizing services can be enough to wipe out profits—and then some. If the population has a higher than usual proportion of females, children, or lower-socioeconomic-status individuals, this can translate into rates of utilization that may be much higher than the group's norms. It is thus common to obtain specialty consultation when preparing bids on capitation contracts and to seek "stop-loss" insurance as part of those contracts to place a cap on losses that would stem from unanticipated high utilization.

3. **When contracting at risk, it is vital that you and the insurer are clear on the nature of the services to be covered.** In our example, the capitation rate was $2 PMPM for outpatient services. Does this include outpatient chemical dependency detoxification programs? Does it include services that are accessed outside the group's geographic coverage area, such as when clients are away at college? Does it include the cost of behavioral consultations given to covered individuals while they are in medical treatment? Such gray areas must be addressed during the contracting process or the group may be left with unanticipated expenses and dwindling profits.

CHAPTER SIX

Designing Collaborative Clinical Services

with Albert Villapiano and Stephen Butler

Acts have power, especially when the person acting knows that those acts are his last battle. There is a strange consuming happiness in acting with the full knowledge that whatever one is doing may very well be one's last act on earth. I recommend that you reconsider your life and bring your acts into that light.

—don Juan to Carlos Castaneda, *Journey to Ixtlan*

INTRODUCTION

The central purpose of most behavioral practices is the provision of high-quality clinical services to those with social, emotional, and behavioral problems. As we saw in Chapter 1, this requires the multispecialty integration of a wide range of services. The trend toward collaboration is an acknowledgment that services are most effectively provided when they are coordinated in a thoughtful manner.

What is the glue holding together this coordinated effort? In this chapter, we present an overarching conceptual framework for services delivered through collaborative practices. The model is integrative and makes use of ideas drawn from many rich theoretical and research traditions. We also describe the range of ser-

☆ IN THIS CHAPTER

- Presenting a time-effective framework for the delivery of clinical services
- Defining a service menu for the group practice
- Creating linkages among clinical services for cost effectiveness *and* quality
- Assessing the quality of your clinical work

vices that can be offered at a behavioral practice and how they may be seamlessly interwoven. Most of all, we help you make an important shift in your thinking, from fragmented services to integrated, programmatic, team-based care.

THE TIME-EFFECTIVE TREATMENT MODEL

For your practice to offer and deliver a coherent set of services, there must be an overall, unifying clinical perspective that permeates the system and guides clinical decisions and program development. It is crucial that this perspective not become a straitjacket that constrains practice but one that can flexibly draw on the diverse strengths of multiple disciplinary and theoretical traditions in mental health. The core model that we employ is the "time-effective" view of behavioral treatment. This model is an integrative approach that embraces certain values on the part of the clinician and the system and an overall perspective about how treatment is carried out (Budman & Gurman, 1988).

Time-effective treatment is oriented toward efficiency *and* effectiveness but is *not* always brief or short term. Rather, time-effective work seeks to maximize effectiveness in an efficient manner. Although managed behavioral health care has been most often associated with "brief therapy," there are numerous problems with this term. These problems include the fact that much outpatient clinical work is already considerably *briefer* than the treatment advocated by many short-term therapy experts. For example, whereas the average length of therapy across various outpatient settings is approximately four to eight visits (Garfield, 1994; Phillips, 1992), Strupp and Binder (1984) and Davanloo (1980) advocate "short-term" therapies of 25 sessions and more. Even the cognitive behavior therapy approach of Beck and his colleagues (Beck, Rush, Shaw, & Emery, 1979) commonly extends to 15 or more visits.

Although it has been assumed that brief treatment is 20 sessions or less (Koss & Shiang, 1994), this definition runs into problems if one assumes that these 20 visits can be divided and applied over differing periods. For example, if one took 20 visits and "cut them in half," one would have 40 half-sessions. Would this still be brief treatment? What if you then took these 40 sessions and allocated them over a 2-year period? Still brief? It is our view that one cannot easily define time-effectiveness by a particular number of visits.

One final complexity in defining brief work is that the course of treatment for most people is much different from that described by textbooks and managed care guidelines. (For a review of factors mediating duration and outcome in psychotherapy, see Steenbarger, 1994.) That is, most people who enter a course of treatment—be it very long or very short—return for additional treatment at a later point (Cummings & Sayama, 1995). Indeed, more than 50% of those seen in an episode of treatment are likely to again seek professional help within 1 to 2 years of "termination" (e.g., Kovacs, Rush, Beck, & Hollon, 1981). Thus, simply to encourage brevity says little about what one is actually advocating.

Although much of the original work on time-effective treatment related to outpatient psychotherapy for a relatively healthy population, recent work has focused on populations with more severe presenting problems (Budman et al., 1996). It is our belief that this model is applicable to any type of behavioral intervention, including psychopharmacological treatments. Rather than referring to a particular therapeutic approach, the model is an overarching way of viewing the intervention process and attitudes about this process.

Drawing upon Cummings's (1977) discussion of "ideal" versus "realistic" views of treatment, Budman and Gurman (1988) coined the term "time-effective" because it more clearly describes a way of practicing that is useful and realistic in the world of accountable health care. It also does not make the rigid and impractical assumptions that seem to us to plague familiar "brief" therapy models. We see time-effective treatment as a set of attitudes present for the therapist, patient, and clinical setting that draw on research and an understanding of "best practices" in behavioral treatment. The clinician must assume some important attitudes.

Think with a Beginner's Mind—Think with Flexibility

Shunryu Suzuki, a Japanese Zen master who emigrated to the United States and taught in San Francisco until his death in the early 1970s, stated: "In the beginner's mind there are many possibilities, but in the expert's there are few" (1970, p. 21). Working time-effectively may require that the clinician think with a beginner's mind about his or her interactions with patients. Rather than assuming a perspective that is closed to new possibilities (and locked-in to particular "truths" about intervention), the therapist is encouraged to approach his or her clients in a flexible, open manner that allows for a variety of hopeful possibilities for change and improvement. What also follows from this beginner's-mind perspective is that integration of methods and approaches is encouraged. Adherents of particular approaches to psychotherapy can become rigidly locked in to their points of view and are sometimes antagonistic toward other schools of treatment. In our view, many developments in the areas of psychotherapy, substance abuse treatment, and psychopharmacology can be readily and thoughtfully integrated into an amalgam that is far more powerful, resilient, and efficient than the "pure gold" of the individual approaches considered in isolation.

Parsimony and Small Changes Are More Important Than "Cure"

If one can use a parsimonious, "minimalist" intervention to achieve even a small change, this may have major implications for the individual, couple, or family. This is due to a process described by chaos theory experts—chaologists—as feedback (Briggs & Peat, 1989). Such feedback processes in nature are self-amplifying, leading to large changes. It is also highly unlikely in our view that most psychological disorders—at least those that do not just involve very specific and discrete systems, such as a simple phobia—can be "cured" (i.e., eradicated permanently). We know for example, that depression tends to have a repetitive course and that even following an episode of treatment with excellent outcome there is a tendency toward relapse if some type of maintenance intervention is not provided (Frank, 1991). Also therapy is not, for the most part, prophylactic and will not ensure a happy trouble-free life forever after. In trying to achieve such prophylaxis, the therapist may search for "therapeutic perfectionism" (Malan, 1976) and, in this search, unnecessarily lengthen treatment. From our perspective, **the only thing that cures life is death**. (With an interest by some in "past lives therapy," even this is no longer true.)

Viewing Patients from a Lifespan Developmental Perspective Is Encouraged

This perspective assumes that people are already in the process of change when they come to see us. Adults continue to change throughout the life cycle and are not seen as lacking an internal momentum toward improvement (Gilligan, 1982; Vaillant, 1977). Because we are all continually changing, there is an increased possibility for patients to move forward and improve their lives. Stone (1992) reviewed several longitudinal studies that followed the life courses of patients diagnosed with severe borderline personality disorder. (Most of the patients had entered these studies as inpatients.) He found that two-thirds of the patients, after an interval of 10–25 years, were doing "fair" to "well." This was the case regardless of the types of treatments they had over this period. These improvements occurred even for those patients who had the most severe pathology and debilitating impairments when they entered the study. For some patients, the central treatment issue may be how to keep the patient alive until developmental processes can take over.

Patient Strengths and Resources Are Emphasized

In the past, many treatment models were strongly oriented toward patient pathology. With advances in solution-oriented treatments (e.g., de Shazer, 1985) and cognitive behavioral approaches (e.g., Beck et al., 1979), client strengths are becoming more central to our views of helping. Therapy thus becomes an identification and cultivation of existing assets, not simply the remedial treatment of deficits. Work by Ricks (1974) underlines the importance of a strength and resource-based approach. Ricks compared the process notes of two doctoral-level child clinicians, one of whom had excellent outcomes with the very disturbed adolescents when he treated (Ricks called him Supershrink) and another whose outcomes were uniformly poor working at the same clinic with a similar population of adolescents (whom we will call Pseudoshrink). Ricks found that Super-shrink tended to have an optimistic and hopeful, strength-oriented approach to therapy despite the difficulties of his patients. Pseudoshrink, on the other hand, was most often negativistic, hopeless, and despaired about the future for the patients he saw. For example, a quote from Pseudoshrink's notes about one patient read: "I tell him my impression is that his spirit has been broken. . . . At the present time it is certainly impossible to get him interested in any occupation and there doesn't seem to be anything else to do but have him come in for psychotherapy. . . ." (Ricks, 1974, p. 282).

The patient then fails to come to the next two sessions. When he returns, Pseudoshrink notes: "He is still very depressed and hardly said anything to me at all. The case certainly has an ominous aspect" (p. 282).

After this session, the patient (fortunately) stopped coming. It is not difficult to predict the outcome of therapy that goes on with such a hopeless and dismal tone.

Encourage Changes between Sessions

There are many more hours between therapy sessions than within sessions. The therapist needs to find ways to help the patient "carry" the therapy/therapist outside sessions with him or her. A posthypnotic suggestion that was frequently used by Milton Erickson was, "My voice will go with you." It is an important task of the time-effective therapist to have his or her voice go with the patient. Homework assignments and between-session tasks are very important elements of time-effective treatment and allow the work to continue outside the consultation room.

Change Is *Not* a Linear Process

If you put popcorn into your microwave oven and turn the microwave on, you will observe a nonlinear process. There is not a smooth flow with each kernel getting bigger and bigger before it pops. Rather, as the heat is absorbed, one kernel after another becomes sufficiently hot to suddenly explode into a full-size piece of popcorn.

Countless significant processes in nature tend not to be uniform, smooth, or linear (Briggs & Peat, 1989). Weather fronts arrive and depart in seemingly unpredictable ways; earthquakes strike with little or no warning. A peaceful snow-covered mountain valley may suddenly become the scene of an avalanche. Although patient change processes in psychotherapy are often discussed as if they were gradual and linear, this is rarely the case. Often, extended periods occur for the patient during which little or nothing appears to be happening (on the surface). Then, suddenly, "something clicks" and the patient is able to do things, act, and think in ways that he or she could not or did not do previously. We believe that change processes are cumulative and that patients take different things from different episodes of therapy. It may appear to the therapist that a particular episode of treatment was not useful or helpful to the patient. It is only years later that with additional episodes of treatment and with certain life events occurring that the patient is able make use of the earlier information.

Gunderson et al. (1989), studying a group of hospitalized patients with diagnoses of borderline personality, tracked these patients over an extended course of follow-up outpatient treatment. The single best predictor of a patient sticking with the index course of outpatient therapy was the number of previous episodes of therapy and the number of different therapists the patient had seen. Thus, the patients who stayed with the index episode of treatment were more likely to have had other prior treatment that they had dropped out of. Seemingly, though the patients might not have seen the value in these previous abbreviated therapies, he or she might have cumulatively and covertly learned and gained something from these encounters. When this latent learning reached a critical mass, the patients could continue in treatment and, it is hoped, make some positive changes.

Financial and Resource Allocation Issues Are Critically Important in Time-Effective Therapy

For the most part, clinicians tend *not* to operate in time-effective ways by choice (at least initially). To do so requires a high degree of thoughtful organization and planning. For a group practice, moving clinicians in a time-sensitive direction may engender conflict and incur training and reorganization costs (Budman & Armstrong, 1992). For some organizations, the move toward time-effective mental health care is related to cutbacks in resources, large waiting lists, and/or attempts by an organization to be "managed care friendly" and thus receive more business from managed mental health companies.

The movement toward risk contracting is requiring clinicians to actively factor cost into their treatment planning decisions. Even practitioners operating outside managed care systems find themselves needing to be cost-effective, as they market themselves to a price-sensitive, cash-paying clientele. We believe that concerns over cost and quality can best be addressed by avoiding "one-size-fits-all" treatment planning (i.e., X number of sessions per patient) and relying on a sophisticated clinical MIS to identify the unique needs of each client and guide the flexible, judicious allocation of time in treatment. This allows a meaningful number of clients to be seen briefly while preserving resources for patients who need a "higher dosage" of therapy (Steenbarger, 1994).

Patient Readiness for Change: The Prochaska and DiClemente Change Process Model

In our view, one of the most important developments in applied psychology with major implications for time-effective treatment is the work of Prochaska and his colleagues (Prochaska, Norcross, & DiClemente, 1994) at the University of Rhode Island. Prochaska and his team, working with smokers, developed a model of how people change, with or without professional intervention. The stages-of-change model appears to have applicability across all varieties of change, such as losing weight (O'Connell & Velicer, 1988) and going for a mammogram (Rakowski, Dube, & Goldstein, 1996) (see Figure 6.1).

The stages-of-change model identifies five levels of readiness to engage in life changes. *Precontemplation* is a level prior to the recognition of any problem. The most common example would be clients in denial of their addictions. When the client in precontemplation appears in treatment, it is often because someone else has initiated the request for change: a spouse, parent, or representative of the judicial system.

The next step on the route to change is the phase of *contemplation*. This stage of change is characterized by ambivalence and uncertainty about whether the individual wishes to make the particular change being addressed. For example, the woman who is a substance abuser in a state of contemplation is beginning to see that drugs are having a destructive effect in her life, though there are also many issues pressing her to keep using drugs. Often, clients in contemplation are dealing with an approach–avoidance conflict, caught between the pros and cons of

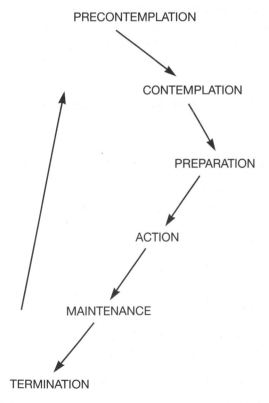

FIGURE 6.1. Prochaska and DiClemente stages-of-change model.

making a commitment to change. As a result, they are usually highly ambivalent about change and may remain so for very extended periods.

In the *preparation* stage the potential changer has not yet acted but is preparing to do so. The individual has somewhat resolved the ambivalence around making the change but has not yet taken the step of acting in a way that will facilitate the process directly.

Action is characterized by the person vigorously moving toward taking change steps, with obvious interest in modifying his or her behavior. The changer is clear about his or her desired direction and has probably tried to achieve that goal. These attempts may or may not be immediately successful. At this phase, however, the client has a clearly identified problem, goal for change, and motivation to begin work.

During *maintenance* the person attempts to hold on to his or her gains. This is often done in a very effortful way. Thus, the nondrinking alcoholic may feel great temptation in many circumstances in which he or she would have drank previously (at parties, to relax, etc.). Maintenance may continue for very extended periods, as in the case of recovering persons who attend Alcoholics Anonymous on a lifelong basis.

There are two very important implications of the stages-of-change model:

1. **Change is a nonlinear process in which periods of high motivation and significant process are interwoven with periods of doubt and relapse.** Rarely is it the case that one enters treatment and makes a change once and for all time. Relapse is not necessarily a treatment failure and may be central to the change process (see Table 6.1).

2. **The approaches that are most likely to be helpful for patients may be a function of their readiness for change.** Clients in precontemplation

TABLE 6.1. Stages of Change and Therapist Tasks (Prochaska et al., 1994)

Stage of change	Therapist task
Precontemplation	Raise doubts: Increase the patient's perceptions of the risks and problems with the current behavior. Educative interventions may be useful here. Emphasize pros.
Contemplation	Tip the balance: Weigh reasons to change and reasons not to change. Look at small steps that have been taken toward change already and what has allowed these to work. Paradox may be useful here. Look at cons.
Preparation	Help the patient think about the ways that he or she can now move toward taking steps to change.
Action	Help the patient look at change strategies that he or she might use.
Maintenance	Help the patient maintain change and prevent relapse.

may require psychoeducational input from the clinician to help them come to some realization and recognition about their problem and why change might be useful. Those in contemplation may need insight-oriented work to help them explore the pros and cons of attempting to change. Those in an action mode might be ready to jump right into solution-focused and/or cognitive-behavioral modalities. The time-effective therapist factors such differences into treatment planning.

In sum, the time-effective model of treatment is a framework for identifying the unique needs of patients, defining the helping approaches most likely to be helpful for those needs, and allocating resources based on those assessments. Rather than focus on quality at the expense of cost or cost at the expense of quality, it is an effort to deliver *value* to consumers: the highest quality of care at the most reasonable cost.

☞ LOOKING AHEAD

If you are practicing in a cost-competitive market under risk contracts, how can you best determine needs for shorter and longer-term treatment?

Our DISCUS model at the end of this chapter (Reader's Resource 6.1) may help you become more time-effective!

THE CONTINUUM OF CLINICAL SERVICES

The integrated delivery system (IDS), in which a single provider organization offers a full array of services, is an unrealized vision in most parts of the United States. The services offered by such a system are (1) integrated across levels of care (from inpatient or partial hospital to intensive outpatient and ultimately to standard outpatient), (2) multidisciplinary, and (3) capable of servicing a wide variety of presenting problems (mental health, chemical dependency, child and family, geriatric, etc.). Given the potential of integrated systems to more firmly control cost and quality, it is likely that collaborative practices over the next decade will expand their scope and move toward this vision.

The IDS

Table 6.2 provides a lengthy description of the services offered by an integrated system. Most practices will not have each and every service available. The table, however, offers a menu from which groups, networks, and integrated systems can choose in developing programs.

TABLE 6.2. Continuum of Care: A Comprehensive Array of Services

Triage/assessment	Outpatient	Intensive outpatient	Partial hospital day treatment	Residential	Hospital
• Single point of entry into the delivery system	• Least intensive service with client contact typically less than 2 times per week	• Intensive IOP meeting more than 2 times per week	• Most intensive outpatient service, meeting more than 2 times per week and more than 3 hours per day	• Residential care with staff supervision	• Residential care with 24-hour medical supervision
• Rapid assessment and referral to level of services required	• Traditional individual, group, couples, and family counseling	• Psychoeducation, group-based programs often with a psychosocial and rehabilitation focus	• Psychoeducation, group-based programs often with a psychosocial and rehabilitation focus	• Usually no treatment program as residents often work or access other treatment programs	• Primarily accessed to stabilize a crisis or medically complicated situation
• Often has mobile capabilities	• Offers psychopharmacology services and medicine clinics	• May include community or in-home services such as visiting psychiatric nurses		• Often a "step-down" from inpatient level of care	• Some psychoeducation, group-based programs often with a psychosocial and rehabilitation focus
• Has access to in-home psychiatric services, especially for children and those who are seriously mentally ill	• Able to provide high-frequency outpatient services to avert the need for more intensive services			• Support stabilization and recovery when a client's home cannot	• Patients often "step down" in less than 1 week to ambulatory levels of care
• Often the location of a 24-hour emergency capacity	• Often offers school and community consultation				
• Maintains up-to-date knowledge of and access to treatment and community resources	• May include preventive interventions such as community education				

Case management and specialized case management: In larger systems and especially those that manage clients with severe and persistent mental illness, it is very important that case management be included. Case managers follow patients in their tenure through the system regardless of level of care at which the patient is being treated at a given time. In this way they represent the "glue" that keeps the patient's care integrated and unified. Without case management, more difficult patients will "fall between the cracks" at the various boundaries of the system.

The following four characteristics cut across the continua of care found in integrated practices:

1. Rapid assessment, triage, and referral of patients to the level of care best matching their needs and acuity.

2. Treatment and intervention resources at varied levels of intensity.

3. Efficient movement of patients within the system in response to their individualized treatment plan needs, with the objective of providing the necessary services at the *least intensive* and *least costly* level of care.

4. Case management (patient care coordination) functions which monitor utilization of services, treatment compliance, and linkages to community resources.

How far does your practice need to go to actualize this continuum? That depends in large part on the needs and demands of payers and referral sources in your region. In highly managed environments, such as major urban centers on the coasts, a practice should be prepared to offer a broad outpatient continuum with strategic linkages to programs and facilities. Less managed settings may simply require a commitment to cover and coordinate basic psychiatric and psychotherapeutic services, with linkages to substance abuse providers. In most settings, however, collaborative efforts should be prepared to offer the following:

- **Multidisciplinary/multispecialty/multimodal care.** It is especially important to link psychiatric and psychotherapeutic services and provide a range of individual, family, and group services for clients.

- **Prompt intensive outpatient care.** Part of the commitment that practices make to cost containment is to keep patients out of the hospital wherever possible, by intervening early and often at the outpatient level.

- **Dedicated clinical management.** Practices are expected to have medical or clinical directors who oversee services and ensure that the proper care is delivered in a timely fashion to all clients.

Note that a practice can offer all these features without having to offer them by themselves. Collaborations occur among practices as well as within them and can form the backbone of fledgling integrated systems. Thus, Practice A might specialize in child and family therapy, Practice B in adult work, and Practice C in chemical dependency programming. The three may form an alliance to coordinate and market their services, with representatives from each organization participating as members of an overarching team. Such integration can also occur through alliances of facilities and outpatient groups. It is our experience that collaboration first takes root within the group or network, then expands to embrace other practices.

The Collaborative Management of Clinical Practice

Organizations that make the transition to clinical integration become *process-oriented* and *program-oriented.* They look not only at the services provided but at the manner in which these services are programmatically linked and the ways in which clients can move among the services. The opposite of an integrated practice is a collection of practitioners, each offering care in their own way. Collaboratively managed practice, as we saw in the last chapter, is team-based and program-centered.

Let us explore the ramifications of collaborative management for the design and delivery of clinical services. Figure 6.2 describes a matrix of programmatic services. A program is defined for each major set of presenting concerns, with membership consisting of professionals from the major specialty areas of practice. Within each program are several defined levels of care, each corresponding to a particular acuity of patient need. Thus, for example, levels may be set for maintenance, routine, urgent, and intensive care (see below). Practice guidelines defined by each team determine when clients are assigned to a given care level and when they move between levels. Each clinical team embodies the elements of Jamieson's (1996) model (see Chapter 5), with an overall strategy for delivering cost-effective, high-quality services. Information flows into the team to assist with decisions regarding delivery of services at specific care

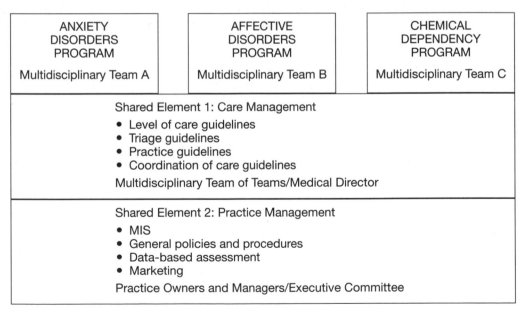

FIGURE 6.2. The programmatic organization of collaborative clinical services. Distinct multidisciplinary clinical programs are linked by shared clinical and management elements.

levels; it flows back to the team to aid ongoing treatment planning and quality assessment.

Note, however, that there must be collaborations among programs as well as within. A client with complex Axis II concerns may require a unique, coordinated set of interventions addressing overwhelming anxiety, depression, family conflict, and substance abuse. At such points, members from each relevant team can be deployed to coordinate efforts and define an integrated treatment plan that draws on components from each of the programs. The client thus might participate in psychoeducational and treatment groups for substance abuse, anxiety management groups addressing posttraumatic stress disorder symptoms, cognitive therapy and medication management for the treatment of depression, and intermittent family therapy. These might be packaged as a modular set of time-effective interventions with multiple professionals rather than a time-unlimited therapy with a single provider.

Anchoring all the treatment programs is an overarching "team of teams" led by the clinical/medical director of the practice. Such coordination is necessary if each program is to collect comparable information, link to a single triage point, and present itself in a unified way to referral sources. The coordination also assists with the reconciliation of overall practice goals and specific programmatic objectives. For instance, if the practice as a whole sets a strategic objective of a 20% annual increase in managed care referrals, each program can formulate substrategies for increasing its enrollment and managing the expanded patient flow. Similarly, if the practice decides to move into a managed Medicaid market, each program may need to augment its clinical services, perhaps by defining additional levels of care and review mechanisms.

This discussion should make clear the supreme importance of communication systems within collaborative practices. True collaboration requires an ongoing stream of communications within treatment teams, among teams, and between teams and practice leadership. If each of these communications requires face-to-face meetings, there will be little time for the provision of clinical services. Voice and electronic mail systems, workgroup software, and the judicious use of fax modems and scanners can greatly speed communication flows and deliver timely data for decision support. **There can be no time-effective clinical services without time-effective management**.

☞ LOOKING AHEAD

How are communications technologies helping to shape clinical services?

Check out our interview with Michael Hurst, PhD, president and CEO of Instream, Inc., at the end of this chapter (Reader's Resource 6.2).

THE ORGANIZATION OF CLINICAL SERVICES

Once again, we can think of the collaborative practice as an integrated system consisting of interwoven subsystems. The subsystem components represent (1) programs of treatment for particular populations and/or disorders and (2) organizations of treatment programs into various levels of intensity. The goal is to facilitate the client's movement through various stages of change by identifying and addressing needs at each phase. The collaborative practice is thus highly process oriented, relying on real-time data to continually monitor and shape treatment outcomes and plans.

Defining the Site of Collaboration

As practices move further along Chapter 1's Collaborative Cube (see Figure 1.1), the sites of collaboration and the team of collaborators change radically. In a small practice, collaboration may mean creating closer linkages between psychiatrists and nonmedical therapists to better coordinate treatment planning. In larger systems, there may be an awareness that a sizable percentage of primary care visits are for nonmedical, emotional problems, requiring tight collaboration between primary care providers and mental health professionals in an overarching biopsychosocial model of care (Doherty, McDaniel, & Baird, 1996). At a broader level still, we are beginning to see closer integration of behavioral services and social services programs for special-needs populations receiving care within the public sector (Egnew, Geary, & Wilson, 1996). Given that there is a significant overlap between high utilization of medical services and the presence of diagnosable psychosocial problems (Katon et al., 1990), we are confident that the days of dividing the person into organ systems and compartmentalizing his or her treatment are numbered. Increasingly, we will see interdisciplinary sites of collaboration that embrace medical and social services—not just mental health treatment.

This has important implications for group practices—and practitioners—seeking to implement time-effective models of care. If you are a mental health professional seeking to maximize your attractiveness to a group practice or if you are contemplating starting your own group, **one of the very best strategies for success is to identify the gaps in the health care delivery system and create collaborations to fill these.** It is *very* likely that such collaborations will create value for consumers, insurers, and community referral sources. Once you begin to view your market from a systems perspective, these gaps become clear:

- The absence of intensive outpatient services to serve as a bridge between traditional outpatient and inpatient care.

- The absence of readily available behavioral services to patients seen in primary care settings.

- The absence of intensive programs of coping and support for patients with serious medical problems, such as cancer and heart disease.

- The absence of solid behavioral medicine programs to control weight, smoking, and other health risks.

- The absence of coordinated programs of individual therapy.

- The lack of coordination among psychopharmacology services, individual and family therapy, and school programming for at-risk children and adolescents.

- The absence of integrated medical, behavioral, and social programs to address complex behavioral health needs, such as sexual abuse.

Once you have made the transition to collaboration *within* the group practice, your journey has not ended. Some of the very best opportunities in mental health lie in broader collaborations with other helping systems.

Entry into the System: Triage

Whether the site is a mental health clinic or a multidisciplinary medical setting, your delivery system will have a common set of components. The *triage component* is the "hub," or "front door," of many behavioral health care delivery systems. This part of the system must be able to rapidly respond on a 24-hour basis to emergencies and acute cases. At other times, this component determines that incoming cases can wait for care and enter the system in a more routine manner. Accomplishing these functions generally requires a 24-hour central phone line with a "live" screener. The person who answers the phone either needs to be a credentialed clinician or a well-trained receptionist/technician who can easily access a credentialed clinician (usually in 10 minutes or less). The triage clinicians are responsible for screening, assessing, making referrals, and providing information to all callers coming into the system who cannot be serviced by the technician alone. This includes:

1. Accurately assessing the acuity of presenting problems.

2. Triaging referrals to appropriate levels of care.

3. Understanding the admission and discharge criteria of each service within the practice.

4. Keeping up-to-date regarding the availability of system services and staff participation in managed plans.

5. Developing effective working relationships with key staff to facilitate the flow of referrals and smooth transmission of paperwork.

6. Developing effective working relationships with key referral resources outside of the system.

7. Developing and managing a continuous quality improvement process to track referrals.

8. Responding professionally and thoroughly to all calls and representing the system to the "outside world."

Ideally, this triage component should be able to present itself as a "one-stop shopping" resource for mental health and chemical dependency referrals. By responding rapidly, effectively, and thoroughly to all callers, this component also becomes a powerful marketing function for the entire system.

Crisis Coverage

The lion's share of MCO contracts for group practices require 24-hour crisis coverage, 7 days a week. Such coverage is necessary if the practice is to make a full commitment to keep patients out of costly inpatient settings.

There are numerous ways to structure crisis services. Generally, there will be a telephone number that is publicized to patients, referral sources, and care managers. After hours, the number may be answered by a professional answering service, which can screen nonemergent calls. Callers who are simply requesting information or a routine visit, for instance, can be told to call back when the office opens. Callers who have more urgent needs are told that a clinician will return their call within a few minutes. The on-call clinician can then be paged and the crisis intervention can begin.

A good telephonic crisis intervention consists of an assessment, provision of support and reassurance, and development of an action plan. Not infrequently, practices will follow structured guidelines in conducting crisis work. At the very minimum, the crisis clinician should obtain a brief, relevant history (useful in determining potential for acting out or suicidality), a description of current stressors and supports; an idea of current functional impairment and symptom patterns; a brief history of current and past medical and mental health utilization; and an idea of mental status and potential danger to self or others. It is extremely helpful if the crisis clinician can schedule a meeting with the client for the following morning if the call comes at night and if needs are not emergent. Many times, simply having the reassurance of an upcoming meeting is enough to calm callers and get them through the night.

Should a telephone assessment prove inconclusive, a face-to-face intervention to determine risk and capacity for functioning will be necessary. Many groups at this juncture simply refer the client to an emergency room and thus lose control over the case. This will clearly signal any insurer that the practice is halfhearted in its commitment to contain costs. If the practice can conduct the face-to-face assessment, it will find that a significant number of cases can be seen within intensive outpatient settings (see below) or triaged to 23-hour observation beds for crisis stabilization and reevaluation. Working closely with care managers on these occasions will engender considerable goodwill for the practice. It also serves as useful preparation for the time that the clinicians will themselves be at financial risk for the costs of care and will need to divert inpatient admissions wherever prudent.

Especially helpful are alliances between outpatient practices and inpatient facilities to coordinate emergencies that present at triage. These alliances can smooth the path of cross-referrals and help both organizations with communications and treatment/discharge planning. A major problem for the information-based group is the loss of data that results from referrals outside the practice. Alliances with other provider organizations can help the participating organizations coordinate data collection and assess treatment outcomes. For example, if data on symptom intensity and functional impairments are collected by both the outpatient group and the hospital, a sharing of information can enable both organizations to tailor treatment plans and track progress. This can become especially useful in discharge and treatment planning once the patient is ready to leave the inpatient setting.

Standard Outpatient Services

Standard outpatient services provide counseling, psychotherapy, psychiatric assessment and treatment, support, education, and consultation in the least intensive setting appropriate for a given level of need. Sometimes these services can be mobile and provided in alternative community settings, such as schools, churches, courts, and businesses. Preventive resources may be offered, especially through community educational initiatives. Unless there is a crisis, individual, group, couple, and family treatment is generally provided with an intensity of less than two sessions per week.

As we indicated earlier, a major threat to the delivery of high-quality services is the extreme variability in practice patterns among providers. Take panic disorder, for example. Some practitioners view psychotropic medication as the treatment of choice, with psychotherapy as a possible adjunct; others first rely on talk therapy and only look to medication if verbal treatment does not yield progress. Even within the respective groups there is great variability. Some therapists emphasize the use of cognitive-behavioral techniques, such as exposure methods, in the treatment of panic; others lean toward insight-oriented approaches. Among psychiatrists and primary care providers, there is a discrepancy between those who prescribe anti-anxiety agents for panic and those who rely on antidepressants. Which approach and treatment a given client receives becomes a matter of "luck of the draw," not a function of careful consideration and research understanding.

To address this situation, there is a growing trend toward the use of practice guidelines in treating various problems. These may be fairly loose and informal, offering general guidelines regarding criteria for psychiatric consultation and treatment, specialized referrals, and so on, or rather specific, suggesting treatments for given problems based on research findings (see Barlow, 1993). The purposes of the guidelines are severalfold:

- **Standardization of care.** Practice guidelines offer a consistent level of quality to the public.

- **Coordination of care.** Guidelines help clinicians know when to access multidisciplinary options and ensure that services are properly coordinated.

- **Benchmarking.** Guidelines can provide targets for quality improvement efforts, allowing groups to assess the degree to which their work follows accepted standards of care.

An excellent way to assess the clinical sophistication of a practice is to see its practice guidelines and triage protocols. These should cover routine outpatient services as well as less frequent circumstances that can be challenging (e.g., handling the acutely suicidal client). As we've seen, NCQA accreditation criteria require behavioral MCOs to operate under such guidelines, which means that accredited MCOs will need to contract with guideline-based groups. The absence of guidelines is a sure sign of a practice that will have difficulty remaining competitive in coming years if it hopes to garner business from major insurers.

In evaluating or designing standard outpatient services, we encourage you to be especially cognizant of the linkages between medical and nonmedical providers. The behavioral health problems that are associated with greatest cost—including major depression, eating disorders, psychosis, and the behavioral care of patients with chronic medical problems—are also those that tend to require psychiatric consultation and treatment. Often, keeping clients with such problems out of the hospital depends on rapid intervention, especially by a medical professional. Outpatient services should be structured so that there is ready access to medical/psychiatric expertise and built-in mechanisms for communication and consultation between medical and nonmedical providers. The same is true between mental health and substance abuse providers in dealing with the needs of dual-diagnosis patients. Coordinated care equals quality care.

Group Therapy Services: A Critical Component
of the Continuum

Challenges to many traditional outpatient services are accurately assessing the needs of their customers and developing efficient, time-effective interventions that adequately support the other components of the continuum of care. For many settings this involves the development of comprehensive group therapy programs to provide the support, skill development, education, and insight that previously may have been offered only in individual sessions (Steenbarger & Budman, 1996). Group treatment is perhaps the most underutilized modality in the effort to deliver extensive, high-quality, time-effective treatment across the continuum. Indeed, it is rare to find behavioral practices with ongoing group programs that are well integrated into the menu of other clinical services.

Nonetheless, we believe these programs to be critical for a variety of reasons:

1. **At every level of the continuum they support the delivery of high-quality, good-outcome care.** Research has demonstrated repeatedly that group therapy tends to have as good or better outcomes than individual treatments for a variety of presenting concerns (Steenbarger & Budman, 1996).

2. **Group therapy programs support the work of individual clinicians in the practice.** Clinicians do not need to feel that with very difficult clients they need to "do it all themselves." Clients can be referred to one of a variety of different groups which can enhance their care and take the pressure off the primary clinician.

3. **Group therapy programs dramatically illustrate themes that are central to the practice.** Therapy group programs by their nature work best when they are receiving a steady flow of referrals from different sources. They require cooperative work among clinicians and are often formed to deal with shared and difficult problems.

In our consultation work, a problem that we see repeatedly is a deemphasis of group treatment. In one very large HMO with several dozen linked behavioral group practices, the group therapy program was nearly nonexistent. Although these group practices had tens of thousands of visits and referrals each year, patients seen in the outpatient centers were nearly always seen individually. Those few groups that did exist represented groups that a given clinician found interesting and wished to run. For example, many of the clinicians on staff were in their 40s and 50s. The female therapists who did run groups had a tendency to run groups with names such as "Women and menopause," or "Women alone in their middle years." The male therapists ran such groups as, "Men at midlife." There is nothing inherently wrong with these groups. The problem was that the population of clients dealing with adjustment issues related to midlife were not the biggest concern to the HMO. These clients could often be treated relatively rapidly and successfully in any mode of treatment. There were, however, other populations that represented enormous cost and resource difficulties for the practices that were not being addressed. For example, there was no systematic program that had been developed for patients with serious personality disorders, despite clear research indications that these have value (Piper, Rosie, Joyce, & Azim, 1996).

The clinical director of a practice may have great difficulties launching and maintaining a strong group therapy program for several reasons. This is especially the case when dealing with a salaried staff. Some of the resistances to group therapy on the part of clinicians are:

- **Poor incentives for clinicians and clients to form or enter groups.** A salaried therapist may get the same amount of money working with eight difficult clients in a group or one "easier" client in an individual session. If clients' benefits are charged in the same way for group or individual treatment (i.e., "a session is a session regardless of modality"), most will choose to be seen individually (Steenbarger & Budman, 1996).

- **Inconvenience of times for group therapy.** For the most part groups must be run at times that the most people can be present. Therefore, most groups are run very early in the morning or in the evening after work. This poses scheduling difficulties for clinicians.

- **Long "downtimes" between groups.** We have seen instances in which a 12-week therapy group could only be run once or twice per year. By the time a clinician had screened all the potential clients for the group and was prepared to start the group again, holidays intervened or some members who had planned to start the group dropped out. By the time the group actually began, months had gone by.

- **Lack of skills and training in group therapy.** The majority of mental health professionals lack specific training and skills in group therapy. Administrators can push clinicians to run groups, but they cannot force them to run them well.

Fortunately, steps can be taken to address each of these issues:

- **Poor incentives for clinicians and clients to participate in groups.** Clinicians must be given incentives for running therapy groups. Exactly how this is accomplished may vary. However, clear financial incentives for running groups and for maintaining the size of groups must be built into the system. In regard to patients, behavioral health care coverage must offer them incentives to participate in therapy groups. The client needs to be charged fewer benefits for a group session than for an individual session. In a private, fee-for-service practice, group therapy usually costs between a third to a half as much as individual therapy.

- **Inconvenience of times for group therapy.** If therapists are given incentives to run groups, they will run the groups at varied hours and hours that are less convenient to the therapist and more convenient to the clients.

- **Long "downtimes" between groups.** It is our recommendation to offer many groups that are time-limited *by member* rather than end the entire group at a given point. This method would allow members to enter an ongoing group and stay for a fixed period. When this is not possible, dates should be set every 6 months for the start of particular groups. Even if relatively few members are available at the starting date of a group, the group should begin. Once this has happened several times and referring clinicians are aware that groups begin when they are supposed to begin, referrals will be made in a timely way.

- **Lack of skills and training in group therapy.** To run groups well and comfortably, clinicians need to be trained in group psychotherapy. We generally believe that not every therapist is inclined to run groups or is interested in group treatment. Therefore, we generally recommend that each behavioral practice have a set of specialists in group therapy approaches who enjoy running groups and want to do group treatment. Efforts should then be made to thoroughly train and support these people in the delivery of group services.

The Coping Skills Group

Although it is beyond the scope of this book to delineate every single type of service or therapy group that could be offered through a standard outpatient program, we will describe a program that we believe would add value to almost every group practice to which we have consulted. It is what we call the coping skills group (CSG). The CSG can be used with clients regardless of their diagnoses and problem areas. Clinicians can be taught its format easily, and clients enjoy it and find it to be most valuable. The CSG can be seen as preparation for treatment for some patients and for others is the therapy itself. In many systems, clinicians and administrators come to view it as the prerequisite for other treatments within the system.

As can be seen from Table 6.3, the CSG offers a variety of generic psychosocial skills that are practical, useful, and of value to most treatment populations. The specific skills emphasized by any single group will depend on the client population. For instance, clients with unifocal anxiety or depressive complaints could use the group as a self-contained treatment, as they learn to identify, challenge, and modify maladaptive beliefs and expectations. Clients with more significant Axis II and dual-diagnosis complaints could utilize the group as an adjunct to individual work, to develop self-control and affect-modulation skills (Linehan, 1993).

The group format allows for considerable social support and modeling and rehearsal of skills. The extensive feedback that clients provide one another in these groups also can be a powerful prod toward change. Among groups operating on a risk basis, the allocation of routine skill development to group formats also helps clinicians free up their individual session time for clients who most need it.

TABLE 6.3. Coping Skills Group

Session 1: Cognitive-Behavioral Skills
Managing our thoughts and feelings
1. What are cognitive skills?
2. How we fool ourselves
3. Correcting our thinking problems

Session 2: Assertiveness Skills
Asking for what we want
1. Why be assertive?
2. What is assertiveness?
3. Three-part assertive messages
4. The art of saying "no"

Session 3: Anger Management Skills
Minimizing the negative effects and maximizing the positive ones
1. What is anger?
2. Risks involved with anger
3. How to manage anger

Session 4: Communication Skills
Effective listening and expression of thoughts and feelings
1. What is effective listening?
2. How to express your ideas effectively
3. Exploring alternative ways to respond

Session 5: Stress Management Skills
Understanding and managing the impact of stress
1. Body awareness, exercise and nutrition
2. Relaxation
3. Coping skills

Session 6: Depression Management Skills
Overcoming the vicious cycle of depression
1. What is depression?
2. The role of our thoughts
3. The importance of structure and activity
4. Improving relationships

Session 7: Anxiety Management Skills
Understanding and managing the anxiety response system
1. What is anxiety?
2. Steps in managing our thoughts
3. The role of rest and relaxation

Session 8: Resource Development Skills/Where to Go from Here
Developing natural/community resources and personal goals
1. What is self help?
2. Identifying helpful community resources
3. How to involve family, friends and coworkers

The CSG is a good example of thinking *programmatically* in a collaborative practice. Too many times practices are collections of clinicians working near one another but doing little differently than they would if they had rented office space in the same building. If this is the case, the collection adds little value to any of the practices. If, on the other hand, clinicians develop, maintain, and expand programs, the practice becomes greater than the sum of its parts.

☛ **LOOKING AHEAD**

When you develop services along a continuum, how do you know if you are really providing value to a community?

Our Quality Crash Course at the end of this chapter (Reader's Resource 6.3) can help you evaluate your services!

Intensive Outpatient Treatment

Intensive outpatient programs (IOP) originally developed out of the recognition that patients in day programs often progressed to the point where day-long treatment was not necessary and that they would be better served by even more rapid integration into their natural networks. Most IOPs allow patients to continue to work and attend to family and other responsibilities outside the program while providing a more intensive treatment experience than can be achieved through traditional outpatient services. Many times, IOPs can be successfully developed within outpatient settings and thus optimize the use of staff, space, and programmatic resources.

Typically, an IOP patient participates in treatment up to three times per week for 2 to 4 hours each session. Treatment includes a focus on psychosocial factors with the necessary attention to skill development, medication management, and case management to help the patient integrate into the community as smoothly as possible. Well-designed programs usually expect family or significant other involvement to educate and aid in the mobilization of natural resources. Group therapy programs are common components of IOPs, providing support and structure in a cost-effective manner. Indeed, any time a group practice coordinates individual and group therapy services with psychiatric care, the practice essentially has an IOP.

Practice managers who attempt to implement an IOP will inevitably run into an unfortunate fact of reality: Many MCOs either do not reimburse IOPs on a programmatic basis or only do so with facilities. If the MCO does not bundle the reimbursement for an IOP (e.g., offer a single, per-patient all-inclusive fee for IOP services), it is necessary to seek separate authorization for each IOP component. Thus a patient may start with individual therapy and only later receive authorization for psychiatric consultation and concurrent group treatment. This can make it difficult to implement the IOP on a time-effective basis for clients who are in crisis. In our experience, this is especially problematic among HMOs, which generally have limited benefits for outpatient behavioral health services that do not readily accommodate intensive intervention.

When an MCO does reimburse for an IOP, it often will do so with facilities, not outpatient groups. The IOP is used in such circumstances to divert inpatient admissions or to abbreviate their duration. Reimbursement of IOPs on a facility basis are often at rates unfavorable to outpatient groups. For instance, a week's participation in an IOP might be reimbursed at roughly one-quarter of the per diem inpatient stay rate, which would not cover individual, group, and psychiatric services on a fee-for-service basis. Such facility IOPs really amount to milieu stays with group treatment and medication management. Because facilities often have sufficient underutilized space and staff to accommodate patients for several hours at a time, it may make sense for them to contract at these lower rates of reimbursement. Outpatient practices, on the other hand, would not find such a bundled rate to be attractive.

Because of the funding problem with MCOs, most outpatient practices do not build IOPs and thus cover a limited portion of the care continuum. This is understandable, but in our estimation it can be a mistake. If your practice's strategic plan calls for significant business with managed insurers, you will be expected to contain costs **regardless of whether the marketplace has developed sophistication in the financing of IOPs.** This is especially the case as your group moves toward bonus and/or risk-sharing arrangements. Developing an IOP can be an excellent way of building the programs and skills needed to succeed financially under case rates and subcapitation.

So, how do you develop an IOP if insurers operating in the region do not have an adequate reimbursement structure in place? We were afraid you'd ask that question. Many times, it means starting off on a piece-by-piece fee-for-service basis, soliciting authorizations for each component of the IOP when needed. Over time, as you develop a positive, trusting relationship with the MCO, such authorizations will become easier and more streamlined. If the MCO is assured that the group practice will not abuse the IOP and is truly committed to keeping patients out of the hospital, it will have an incentive to authorize necessary services in one fell swoop.

This, however, still does not address the limitations of the average HMO, which may only have 20 sessions available to clients in the annual benefits package. Occasionally, such an HMO will be liberal in allowing your group to access the chemical dependency benefit; trade inpatient days for outpatient visits (on a two-for-one basis or better), or trade outpatient visits for group sessions (on a two-for-one basis or better). Such steps can help fund an IOP even if the components need to be authorized separately. If the HMO has no such mechanisms for funding (and most in our experience do not), we say: *Do the IOP anyway.* As we note later, we would go so far as to run a time-effective group treatment program *for free* to patients currently enrolled in the group practice. That way, ongoing support could be provided to any patient who needed it and a de facto IOP could be constructed for any patient currently receiving medication and psychotherapy. Such a loss leader may more than pay for itself in the form of marketing potential to MCOs and internal benefits to the practice.

Facility-Based Programs

The dramatic impact of managed care on inpatient psychiatric programs has forced hospital facilities to offer their own continua of treatment. As a result, much hospital-based work is not being conducted on a 24-hour, inpatient basis. This creates unusual opportunities for alliances between outpatient practices and facilities in creating intensive inpatient alternatives.

At the front end of the facility-based continuum is the observation/respite (23-hour) bed. This is a place where a patient can stay for observation, evaluation, crisis management, and support. Many times, a presenting crisis can be dealt with in the 23-hour bed and followed by a referral for intensive outpatient treatment. This makes the observation bed a useful mechanism in diverting inpatient admissions. The bed is also helpful in those situations in which it might be difficult to assess lethality due to a patient's intoxication, extreme exhaustion, or acute emotional distress. Although most observation beds are located within hospitals, there is a growing trend to integrate these into community-based triage centers. Such structures create a closer linkage between outpatient services and the front ends to inpatient care.

Day and partial hospital programs were originally developed as "step-downs" from inpatient programs and often were indistinguishable from the inpatient program, where they were located, until the patient went home at night. Today these programs are offered in a variety of sites, including hospital and community mental health settings. With the growing privatization of Medicaid and accompanying pressures for cost containment, this promises to become an increasingly competitive segment of the continuum. This is because Medicaid recipients utilize inpatient services at approximately four times the rate of privately insured individuals (Freiman et al., 1994). Organizations with well-developed alternatives to inpatient care will be especially attractive to payers insuring Medicaid populations.

Patients usually attend partial programs from 3 to 7 days per week, from 4 to 8 hours per day, depending on their treatment plan. As with IOPs, the treatment includes a focus on psychosocial factors affecting stabilization and integration back into the community. These programs are more intensive than IOPs, however, and usually involve medical and nursing supervision as well as individual, group, and psychiatric treatment. It is not at all unusual for average lengths of stay in inpatient treatment to decrease from double to single digits as partial programs take root. Increasingly, therefore, inpatient services are used for stabilization only for those clients at acute risk to self or others or wholly unable to care for themselves. Clients with greater adaptive capacities are preferentially routed to partial programs or IOPs. This is especially true in chemical dependency treatment, where outpatient detoxification programs and intensive outpatient group programs often substitute for traditional 28-day inpatient stays.

Residential care is often used as a step-down from inpatient treatment for clients who are not a safety risk. It is a primary alternative to inpatient care when a patient's home environment would not be conducive to supporting stabilization and recovery. Staff supervision is 24 hours per day, but medical and nursing supervision are only available as needed and usually not on site. Many programs encourage residents to gradually begin to return to work and attend to other responsibilities, as they solidify their gains, identify barriers to successful community integration, and develop effective coping skills to overcome these barriers. Lengths of stay typically are up to 30 days for adults and up to 60 days for children. However, length of stay depends on the availability of other effective community supports and services. Residential programs typically combine group, milieu, and psychosocial programs with individual counseling and medication management to create a high degree of potential structure for patients needing support.

Programming in a residential setting tends to be skills-based to help clients cope with anticipated difficulties in returning to home. During a residential stay, clients can also be connected to needed social services programs and vocational and educational resources. It is common for immediate family members to be included in some of the counseling sessions, to mobilize their assistance as supports to the patient. It is also common, as residential stays come to a close, for clients to conduct trial stays of limited duration at their homes. For these reasons, residential placements near clients' homes are preferable.

As we noted previously, *inpatient care* is at present the referral component of last resort, due to its cost, its disruption to other parts of a patient's life, and the availability of other more efficient and effective ambulatory treatment alternatives within the patient's community. Patients are referred to this level of care when acute stabilization, with 24-hour medical and nursing supervision/monitoring, is needed. Typically, this occurs when patients are assessed to be a risk to themselves or others, or when they have a medically complex condition, such as acute substance abuse withdrawal.

When inpatient lengths of stay were 30 to 90 days, such programs included intensive milieu treatment as well as group, family, recreational, occupational, and expressive therapies. However, as lengths of stays have decreased to the single digits, many of these treatment resources were eliminated or streamlined to accommodate the demand for rapid assessment and stabilization process. Today, many of these same services can be accessed in the non-hospital-based programs described earlier.

What the Continuum Means for Your Group Practice

Understanding the full spectrum of clinical services can help a group practice decide on its scope and service menu. In smaller markets less dominated by managed behavioral health care organizations, much of the group's collaborative work will be internal, linking the efforts of clinicians from differing specialties. Groups in larger, competitive markets will find greater pressure to link with other helping entities: hospitals, medical practices, and community agencies. At the very least, your group will experience pressure to do the following:

- Create or link to outpatient alternatives to hospitalization.

- Expand links to primary care providers.

- Expand links to chemical dependency programs and other specialty treatment sites.

Remember: You are marketing programs and processes, not just individual clinicians. Your distinctive advantage can come from the manner in which you link services and manage an entire course of treatment. The content and organization of your clinical services are your real "products."

If you are an individual clinician seeking to join a group practice, your understanding of the continuum can help you identify where you might best fit within the group and how the group you are considering fits into the larger picture of community needs. For example, if you detect that the community lacks integrated services for Axis II clients in acute crisis, you may want to market your ability to design and deliver such services for a group. Just as the group must market itself to the community with distinctive advantages to clients and referral sources, you want to think about the distinctive services that you would bring to a group. Where are the gaps in the group's service menu? Which populations are not being served in a coordinated, programmatic way? These may be the openings you need to build your career as an all-star clinician in a successful collaboration.

SOME BUSINESS ASPECTS OF DELIVERING CLINICAL PROGRAMS

It is important to keep an eye on costs when developing clinical programs. It is also necessary to market these services effectively. In a sense, each new clinical program deserves its own business plan. This will ensure that each program becomes a profit center to the group and an effective use of the group's time, money, and energy.

A Note about Reimbursements

Although the delivery of services across levels of care can be cost- and clinically effective, we must warn behavioral practices to exercise extreme caution before developing IOPs, day programs, and other inpatient alternatives. These programs are staff-intensive and thus can represent a significant source of overhead. The group must be assured of a relatively steady and significant demand for these services before sinking resources into program development. We recently encountered a group practice that leased an extra suite of offices to accommodate a planned day program. The program was nicely conceived but was unable to generate sufficient referral flow from the community due to spotty marketing and low MCO interest. Consequently, the group experienced major cash flow problems as it faced stiff monthly bills for the leased space.

It is imperative to research your market before developing clinical programs, but especially costly, intensive ones. Many MCOs pay lip service to the concept of hospital alternatives but lack the reimbursement flexibility and care review mechanisms to fund and gatekeep these services. Quite a few MCOs in our experience, including a number of smaller HMOs, have no provisions for, say, trading inpatient days for outpatient visits. As a result, patients with a 20-session outpatient benefit cannot be easily accommodated in an IOP. If a majority of MCOs in your region have such limitations, it would be imprudent to sink significant resources into intensive outpatient programs.

We strongly suspect that alternatives to hospitalization like outcomes assessment make for great talk among MCOs but are not always accorded meaningful financial incentives. Themselves hamstrung by tight premiums from purchasers, many MCOs cannot afford the clerical infrastructure that would be needed to adequately gatekeep and review a variety of new clinical services. Such initiatives may only blossom once practice organizations are themselves reimbursed on a risk basis and have the patient flow and financial incentive to define and monitor their own continua of programs.

In rural areas, collaborative practices may never cover a sufficiently large number of lives to justify ongoing intensive programs. When this is the case, the best choice is to develop a well-rounded set of group therapy services that can be appended to individual therapy and medication management on an as-needed basis. By yoking these stand-alone services, groups and networks create de facto IOPs without investing extra resources in staff or space. Data could be collected regarding the effectiveness of such informal IOPs as one means of selling MCOs on the concept of more formalized programs.

Selective Programming

One of the major problems in behavioral health is that everyone seems to be a generalist. Dr. Steenbarger fondly recalls starting a provider network and wading through credentialing forms that asserted that the clinician "specialized" in the individual and group treatment of children, adolescents, adults, couples, and families. It called to mind the story of the overinclusive student who submitted a term paper on "Lincoln: The Man, The Car, and The Tunnel"!

If you are just beginning a practice or expanding a small one, we strongly encourage you to (1) think selectively and (2) think programmatically. As we mentioned earlier, *programs*, rather than isolated and uncoordinated services, can very much help to differentiate a group from its competitors. These must be developed selectively, however, to capitalize on the distinctive strengths and interests of the clinical staff. Too many programs water down the value of any particular offering. A successful program matches the talents of clinical staff with the needs of a community. As a rule, program development should be limited to the several most common diagnoses presenting to the practice, as well as the most common sources of emergencies.

Beginning practices might think about starting just one well-developed clinical program and executing that *very well*. This is a version of our aforementioned "specialty expertise" strategy. For example, individual and group therapy services, along with medical consultation and management, could be integrated and packaged as a treatment program for eating disorders. Data collection would establish such program parameters as average duration of treatment, patient satisfaction, and outcomes. These data could be marketed to insurers and other referral sources and the program could even be tailored for particular patients as an IOP. Over time, the group might develop a favorable reputation for this work, facilitating related referrals in such areas as addictions and trauma. The idea is to develop the program as a *marketable product*.

In some cases, your group won't have the staff resources to develop and deliver a full product. An outpatient dual-diagnosis treatment program, for instance, would have to draw on the expertise of medical, substance abuse, and psychotherapy providers. If your practice does not have all these components in place, it may be possible to team up with a complementary practice to deliver the desired program. By facilitating communications and referrals across groups, a group specializing in substance abuse and one specializing in psychiatric services might be able to jointly market their collaboration, creating a service that is more attractive than any of the individual offerings of the respective groups.

Larger, more established groups should have entire product lists that embrace unique services in such areas as child treatment, substance abuse, geriatric services, women's issues, and Axis II disorders. Each program/product would have its own triage criteria, service array, treatment guidelines, outcomes assessment, and clinical supervision/oversight. These might be written up in summary form and made available to referral sources and insurers as marketing tools.

Approaching Clinical Care with a Business Mind

Earlier we spoke of the value of approaching clients with a "beginner's mind." We also approach practice with a business mind. This means having the flexibility to design and market collaborative clinical services in ways that create unique advantages for the patient, the insurer, and the group practice. Not infrequently, this is some of the most creative work of practice managers and clinical teams.

Consider an example drawn from our recent experience. A behavioral group head sent us an e-mail requesting advice regarding the development of his practice. He recognized that MCOs were taking an increasing share of business in the region and worried that his group was too small to attract their attention. He also realized that he needed to do much more to document the quality of his group's work. To this point, the group had undertaken little data collection, given the full caseloads of the practitioners and his own time demands managing the enterprise. Finally, he wondered how he could accomplish all of his MCO marketing and data collection cost-effectively because margins were becoming alarmingly thin.

The good news, he reported, was that business was strong and that his current group of MD and non-MD providers were a cohesive bunch who worked well together. A number of his group members had experience in both inpatient and outpatient settings with adolescents and adults. He felt that the group really did have a lot to offer MCOs and other referral sources. His sense, having talked with several representatives from area MCOs, was that they were not overly impressed with the other groups in town—especially their ability to gatekeep inpatient utilization. In sum, he said, things were going well, but there were signs that they wouldn't remain that way for long.

Here, in somewhat abbreviated form, was our advice. We offer it not as a blueprint for all practices but as an illustration of the collaborative management mind-set in designing clinical services:

- **Step one.** Hire an unlicensed clinical or counseling psychologist straight out of an accredited predoctoral internship. Structure his or her experience as a postdoctoral one that will provide (1) significant clinical experience, (2) an immersion in behavioral health care practice and administration, (3) free supervision toward licensure, (4) a salary meaningfully ahead of their internship stipend (but below your prevailing staff rates), with health benefits, and (5) possible staff appointment at the end of the year.

  Our reasoning: This is a win-win. The group practice will get a talented, hustling practitioner for about $25,000. The graduating intern will have a secure position for a year, with benefits, solid experience, and guaranteed supervision toward licensure. Even if the post doesn't lead to ongoing employment with the group, it will provide great references and experience, which can be difficult to obtain for an unlicensed PhD.

- **Step two.** Beat the bushes for cash-paying clients. Announce a sliding-fee scale, with rates going as low as $35 an hour. Go after HMO clients who may have run through their benefit. Market to primary care physicians and school systems, letting them know that cost will not be an issue. Feed all cash cases to the newly hired staff person.

  Our reasoning: If you can secure 15 face-to-face hours a week of business for the new clinician, you can basically cover his or her salary. Most markets have an underserved population that lacks both Medicaid and good health insurance. It is often possible to get good word of mouth and community visibility by offering flexible rates. Eventually, this will also help to bring in other, full-pay and insurance cases.

- **Step three.** Make the new clinician your coordinator of practice assessment. (Hence, you'll want to choose someone with research and computer skills.) Start collecting a minimum data set on all patients, including client satisfaction and functional status measures, length of treatment, and diagnoses. Data should be collected on scannable forms and scanned into analytical software (database or spreadsheet). The new clinician would be responsible for collecting and summarizing the data.

Our reasoning: This arrangement makes data collection minimally burdensome for the clinicians because they won't need their own computers and will only have to blacken in circles to complete forms. It ensures, however, that data will truly be collected because a person is directly responsible for this function. The data could even form the backbone of a publication that you could pursue with the new professional, creating yet another win-win.

☛ LOOKING AHEAD

Data collection has become a core component of marketing and managing group practices.

At the end of this chapter, Mark Maruish, PhD, offers his perspectives (Reader's Resource 6.4).

- **Step four.** Begin an ongoing support group for clients of the group practice. The group would be run by the new clinician and would be held twice a week in a late afternoon/early evening time. *There would be no charge to patients or insurers for the group services.* It is purely a skills-oriented support group, offering discussion, rehearsal, feedback, and work on coping. Any client in the group practice needing extra support and/or going through a crisis could participate in the group. Include the group therapy service in data collection efforts. Market the group to community referral sources (but not MCOs at this point) as an extremely cost-effective way to get patients seen three times a week. (Note: the client *must* be seen in individual therapy within the practice to be eligible for the support group.) Consider running two groups simultaneously: one for higher- and one for lower-functioning clients.

  Our reasoning: The group is going to be a loss leader. You won't bring in revenue from it directly, but it's going to score a lot of points in the community and may very well attract enough cash-paying clientele to cover your new staff member's salary. It will generate a quick flow of referrals and get the practice off the ground quickly toward an ongoing group therapy program. Eventually, word of mouth will bring other clients into the practice and the free group will more than pay for itself.

- **Step five.** Armed with data from the individual and group therapy within the practice, approach MCOs with your results. Show them your low rate of hospitalization and your ability to work with difficult clients cost-effectively. *Package your combination of individual and group therapy as an IOP that costs the MCO nothing!* Because the group is a free support service, it does not have to be authorized by the MCO and will not be reimbursed. Your pitch to the MCO is that you know very well who needs additional support and you are going to provide it free of charge as part of your commitment to keeping patients functioning in the community. If the MCO will contract with your group practice and preferentially route referrals your way, you'll provide a full array of cost-effective outpatient services.

Our reasoning: You've just outmaneuvered the competition and created a unique selling point for your group. In one fell swoop, you have (1) established your group's accountability with hard data, (2) aligned your group with the MCO's cost-containment goals, (3) offered a service (IOP) not currently available to the MCO, and (4) offered it free! Again, you've created a loss leader. You won't collect money from the group, but as a marketing tool it will bring in more than its share of business. If it gets very popular, add groups. (Note: carefully gatekeep the use of the group and make sure that any contract with an MCO doesn't simply result in their dumping only the most severely impaired cases on your practice! If more than 20% of your MCO referrals qualify as needing elements of the IOP, someone else is probably skimming the cream.)

Elements of the Business Mind-Set

Our vignette illustrates several key facets of the business mind-set underlying successful collaborative practice:

1. **Efficient *can* be effective.** By creating programmatic services that link group and individual care, the practice will be in a position to offer care with documented quality in a cost-effective manner.

2. **You have to invest money to make money.** The group's owner is taking a risk by funding a new position but will get quite a bit for the investment, including a mechanism for data collection, a groups program, and a marketable service to MCOs. Given that the position is funded modestly, at a salary level that can be covered by a doable flow of cash-paying patients, the rewards outweigh the risks.

3. **Create win–win situations.** The strategy outlined above works for all parties involved. The new staff member will gain valuable experience, credentials, and references. The group practice will have entered the world of data collection and programmatic services. The community will get affordable services. The MCOs will have an eminently affordable IOP. And the referrals flow.

4. **Meet the need.** The group practice identifies a critical need in the community—the lack of control over inpatient utilization and the relative absence of sliding-fee services—and uses this to create a strategic advantage.

5. **Be creative.** The group's strategy can be implemented in creative ways.

Staff members could be enlisted to assist with the supervision of the new clinician, creating valued and varied roles for them. Over time, it may be possible to hire postdoctoral professionals on an ongoing basis to staff new services, creating a respected training program within the group practice and enhancing the recruitment of clinicians.

The collaborative mind-set is one which is programmatic and data-based. It entails a fundamental shift in the view of professional services, from clinician-based care to team-based, standardized treatment. Groups and networks able to make this shift of mind-set will find that it opens new vistas for the creative delivery of high-quality care.

CONCLUSION

This chapter has encouraged behavioral practices to think of their clinical services in time-effective and programmatic terms. Time-effectiveness bridges quality and cost, delivering needed services as efficiently as possible. Programmatic clinical services provide the practice with marketable products across a continuum of client needs and practice specialties, integrating care that traditionally has been fragmented. Successful outpatient organizations deliver packages of team-based services tailored to the needs of patients and diagnoses, not just "me-too" clinical services conceptualized and delivered in isolation. Ultimately, the structure, function, and content of clinical offerings are expressions of the overall strategic vision of the practice and its blending of cost and quality mandates.

✔ SUMMARY

- The time-effective framework can be helpful in creating an overarching philosophy of treatment that delivers high quality at affordable cost.
- The group practice draws on individual therapy, psychopharmacology, and group treatment to cover a continuum of needs across a range of clients and presenting problems.
- Opportunities for groups and individual clinicians can be created by identifying gaps in the local service continuum and developing programmatic services to fill these.
- A central challenge to group practices is the design, delivery, and linkage of clinical services as marketable products that address the needs of referral sources.

We hope this chapter has illustrated for readers that collaboration is more than a buzzword. It is a distinctive way of defining the services offered by mental health professionals, linking those services into coherent programs, and continually evaluating the success of those programs. The collaborative culture that we have observed in the successful practices we've interviewed is distinguished by teamwork and an atmosphere of continual innovation. In these "learning organizations" we believe we have located the future of mental health.

READER'S RESOURCE 6.1
The DISCUS Model:
A Guide to Utilization Management

Utilization management begins with the recognition that a group practice has finite clinical resources and that these must be allocated to clients—or an entire population—as judiciously as possible. This becomes an increasing concern as groups move toward risk contracting. In our capitation exercise at the end of the previous chapter, for example, we found that a $2 PMPM reimbursement for outpatient services roughly translated into an average of six sessions per client. The task of utilization management would be to keep the system as a whole to that average, allocating the greatest resources to clients with the most extensive needs.

How do you determine priorities for your allocation of clinical resources? We have assembled a model, which we refer to by its acronym (DISCUS), that can be a useful start for clinicians and groups needing to make the tough choices regarding brief versus longer-term treatments. Each variable in the DISCUS model helps the clinician assess the needs of a given patient:

- **D = duration.** The duration of a client's problem will give a clue as to its chronicity. A problem of brief duration may very well be situational and amenable to short-term intervention. A problem that has recurred through the client's lifespan is much more likely to be chronic and susceptible to relapse. Indeed, the presence of a high-duration problem is an important clue that (often group-therapy-based) relapse prevention programs might be helpful for the patient.
- **I = interpersonal history.** A client with a favorable interpersonal history (i.e., who has a history of positive, ongoing relationships) is much more likely to be able to bond quickly with a therapist (and hence receive help briefly) than a client with a history of chaotic or traumatic relationships. In the latter circumstance, a patient may need months of visits before sufficient trust is established to work on core problems, clearly ruling out traditional brief therapy.
- **S = severity.** Severity is the degree to which a problem or set of problems interferes with the life functioning of the individual. It is generally assessed in several domains, such as work functioning, home functioning, relationships, emotional functioning, etc. A high-severity problem generally requires crisis intervention and the coordination of several helping modalities (coping groups, individual therapy, psychopharmacology). When high severity is combined with

(cont.)

READER'S RESOURCE 6.1 (*cont.*)

long duration, it is almost always a sign that ongoing support and intervention will be needed.

- **C = complexity.** The complexity of a problem refers to the breadth of its symptomatic manifestations. A very complex problem manifests itself through multiple, interwoven symptoms and difficulties, such as concurrent somatic complaints, substance abuse, depression, anxiety, interpersonal conflicts, and self-abusive acting out. A low-complexity problem may be limited to a single manifestation, as in the case of, say, test anxiety. On average, a high-complexity problem tends to require multiple interventions to address each of its components and hence cannot be treated in very brief modalities.

- **U = understanding.** Does the client demonstrate an understanding that there is a specific problem or problem set that needs to be worked on and the motivation to do so? This reflects the stages of change discussed earlier in the chapter. A client with an understanding of the problem and who is motivated to deal with his or her difficulties has a clear idea of what needs to change and is ready to take action. A client lacking understanding may be in denial with respect to problems and may not be prepared for the steps needed to change. It will be difficult to conduct brief therapy if the client needs multiple sessions just to identify a focal problem and achieve the momentum needed to tackle the problem. Also implicit in this idea of understanding and motivation is that the patient's view is that he or she is an integral part of changing the problem. Someone who sees the problem as everyone else's fault and responsibility will be unlikely to make appreciable changes.

- **S = social support.** What is the patient's current level of social support from friends, family members, and significant others? Many times, therapy is elongated simply because the client needs the therapist as an ongoing support, not just as a change agent. It is generally easier to work on change between sessions and sustain change after treatment if the social support network backs the client's efforts.

Although the DISCUS variables can be assessed through informal clinical interview, groups may choose to use them to form the backbone of clinical data collection efforts. By monitoring DISCUS and correlating the variables to outcome and utilization data, the group can begin to form its own profiles of clients who benefit from briefer versus more extended intervention, psychotherapy alone versus with psychopharmacology and so on. Such profiling permits a group to monitor cases as they progress, to determine the degree to which changes are occurring at the expected rate. Utilization management efforts can then recommend changes to treatment plans when necessary as a way of making optimal use of limited resources.

READER'S RESOURCE 6.2
Interview with Michael Hurst, EdD, President and CEO, Instream, Inc.

"We value our time too little. . . ."

Michael Hurst, EdD, has had an interesting and varied professional history in behavioral health. He began his academic career as a major in aeronautical engineering at MIT, switching later to history and psychology. His background in statistics and engineering, however, has continued to influence his work in the area of communications systems for behavioral group practices. He founded and led Hurst Associates in Boston during the 1980s, building it from a group practice to a major provider of EAP and consultative services to industry. After selling his business, he worked for a while in managed behavioral health care before once again striking out on his own with Instream, Inc. In a few short years, Instream has become a major provider of communications systems for group practices, linking practitioners to one another and to MCOs for the purposes of case consultation, billing, eligibility checking, authorizations, and so on. Dr. Hurst generously gave of his time to talk with Brett Steenbarger about lessons learned over his career and the coming boom in communications.

Steenbarger: Tell me how your business evolved.

Hurst: In 1980 I had to decide what I was going to do. I was running three research projects and a group practice and I said, "To hell with it! I'll do the group practice."

Steenbarger: How large was the group practice at that point?

Hurst: It was just myself and four part-time people. That was pretty scary in May of 1980 . . . I had a big shock because as people came on, they said they wanted to do more, and I said, "OK, fine!" Then the state insurance commissioner made a ruling saying that any licensed professional working for another licensed professional had to draw a salary and could not be paid on the basis of proportion of fees received. He defined that as fee splitting, which is illegal. So I put everybody on salary and promptly lost about $28,000 in the next 6 months!

They no longer cared if their patient came to appointments, they no longer cared if they filled their hours. My full-time job became doing all the marketing for the practice to try to keep everybody's time filled. That became a super drag!

Before my partner joined me, I had already decided that I wanted to get into this EAP business and industrial consultation business be-

(cont.)

READER'S RESOURCE 6.2 (*cont.*)

cause sitting here hour after hour gets to be a drag and lonely. When you take a vacation, you have to pay twice: You lose your income and you have to pay for the vacation. So I said, "This is not the way to go."

I drew up five different programs that I thought would be of value to industry and promptly got them all shot down. . . . I figured banking would be a good industry segment to look at; maybe they'd be interested in psychological consultation services. I went to the 15 largest banks in this area and started a cold-calling campaign over the summer. I didn't know what phenomenal success I had until later. Of the fifteen, I got on the phone 13 VPs of HR [human resources] or medical directors. I got in to see 9 of them . . . and 6 eventually became our core customers.

STEENBARGER: Not bad!

HURST: Yeah, that was a helluva strike. At the time, I thought it was terrible. I thought I should have gotten all 15! I didn't know a damned thing about marketing.

. . . All of a sudden our group had a much more stable footing than the simple fee-for-service business. Then over the course of the next twelve years, we developed other divisions. . . . We tried a number of them. . . . We basically would bring in a psychologist and they would have an idea. We were always listening to people's ideas. Everyone wanted to go into business and out of private practice or out of their community mental health center. We'd listen to their ideas and the good ones we'd fund for a year to see whether or not they could make it work as a business. At one point, we had five different business lines going, three of which failed. It was a big shock to the people that after a year's time and we had lost money on the venture, I pulled the plug. Unlike the university or community mental health center . . . , that money was coming directly out of my pockets.

STEENBARGER: You're not running an entitlement program!

HURST: That's right. It was a big shock. We didn't do that any longer. We were much more careful about evaluating an idea before giving a person a year's salary and expenses.

So eventually we had three divisions. One was the EAP and what became the integrated care division. We also did outplacement programs and psych assessment consultation programs. The latter two we ended up selling in . . . 1990. We had four partners at that point. We sat down and said, "Gee, we're very good in each of our areas, but whenever we go to new clients, they think of us as being a jack of all trades, master of none." So we decided we'd better start focusing before we lose credibility. We had gotten at that point up to about a million and a half

(*cont.*)

in sales and we had 15 clinicians and 2 clericals. So we sold the assessment division and we sold the outplacement division to other companies. We focused on building the managed care into the EAP business and turned it into integrated care. We ended up doing case management, utilization review on a contract basis, and all of our work was capitated. I find at this moment everyone is saying, "You have to be so careful with capitation." We were doing that 10, 15 years ago!

STEENBARGER: Wow!

HURST: Part of the way we were able to control that was [with] a database program called DataEase, in which I created a large database along with electronic forms. Then I installed the LAN—I actually did the wiring myself—and got this whole system running where if they answered the phone, they literally had the intake screen in front of them and then it would pass along to the other screens. . . . It was all stored in the database. Eventually I figured out: I can use all of this data for more than just reporting on our clinical practice and our billing. We can use this for studying how we operate. So I wrote up scripts . . . to follow everyone's service logs and see what proportion of their contractual level they were doing and in what area. Were they doing it in supervision, in training, EAP evaluations, mental health visits, or whatever? Then I went around to everyone and said, "Gee, here's what came out of the computer when I compared what you're supposed to do with what's in there." And a few people were shocked! . . . That worked out well. I started that particular program in 1988.

[Note here the creative use of information technology to monitor and manage the practice. Dr. Hurst's experience—needing to stay on top of overhead and cut cost centers that are not yielding adequate revenues—was a major driving force behind his computerization of his business.]

STEENBARGER: How did you make the transition to Instream?

HURST: We realized from our experience . . . that communications was a major problem for MCOs and providers. . . . We're in the tenth version of our product. We have 1,700 providers online, 94 groups, and we have 5 major MCOs.

STEENBARGER: What do you see driving the demand for communications products such as your own?

HURST: The incredible inefficiencies of the post-office-and-fax system. And the incredible frustration of providers having to get on the phone to talk to somebody to blow their nose. They really don't like doing that. In hospitals—that part of the provider chain—they have managed care departments. These are just nurses whose job it is to call the managed

(cont.)

READER'S RESOURCE 6.2 (*cont.*)

care company, get the eligibility verified, get a case manager on the line, and then call the doc to get the doc to pick up the phone for permissions. Anything that could short-circuit that process to save people the aggravation, the time, and the money is worthwhile. Unfortunately, however, the comparison becomes, "Well, I can throw a claim in the mail for $.32." They forget that that's not all there is to the cost of doing that claim. . . .

[A few years ago] behavioral health costs had been accelerating more than 35% per year. People didn't realize that until they carved out medical surgical, made that managed care, and then watched their indemnity behavioral rates skyrocket. That's how managed behavioral health came about. What I foresee personally is that . . . they should be integrated. The soma is not separate from the psyche or vice versa. They're inherently related and the care ought to be as well.

STEENBARGER: So you're seeing a carving back in of the behavioral health piece.

HURST: That's right . . . and then there comes a much greater need to communicate and share data.

[The great frontier of collaboration is the electronic medical record and online consultation systems. It is difficult to imagine large-scale integrations of behavioral and medical systems without a communications platform linking multispecialty providers.]

STEENBARGER: Right! One of the things I've run into is that it often isn't cost-effective to put behavioral health clinicians in the primary care space. On a per-square-foot basis, you can't generate the revenues and justify having the body there, so there have to be other strategies to achieve the integration.

HURST: . . . I don't agree entirely. I agree with the economic analysis on a per square foot basis. Obviously, whereas a physician can generate $2,000 a day in a modest practice, it is difficult for anyone in behavioral health to generate that amount. On the other hand, they do have a higher overhead too. They have tremendous equipment costs and much higher staffing ratios per physician than a behavioral health person.

STEENBARGER: That's very true.

HURST: So if you count the entire overhead structure and allocate it properly, the behavioral health person doesn't need the whole infrastructure that a physician does. I'm not sure your analysis is entirely correct when you actually add in all that extra cost on their side.

(*cont.*)

I literally used to practice inside an internal medicine group and that was wonderful. Then later we went outside that group. It became not an economic issue but literally a psychological issue. So we had offices next door to the internal medicine group and with separate entrances, but we had joint staff meetings and it worked out very well.

STEENBARGER: In the future, do you see some of those joint staff meetings and consultations happening online, as opposed to through physical colocation?

HURST: Certainly they could and they should. As we sort through the various means of keeping computerized patient records and security on the records down to the field level, then it's appropriate. But we have some constraints there too. The federal government requires that substance abuse records be maintained separately from medical surgical records. There are certain states—Washington State, for example—that say you cannot comingle claims and administrative data with patient record data. You can't even send them in the same envelope and electronically you're not supposed to send them together either.

STEENBARGER: Interesting . . .

HURST: Here in Massachusetts, there was a big hullabaloo . . . when a secretary in a med–surg unit was able to retrieve the mental health record of a patient. It became front-page headlines that a "clerk" in medicine can get your mental health records. . . . Once all those kinds of issues are sorted out—and one just has to keep their eye on them and do their best until they are—certainly there should be that kind of information sharing. There has to be if you're going to treat a person properly.

STEENBARGER: Does your system have the capability of an entirely electronic record?

HURST: We don't have the record at all. We look to the practice management system vendors to have that and then we provide them with the connectivity. . . . We work with all practice management vendors . . . so that they can create an interface for any of their system users. . . . So you can use the practice management software to run your group and then when you have to do claims or managed care forms that are on our system, you literally just say, "Do that." Actually, it's a print function, "print Instream," and it calls up our program and it populates it with the data from the practice management system.

STEENBARGER: That's very interesting. Are you anticipating offering that for medical group practice software as well as behavioral, to link the docs with the behavioral clinicians?

(cont.)

READER'S RESOURCE 6.2 (*cont.*)

HURST: Yes. There are very serious business competitors out there [for medical practice management services and software]. The med–surg side is an $800-billion segment versus behavioral health, which is 80 to 100 billion, depending on who's doing the estimate. . . . So we're much smaller. Our revenue per hour is much less. Our revenue per case is much less. Every measure that you can use says that we don't have the same economic resources to modernize ourselves. But we should.

I give the example: Let's say that you gross $150,000 a year as an individual or per FTE [full-time equivalent] in your group. If you were a normal business, you would be spending 10% of that gross on information systems and infrastructure. If you were a physician, you'd be spending about 5%. And I will tell you in behavioral health, you're lucky if you're spending 1%.

STEENBARGER: Right!

HURST: So a $150,000 practitioner, when you net it out probably making let's say $110,000—for them to spend $3,000 for [personal computers] and software is a huge deal.

STEENBARGER: But meanwhile they'll take up their time writing letters and sitting on the phone listening to elevator music.

HURST: Which basically tells you we value our time too little. . . . There are many other ways to maximize one's economic value than spending time on the phone and writing out forms.

STEENBARGER: So a big part of your sale is convincing them that the product pays for itself in terms of saving the time and freeing them up to do more of what they're supposed to be doing.

HURST: Fantastically correct.

READER'S RESOURCE 6.3
Quality Crash Course

We have emphasized that the assessment of quality will become an increasingly central activity of clinicians and groups in the years ahead, thanks to the growing demands of the public and purchaser coalitions. But what is quality and how can it be assessed in a valid and reliable fashion? In general, we can distinguish three definitions of quality:

1. **Patient satisfaction.** This refers to measures that assess the degree to which clients are pleased with the services they've received. Satisfaction embraces both clinical variables (Do clients feel they've benefited from their treatment?) and service variables (Do clients feel they've been seen promptly?). A good example of a standardized patient satisfaction tool is the CSQ-8, an eight-item self-report questionnaire (Attkisson & Greenfield, 1994).

2. **Clinical outcomes.** Measures of clinical outcomes evaluate the degree to which clients have actually changed as a function of being in treatment. Hence, they are designed to be administered on at least two occasions: before and after the care episode. There is value, however, in administering these tools on multiple occasions, both during treatment (to evaluate rates of change) and well after the end of treatment (to evaluate the degree to which changes have been maintained). The most common measures of clinical outcomes are *symptom measures*, which evaluate a client's level of depression, anxiety, psychosis, etc., and *functional status measures*, which assess impairments in multiple life domains. Among the more common outcome instruments are the OQ-45.1 (Lambert & Burlingame, 1995), the SCL-90-R (DeRogatis & Lazarus, 1994), and the BASIS-32 (Eisen, 1995).

3. **Indicator performance.** This refers to the degree to which group practices meet or exceed predefined clinical and service benchmarks. For example, the group may decide as a matter of policy that all clients will be screened for chemical dependency at intake and that screening results will be documented in the chart. At periodic intervals, the practice manager can review client charts and ascertain the degree to which clinicians followed the guideline. If the percentage of adherence falls below a threshold level (say, 90%), this may trigger efforts at clinician training and quality improvement. Groups may define several service and clinical indicators and periodically give themselves "report cards" to monitor their quality.

(cont.)

READER'S RESOURCE 6.3 (*cont.*)

Evaluations of quality become formal programs of *continuous quality improvement* when data concerning satisfaction, outcomes, and indicator performance are shared throughout the organization and used as the basis for staff development efforts (Steenbarger et al., 1996). Superior quality is acknowledged and rewarded and used as a model for staff development. Substandard quality is identified and targeted for focused improvement efforts. Managers commonly find that the mere act of giving staff members *supportive* feedback about the quality of their work is helpful in galvanizing change efforts and enhancing motivation. The key is to find what's working and do more of it; find what's not working and, as a team, work toward improvement.

READER'S RESOURCE 6.4
Interview with Mark Maruish, PhD

"Why haven't we demonstrated this?"

Mark E. Maruish, PhD, has a broad and unique perspective on the topics of quality and outcomes assessment. He currently serves as the director of clinical services for Strategic Advantage, Inc. (SAI), in Minneapolis, Minnesota. SAI is the Magellan Health Services subsidiary that provides outcomes assessment and consulting services for facilities within the Charter Behavioral Health System, another Magellan company. Dr. Maruish's background includes serving as senior clinical psychologist for NCS Assessments for nearly 10 years. More recently, he served as instrumentation director and behavioral health care consultant for Health Outcomes Institute (HOI), a Minneapolis-based health care outcomes assessment and consulting organization. HOI has developed and/or distributes numerous condition-specific outcomes instruments for the assessment of both behavioral and medical disorders. The Health Status Questionnaire (HSQ) and its abbreviated 12-item version (HSQ-12) also are distributed by HOI. In addition to his other accomplishments, Dr. Maruish published the edited book *The Use of Psychological Testing for Treatment Planning and Outcome Assessment* in 1994. The second edition of the book is currently due in 1998.

Dr. Maruish kindly shared his expertise regarding quality with Brett Steenbarger in a telephone interview shortly before he left HOI at the end of last year. His perspectives speak eloquently to the forces driving collaboration in behavioral health.

STEENBARGER: Maybe in an open-ended way you could talk a little bit from your perspective about how you see health care evolving, how you see behavioral health care evolving, and the role of outcomes assessment in that evolution.

MARUISH: Well, I've got no great insights here! I do think there has been a little bit of a shift from cost containment. We all know that for the past 10 years, people have recognized that health care costs are skyrocketing. As a result, there have been efforts to contain those costs in various ways . . . including the development of HMOs and other managed health care organizations for delivering health care more efficiently. As I see it . . . the healthcare industry is implementing some control now and, as far as I know, the rate of cost is slowing down. So people have been successful in trying to manage the whole cost issue.

Now I think there has been somewhat of a shift from the focus on

(cont.)

READER'S RESOURCE 6.4 (*cont.*)

that . . . toward the quality of care that's being offered. It's reflected in what we're seeing now with people getting more involved in conducting outcomes studies or implementing some kind of outcomes management program for their organization. These efforts include not only the measurement of clinical and functional outcomes for a patient but also patient satisfaction. . . . My impression is at one point, the people who were most interested were getting involved in doing outcomes early on. I don't want to say that this is the standard, in the sense that everybody everywhere is requiring this, but I do think people are starting to look at this. They need to demonstrate outcomes, that they need to sell their services, to demonstrate to, let's say, third-party payers that they're not just delivering the services, but that what they do is making a difference. That's where outcomes and patient satisfaction measurement both play an important role.

Along with that, being a marketing tool, it also is a means of CQI [continuous quality improvement], if you will. People can use this information to improve the quality of services they offer. They can see that they can determine: "Did that work? If not, maybe I need to start changing what I do. If it did, maybe I need to continue doing what I'm doing."

[Dr. Maruish is absolutely correct. The recent spate of negative publicity regarding quality of care in managed health systems has greatly catalyzed the push for quality, which, as we've seen, is fueling collaboration. Recent federal mandates for minimum lengths of stay for women delivering children are but a first step in the direction of government activism in the area of quality.]

STEENBARGER: Sure.

MARUISH: You know, patient satisfaction is the same way, although people's satisfaction with the outcomes they received from a provider is one thing. There also are other things that are important to patients, like access to the provider—whether it's physical access, how long you have to wait to schedule an appointment, or "Does the doctor sit and talk with you? Do they explain what they're doing?" All of these are becoming important factors.

As health care has tightened its belt, the whole health care market is obviously becoming more competitive and, as in other industries, the service component can become the only edge that a provider might have. We can probably think of several instances in our day-to-day lives where you could go to several different places to buy a product, but if

(*cont.*)

the service isn't there when you need it later on, then you probably aren't going to be going back. . . .

I think that, for the most part, providers are competent to deliver quality services, but there's another component . . . that people purchasing services want. Again, I think that the quality aspect of outcomes, patient satisfaction, and figuring out what works and what doesn't all are coming to the forefront.

STEENBARGER: What do you see as some of the particular challenges for behavioral health care groups and organizations? When we talk about outcomes, those are somewhat different from the outcomes of specific primary care interventions.

MARUISH: . . . From what I can gather, one of the things is that as people start to become lean and mean in behavioral health, they're cutting back on assessment. It's becoming a real challenge to the publishers [of psychological tests and measures] to stay in that market, to convince people that this is something that's beneficial. When you're cutting budgets and a patient is allowed . . . 10 visits and that's it, are you going to spend your money on giving them an MMPI [Minnesota Multiphasic Personality Inventory], SCL-90, or something like that? The natural tendency of a lot of providers is to say, "That's one thing we can cut out. Why do we need that?"

I think that's a challenge to behavioral health care providers to demonstrate that assessment is something that's worthwhile. If you can identify problems up front, you can deal with them quicker and better, and you can make better use of the sessions that are allotted under the health care plan. Assessment can also be used in a follow-up manner at posttreatment to determine, "Did the treatment I rendered work?" Or, at the same time, "What type of treatment works for what type of patient?"

[Dr. Maruish has an excellent point. In an effort to contain overhead, most practices are doing little or nothing to assess the quality of their work. This will leave them poorly prepared for a new environment that rewards such accountability.]

STEENBARGER: How do you see that being done cost-effectively?

MARUISH: I think there almost has to be a demonstration project. . . . That's the real problem. It would be nice if funding from somewhere could be obtained to demonstrate that the use of psychological assessment is cost-effective, especially from the standpoint of medical cost-offset. . . . Sure, you may be paying a little more up front, but you're identifying

(cont.)

READER'S RESOURCE 6.4 (*cont.*)

problems quicker, which hopefully will have some effects down the road. In the short run, it may translate into fewer sessions, less recidivism, and a reduction in total medical costs. . . . I don't think that anybody has actually demonstrated that the use of testing can result in these types of benefits. Clinicians say, "Yes, it helps me out," but nobody has demonstrated that.

STEENBARGER: Do you see HOI getting into this whole area? You have the TyPE [Technology of Patient Experience] measures, you've been doing some work in the field of patient satisfaction. I think the HSQ-12 [12-item Health Status Questionnaire, a general health status measure] is a really interesting instrument. . . .

MARUISH: To a point. That's what I've been trying to do over the past year or so. . . . We do have some behavioral health instruments: the Depression TyPE specification; pretty soon we'll be coming out with a substance abuse TyPE and a panic disorder TyPE. I know that the people who have been developing these instruments for us down at the University of Arkansas are working on two or three other measures: One is for emotional/behavioral disorders of adolescence and the other, I think, is for schizophrenia. So we do plan on having those sorts of instruments to offer providers.

STEENBARGER: Maybe you could comment a bit on your perception of the HSQ-12 and its value as at least a quick and dirty instrument . . . covering some important areas with little time and expense?

MARUISH: We're hoping it will be out the early part of next year. We're in the process of finishing up data collection for that. . . . One of the things that struck me—I don't think it's so much an issue in behavioral health as it is in physical health care, primary health care—is how much you can ask patients to do. For example, in clinical behavioral health care settings, an instrument such as the 53-item BSI [Brief Symptom Inventory] would be considered a brief screening instrument. A screener in epidemiology is more like five items! It's a matter of things being relative here. The impression is that professionals [in medical practice] either don't want to give it . . . or they've gotten a lot of reactions from patients saying, "I don't want to do this." Whereas, in psychology, if you ask a patient to take a 566-item MMPI, they'll take it! It seems to be a different story. . . . At this time, people want something that's short, but at the same time, they want something that's valid and reliable. I think there's a lot of people out there—although they're becoming

(*cont.*)

more educated—that don't quite understand that if you have a short instrument, you're losing something in terms of reliability and validity, not to mention a great deal of information.

The [HSQ] 12 is being developed for uses in which you don't need any fine differentiation of what's going on with a patient. It provides more of a very broad snapshot of the patient in cases where you might want to use that sort of information for case mix adjustment . . . or allowing comparisons across data sets. So it's not intended . . . for day-to-day clinical use, but in those cases where people say, "This is too much; I'm not going to give it." In this case, something is better than nothing. In many of these cases, it will serve the purpose quite well.

STEENBARGER: Are you doing any work in the manner of delivery of the instruments? Computerized assessments, as opposed to pencil and paper?

MARUISH: We've stayed away from that. . . . We've seen that as something commercial vendors can handle. . . . Our mission is just to make those instruments available.

STEENBARGER: A lot of folks who are in the process of starting up groups are so very concerned about minimizing overhead and maximizing clinical hours. If they don't see an activity as immediately producing revenue, they're likely to shy away from it. As you point out, assessment is a classic example. These days, it's difficult to get the authorization for routine psych testing. . . . So a lot of groups are doing without.

MARUISH: I'll play the devil's advocate here. There's no reason that third-party payers should "take my word for it" about the benefits of assessment. Our profession allegedly is built upon some empirical basis of scientific investigation. Why haven't we demonstrated this? The onus should be on us to demonstrate that this does have value and we're not going to come to you and say, "Take my word for it."

[This is a worthwhile observation. Mental health services will be treated as a pure, price-based commodity unless they can be differentiated with respect to quality. This is a particularly acute issue for doctoral and medical practitioners, who aspire to premium reimbursements. One of the great advantages of collaboration is the ability to use the team structure to establish ongoing programs of quality assessment and improvement.]

CHAPTER SEVEN

Triumphs: Lessons from Successful Collaborations

The harder the conflict, the more glorious the triumph. What we obtain too cheap, we esteem too lightly; it is dearness only that gives everything its value.

—Thomas Paine, *The American Crisis*, No. 1

INTRODUCTION

In the preceding chapters, we have attempted to highlight tactics and tools that can guide successful collaborative practices. This final chapter illustrates how practices can triumph by employing these strategies. The following extended interviews are valuable case studies in success, well worth the study of readers. They illustrate that creativity, hard work, and business savvy can be combined to yield thriving and innovative practices that meet the challenge of mental health's future. They also bring to life the qualities that staff clinicians should seek in any of their affiliations.

The first study, with Bret Smith, MEd, LPC, of Relationship Enrichment Center, LLC, and REC Management, Inc., captures the triumphs of a network-model

> ### ☆ IN THIS CHAPTER
>
> - REC Management: An exemplary network-model practice
> - Value Behavioral Health's "Clinical Group" program: A model for MCOs
> - CPG Behavioral Systems: An exemplary staff-model practice
> - Common ingredients of successful collaborations

practice in a highly managed environment. Within a few years, Mr. Smith and his colleagues have built a small start-up group into one of the largest practices in the Southeast, covering more than 400,000 lives in at-risk contracts. Especially interesting is Mr. Smith's technological sophistication, which has allowed him to link more than 30 providers in a comprehensive online network that handles everything from provider communications to billing and data collection.

Our second study, with Julie Bigelow, former executive vice president of provider relations and now chief operating officer for public-sector programs at Value Behavioral Health, Inc., takes us to the managed care side of the aisle for a detailed look at the components of successful practices. Ms. Bigelow outlines the innovative "clinical group" model adopted by VBH, which takes the MCO out of a micromanagement mode and into the role of monitoring and managing quality. We believe that some variant of this clinical group model will become the norm in managed care settings in coming years.

Finally, our last study is with Jeff Zimmerman, PhD, of CPG Behavioral Health Resources, a decentralized staff-model practice of 17 clinicians. From a two-person start in 1985, Dr. Zimmerman and colleagues have built CPG into a statewide practice handling more than 1,300 new cases each year. CPG has introduced a number of innovations with respect to governance and human resource management, linking its far-flung staff in a cohesive culture.

At the end of the chapter, we identify common themes among the triumphs, suggesting possible blueprints for your own organization and yardsticks by which you might assess groups in your region. The interviews were conducted by Brett Steenbarger; annotated comments are by Simon Budman.

CASE STUDY I: RELATIONSHIP ENRICHMENT CENTER, LLC

The Relationship Enrichment Center, LLC, and its management services organization, REC Management, Inc., began from relatively humble and recent beginnings. The founders had no special training in practice management or business administration. Both were master's-level clinicians with few if any connections to managed care organizations, medical practice groups, or other large referral sources. In short, their group possessed no special or unusual advantages; everything was built from scratch.

The Relationship Enrichment Center, LLC, was founded by Bret Smith and Sonia Torretto in September 1991. The group has enjoyed phenomenal success. Two additional therapists joined the practice in Fall 1992; a fifth therapist was added in Spring 1993; and seven more therapists came on board by the end of that year. Since then, the group has added a psychiatrist, a psychologist, and further master's clinicians to reach a staff of more than 30 professionals. These professionals are housed in multiple locations, allowing REC to blanket the greater Atlanta area—and beyond.

Bret Smith, vice president of REC Management, Inc., the management services organization created out of Relationship Enrichment Center, and chief administrator of the center, generously shared time with Brett Steenbarger to describe the group and its approach to a major metropolitan marketplace. The resulting case study touches on a number of facets of group practice, from the lifestyle of managers to the process of assembling an information system.

Development of the Group Practice

STEENBARGER: Maybe you could describe a little bit about your group's growth and the factors behind its success to date.

SMITH: As principals, we felt that our combined experiences and diverse background would allow us to serve a broad spectrum of the community. Our philosophy was simple, "Put the client's needs first."

This commitment, along with our strong marketing and public relations skills, allowed the practice to grow. In the fall of 1992, when two other therapists joined the group, the need for larger office space allowed the practice to move into its present location in Marietta. By spring of 1993, the group had grown to five therapists. The Relationship Enrichment Center was already recognized as a preferred provider by the local community, hospitals, school system, Cobb County courts, attorneys, physicians, and several managed care organizations.

Our decision to be proactive with managed care organizations encouraged us to expand and open facility offices in Fayetteville [Fayette County] and Woodstock [Cherokee County] and bring on additional clinicians to provide services in these underserved areas. By the end of 1993, the group had grown to encompass a multispecialty team of 12 master's-level providers.

[A key element here is that of being proactive. We have seen well-positioned groups with excellent reputations fail because of a lack of proactive leadership. Someone in the group practice must be prepared to knock on the doors of potential customer organizations . . . like managed care companies . . . seeking referrals and contracts. Marketing is not a four-letter word; it is essential!]

In May 1994, the Lilburn office was opened and two additional clinicians joined the group. By this time, the combination of size and distance created a logistics problem which forced us to invest in a network computer system and database billing system, which allowed each office to communicate and centralize patient data directly on the server in the Marietta office. This also allowed the group to track outcomes data and centralize billing for the entire practice.

In 1994, the group incorporated by forming two companies. REC Management, Inc., was established to provide management support services, furniture, equipment, supplies, and facilitate communication between offices and clinicians. The "group" [Relationship Enrichment Center] was incorporated as a limited liability company with each clinician as an equal partner. REC Management, Inc., acting as "manager," holds a majority interest in the company.

By the spring of 1995, the Relationship Enrichment Center, LLC began offering a full continuum of services with the addition of a psychiatrist and a clinical psychologist. This allowed the practice to offer quality behavioral health services with office locations in five counties around metro Atlanta. A joint venture agreement with an area treatment center established an adult psychiatric intensive outpatient program [IOP] in Marietta. To date . . . we have established ourselves as a leader in the market, with over 90 contracts with MCOs and EAPs.

[For Mr. Smith and his group, location and breadth of services appear to be major competitive advantages. These have been achieved by expansion and strategic alliances.]

STEENBARGER: Tell me more about how your group is organized.

SMITH: The Relationship Enrichment Center is a Georgia limited liability company. REC Management, Inc., owns 52% of the company, and the remaining 48% is owned by its partners. Every clinician associated with the Relationship Enrichment Center, LLC, is a partner in the company. Upon joining the group, they pay a capital investment for their ownership share and then pay a monthly management fee to REC Management, Inc. Currently, there are two classes of membership in the Relationship Enrichment Center, LLC: facility members and satellite members.

Facility members are those clinicians who utilize an office suite managed by REC Management, Inc. These members typically work exclusively as providers to REC proprietary referrals. Facility members also depend on the manager to provide phone service, alpha pagers, utilities, and office amenities.

Satellite members are those clinicians who have their own private or group practices and desire to be part of a larger group. Satellite members enjoy the independence of private practice and the marketing support of the group network.

[The arrangement described here is relatively common among some of the group practices to which we consult. Typically, clinicians are required to pay a certain amount to become a partner or member of the practice. The range of charges for such membership or partnership varies greatly from group to group. We are familiar with ranges of cost from $2,000 to $25,000 or more. An important issue that must be addressed by the group practice is that of selectivity. Some practices basically "take all comers," while some are highly selective. Our own inclination is to advise clients to be more rather than less selective. The person you take into your group under these circumstances is becoming a business partner with whom you may continue in practice for many years. Selecting such individuals is a very important decision and cannot be taken too seriously.]

The Work of the Practice Manager

STEENBARGER: Could you describe your lifestyle as a practice manager? How much time is spent on the job? How much time is spent in direct service versus administration? Of your administrative time, how much is spent in internal management (clinical issues, billing matters, supervision of staff, etc.) versus external marketing?

SMITH: I tend to spend anywhere from 60 to 70 hours per week in direct work. Of this time . . . I'm averaging right now between 18 and 20 hours a week in direct service to clients as a therapist. That's a piece I enjoy doing and I feel I need to continue. The rest of the time tends to be spent in just practice management issues which may involve everything from office management, taking care of the billing problems that come up, and training of the therapists. I also maintain our computer system.

One of the things I do not spend a whole lot of time doing is overseeing the clinicians in our office as well as our satellite clinicians. Most of that is handled by our network director and our appointment coordinators. The appointment coordinators handle all incoming phone calls. They input data directly from the client into the computer system, as well as handle our billing and claims filing. If there's a problem they can't resolve, they come to me with it and I take it from that point on.

One thing that I tend to handle is practice management issues. If a clinician needs a particular okay or a definitive clinical answer regarding a contract or specifications of a contract, then I may handle that. An example of this might be [that] a clinician may call me with a client [who] is in current treatment that [the clinician feels] needs to be inpatient hospitalized. The [clinician] will give me the basic demographics and clinicals and from that I will work with the clinician and our care manager to make the best determination of the best means of treating that patient. If it's something that we feel that we can't resolve or if there's a particular billing problem that we can't resolve, at that point I go to our vendor and work with [the vendor] directly.

Probably in terms of external marketing, I spend anywhere from 3 to sometimes 7 or 8 hours a week. . . . This marketing will involve contacting those MCO companies as well as EAP companies that we have network contracts with. I try to contact these people at least once a month. Those that we do a lot of direct business with, I contact probably once a week and some of them I contact every other day, depending on where we are at that time.

[It is crucial that such marketing activities be maintained. "Passive marketing" (waiting for people to come to you because of your reputation, recognition in the community, and so on) is no marketing. Mr. Smith and his group obviously understand the importance of active, ongoing contact with customers. This is the hardest marketing to do and it pays off handsomely.]

STEENBARGER: How do you balance time for yourself and the family versus the business?

SMITH: As you might well imagine, working 60 to 70 hours a week does not leave a whole lot of extra time. I typically get into the office around 9:00 or 9:30 in the morning and I typically try to leave the office around 8 P.M. Most of the evening time is spent in direct client contact, so I tend to use my mornings for marketing and practice management issues. Time for my family is pretty much reserved. I rarely will see clients over the weekend unless, of course, it's an emergency, although I *am* on call 24 hours a day. At times when I'm with my family and don't want to be disturbed, I tend to forward all my calls to the on-call clinician, who can take care of just about every situation that might arise.

STEENBARGER: What are your sources of greatest satisfaction and frustration as a group practice head?

SMITH: I think my source of greatest satisfaction is when a company we're doing work with contacts us and lets us know or lets me know about the work that I or one of our clinicians has done with a client of theirs—particularly one that's been handled quite well, where they feel the client's needs were met in a very positive way. That makes me feel good, because I'm very proud of the clinicians we have and I try to stand up for them and support them and give them all the tools they need to do good work. I believe that our clinicians are very conscientious. They tend to always put the client's needs first, which is something I feel is very important in this age of mental health care. I believe the client needs to be the primary focus, as opposed to the dollar.

My greatest source of frustration is probably when we have trouble getting payment from our vendors! The biggest struggle that I tend to face as a practice manager is the problems we have with collection in terms of our claims filing and claims adjudication. It's amazing how unstructured and unorganized many of the firms are that we work with. They put tremendous amounts of high expectations upon us as well as tremendous pressures to perform at very high levels of efficiency and we are evaluated on a very regular basis according to our outcomes measures. It seems as though the quality which they demand continues to grow more and more difficult; at the same time, often when we are trying to resolve a problem on their end, whether it be getting back an answer from utilization review or case management or even claims questions, it's amazing how easy it is to get lost in the shuffle. . . . We view this relationship as a partnership. We do our job well, they do well. If they do their job well, we do well. So in every step of the way, we feel that we need to maintain good communication.

[Smith's complaint about slow payment is almost universal at the practices we visit. A number of the larger managed behavioral health care companies have recently improved their turnaround times on claims. Small businesses, in general, are

plagued by the problem of late receivables. Our suggestion in this regard is: "The squeaky wheel gets the grease." Call repeatedly. Find out who in the system is willing to be your ombudsman. Don't be reluctant to become something of a pest . . . a friendly pest. It's your money.]

STEENBARGER: What qualities do you feel are essential for a practice manager/ leader?

SMITH: Patience and a commitment to work. I have learned to be patient in this business. I've also learned how to take risks. That's a scary part. I try not to take a risk that I cannot afford to lose. If something is such a strong wager that I can't afford to lose, I rarely will take that risk. An essential piece for practice managers is that they have to make a commitment to the business. You cannot do this working 40 hours a week—**there's no way**.

I think it's very important too that the practice manager have very strong roots to the clinical practitioners. . . . In order to have the respect of the clinicians, you almost have to be a clinician. I think you need to be someone who has experience working with very difficult clients and someone who has had some success in dealing with very difficult clients.

STEENBARGER: How did you first get involved in practice management? Where did you learn the tricks of the trade, especially in the business aspects of the practice?

SMITH: Getting involved in practice management was not something that I realized I was doing until we brought on our third clinician. . . . This was something that Sonia did not enjoy doing, nor did she want to do it, so it pretty much fell upon me. So I began to learn from every source possible. I checked out books from the library, I read every magazine on practice management that I could find, I purchased books and manuals on practice management and developing a practice. I began to subscribe to a number of journals and newsletters to gain as much education as I could. I also started developing contacts in the field, other people who were doing similar types of arrangements with similar practices. And this is pretty much how I learned to do what I did. The rest was by trial and error.

Another thing we did very early on, we identified a very good attorney in the Atlanta area who worked with a firm that had a number of contracts and business relationships with mental health centers, as well as hospitals and university systems. This attorney and his team of attorneys were influential in helping to shape the direction of our practice, as well as the structure from a corporate perspective. We also were able to identify a certified public accountant who understood how a small business needs to operate. Eventually we outgrew his level of expertise by the third year and had to grow to a much larger CPA firm. This firm was very good at helping to direct us to bankers who were very interested in the type of business we had and gave us the type of funding we needed to further our practice.

As you might expect, we don't learn much about the business aspect of practice from our graduate school programs. This has always been something I've had a frustration with. If I could look back, I'd probably go back to school and pick up a second MBA degree. . . . I believe this would help me a lot in retrospect, looking at the decisions we've had to make and continue to make on a daily basis.

STEENBARGER: Could you give a rough sense of how the practice volume of REC has grown, along with the growth in staff?

SMITH: We have found that, particularly in the second and third year of our group, probably from 1992 onward, as we began to really strongly and aggressively seek to get on more and more provider panels, we've seen the volume of referrals begin to grow. . . . One thing that we have noticed is that once providers began to join us, the multiplicity of marketing began to play a role. We're hustlers. There's no question about that. You have to get out there and market yourself and that's a point that we make very evident to our clinicians. One thing that's very difficult is to find clinicians who are good at getting out and marketing their own programs. . . . That's one of the biggest problems that we have.

Right now, in terms of contracted lives that we have, we're somewhere between 420,000 and 475,000 lives that our group does based upon contract numbers that we have. . . . In terms of raw numbers, I know that most of my practice is managed care. I'd say 80%. Across the board, I'd say the providers in our group are seeing 70 to 90% of their business come from managed care. The rest seems to be a mix. Many of them do some consulting, some are involved in other business ventures.

The Structure of the Practice

STEENBARGER: Could you summarize your reasons for setting yourself up as an LLC?

SMITH: The LLC structure of a group is more of a partnership than a corporate structure. One of the advantages of having an LLC is that it gives us the flexibility of a partnership while . . . giving us the corporate veil. The corporate veil is very important to us right now, simply because of the liability risks that are incurred in any type of a group practice. A [unincorporated] group without walls is an accident waiting to happen. It's a very scary proposition in light of the litigation that we have seen just here in Georgia. So we felt very comfortable with this type of a structure.

The idea of the MSO is that we provide a centralized form of management to the LLC. Most corporations will have a board of directors, perhaps a president [and a] vice president. That's the role REC Management provides. We are the managers of that practice.

The advantage of this LLC arrangement is that we only have one tier of ownership. Everyone comes in at the same level, so we don't have different levels or different positions within that company. Everyone comes in at the same level whether they be an MD, PhD, or master's-level clinician. This is a real positive point for our group because it does help to keep us more unified and help to work on the esprit de corps. We don't have profit sharing for our provider–partners and they don't receive any monies at the end of the year, because the LLC primarily is a flow-through company. Whenever we send out billing, it goes out under the LLC tax ID number and all of our receivables come back into that company. These are automatically redisbursed to the providers. Providers receive 100% of all of their billable hours, with the exception of special contracts that we now have where the management company receives a small portion for administrative services.

This is all done under contract, so the providers accept these contracts if they choose to. If they don't choose to work under these contractual arrangements, they don't have to receive referrals from those contracts. That, again, is a choice each provider makes. Interestingly enough, we have some providers who choose *not* to be involved in certain contracts for various reasons. Some refuse due to the paperwork requirements, some may refuse to be involved in certain contracts because they don't like the level of compensation. So we accept that and we respect that . . . but at the same time assume no responsibility for their practice success or failure. That's something we've been pretty straightforward about since day 1.

STEENBARGER: Can a provider for your group be affiliated with other groups?

SMITH: All of our providers are independent contractors. . . . A provider can be a partner in our group and can also be affiliated with other groups or networks. We have established that the provider has no duty to this company, nor does the company have duty to the provider. Most of the providers in our group that are enrolled in managed care panels choose to do so via the group. There are some that were providers as individuals. Many of them, upon joining the group, have chosen to change their tax status with those companies in order to be part of the group. The advantage to them doing this is that they may have been a member of a company's panel for 2 to 3 years and never received a referral. However, if they come in through us, all of a sudden they begin to receive referrals, because we do receive a lot of referrals from these companies. There's no loss to them, since they get paid at 100% either way. The only difference is, if they do it through us, they can take advantage of our management information system.

We have been somewhat successful at getting new providers onto these closed panels. One of the main reasons has been . . . if the group is already on a panel, they will add a new provider, because it's not like they're adding a whole new system. They're just expanding a group that's already on their panel. . . . But that's not true of all companies. Many companies have not been interested.

STEENBARGER: Maybe you could clarify how REC Management, Inc., is compensated. You said earlier that practitioners were taking home 100% of their income.

SMITH: REC Management has a variety of income-producing avenues, chief of which is revenue generated through providing practice management and practice development for the Relationship Enrichment Center, LLC. . . . That brings in probably 70% of our operating revenue.

STEENBARGER: And what does that fee structure look like?

SMITH: The fee structure depends on which class of member they come in as, whether they come in as a facility member or a satellite member. A facility obviously needs everything provided: office, waiting room, computers, et cetera. That fee is less than $1,000 per month. Then the satellite member is a member that has their own office in a remote location or we can locate and put a provider in a regular, established office. Basically, all that provider needs to communicate with us is their own computer system and fax. At that point, they can join us as a partner. There's no duty to this company, but the beauty is that they only pay around $500 a month, because they don't need a roof over their heads.

[The method used by REC Management to generate revenues is not typical of all MSOs. Many MSOs charge participants a small fee of some type to help cover some of their operations but also participate in the larger revenue stream of the provider groups or individuals. Most take a percentage of revenues as their compensation. This supports the growth of the MSO and puts money back into infrastructure development. Under this arrangement, the MSO's compensation is directly connected with how well the participating groups or providers are doing. Although it is clearly working very well for Smith and his group, the biggest problem we see with REC's approach to compensation for the management company is that some unscrupulous individuals running such an MSO might bring more and more providers on board in order to increase the compensation of the MSO without having the business to support these providers.]

STEENBARGER: But they still get the benefit of your computer system.

SMITH: We have a standard list of services that we provide for that rate, which would include the 24-hour/7-day live service, the alpha page system, MIS connectivity, the software, computer training, et cetera: everything that would go along with practice management. The big key, of course, is the marketing.

STEENBARGER: Would it make sense to put a group of your best providers on a salaried basis, both from the vantage point of having more control over their practice and in terms of securing their loyalty and involvement?

SMITH: Absolutely. I'd love to be able to hire all of my clinicians and just put them on salary. I'd make a whole lot more money that way. We have clinicians making $60,000, $70,000, $80,000 a year. If I could pay them $25,000 or $30,000 to do the same work, I could retire in three years! (*Laughs.*)

Unfortunately, the state of Georgia passed a law—because we've unfortunately had a few unscrupulous companies that have been here in the past—called the self-referral law, effective January 1995. The law prohibits companies from having salaried people and independent contractors doing the same type of work. That's also a factor for the Internal Revenue Service, how they distinguish an employee. One of their . . . red flags would be . . . a salaried individual and an independent contractor that are doing essentially the same type of work. The IRS would tend to view them as employees.

STEENBARGER: That's a really good point.

SMITH: Your earlier question was about how we generate money for the management company; 70% of our income is generated through our management fees. There are additional services that must be provided for some of our proprietary contracts. These are high-volume, special contracts that we have with particular managed care vendors. Because of the additional requirements that these contracts require, we have had to expend additional monies [i.e., dedicated phone lines, particular reporting which calls for more man-hours, . . . special filing processes]. We have had in these contracts a special contract rate which goes to the management company, which goes to offset some of the costs of it. That is a minimal amount.

STEENBARGER: So there are a couple of different mechanisms for bringing money into the management company.

SMITH: The third method would be . . . public and private consulting. The management company offers contract management and consulting services to providers and practice groups.

Information System

STEENBARGER: Could you describe your information system? What kind of investment does a group need to make to develop an information system such as yours?

SMITH: Well, that's a big question, Brett! We, as we've grown, have tried to stay ahead of the curve in terms of our communication needs. We realized early on that when we work with a multiplicity of individuals in any organizational structure that communication is going to be the main problem area. We have tried to compensate for this by providing a number of systems to allow our providers to communicate.

At the base of this is a centralized, live answering service. We have relied on that as opposed to a voice mail system simply because of the advantage of talking to a live operator. The managed care organizations that we've worked with seem much more interested in a live answering service than in a voice mail system. It's extremely frustrating for them, particularly when a client gets a recording. They want to talk to a live person.

[In many of the larger systems to which we consult, emergencies are handled in off-hours by the associated partial hospitalization program (which functions during the evening and weekends as well). Voice mail for handling emergencies is not a reasonable alternative.]

Each of our providers is equipped with an alpha pager. This allows the answering service to actually type out a message to the provider, to give them succinct information, and for it to be immediately dispatched. We also have all the pages faxed each day to the Marietta office, so that we have a hard copy of every page that went out to the providers. We also have software on each computer that's loaded onto each provider's computer system. That, by the way, is a requirement of all satellite providers. They must have a computer—PC-based with a modem—on which we can install our proprietary software, allowing them to communicate with our network. We also have alpha software in house in which we can type out messages to the providers.

[Because] we have a network—we have local area as well as wide area network—we have e-mail. So each provider can log on to our network and retrieve the latest e-mail messages. We can send them out individually or can send out dispersed e-mail messages to every provider. We also have built into our e-mail certain instructions about billing procedures for certain contracts. So at any time if [providers have] a question, they can read what we've already uploaded onto the e-mail library and pull this information out. This seems to be working quite well.

[Because] every provider must also have a fax machine, I am able to type up updates from time to time or late-breaking news or information that everyone needs to be aware of and, via fax software on my computer, at 10 o'clock at night, I'll just have this sent out to every fax machine. The nice part about having a computer system, as you know, is that fax software can send the same fax to up to 1,000 or more fax machines one right after the other. So I'm able to keep them updated minute by minute through three different systems: through fax software, through e-mail, as well as through alpha page.

[Smith's move in the direction of making sure that his providers are not technologically challenged is valuable and necessary. We have seen network-model practices without fax machines, computers, or even typewriters in the clinicians' offices.]

STEENBARGER: How do you monitor provider performance?

SMITH: Basically, when a provider sees a patient through REC, that information is then put into our client database, our provider system. We use a brand of billing software called Therapist Helper. Each provider is responsible for inputting [his or her] patient information. If for any reason [providers] are having computer problems or are unable to log on to the network, can fax the information to Marietta. We have a secure fax line with confidentiality provided. They can fax information and then our office staff can input that information for them.

Once the information is on the computer, we are able to pull outcomes reports from these data. This is something I do on a weekly basis. I pull this information, print it out, and see a number of different reports, like the number of sessions and provider patterns for diagnosis. Interestingly, this came up recently [when] I pulled diagnosis and I found that there was one provider who used one diagnosis consistently with almost every client. [Once this was] brought to my attention, I was able to sit down with that provider and discuss this problem with [him]. I find it very unusual that a provider can see 30 different clients at random all with the same diagnosis! So, [once I questioned this], I was able to educate the clinician that these data were being collected and that [the clinician] needed to perhaps get on-going training in DSM-IV [fourth edition of the *Diagnostic and Statistical Manual of Mental Disorders*] diagnosing.

As far as documenting quality, this is something we're monitoring on an ongoing basis. We have clinical practice guidelines which outline formal quality assurance policy and procedures. These clinical practice guidelines are part of a required record-keeping module that all providers must adhere to if they are to continue as providers in this group. This will include everything from the initial assessment, gathering specific information in the patient charts, and also keeping it on the electronic database. [Because] at this point we do not keep progress notes on our computer database, we do require clinicians to maintain certain charting procedures. We also will do spot-checks of provider offices. We have a checklist of expectations that we have of providers . . . everything from signing their charts to using our standardized information forms. . . . If a provider fails to follow our forms or clinical practice guidelines, that provider will be automatically removed from the group. Fortunately, we've never had to do this.

One area that we are very concerned about is the fact that we do promise that we can offer an appointment for routine referrals within 72 hours. Most clients are offered an appointment within 24 hours, whether it be routine, urgent, or emergent referrals. We have found, though, that it is very difficult to document this information. We now have information that we are collecting, which basically stipulates what time the patient called. That is documented by the time the face sheet is entered, because we now have live entering of all face sheets. . . . The patient is offered a live appointment based upon the clinician's schedule in the computer system, and that clinician is paged immediately with that new referral. [Clinicians] must therefore respond back to the appointment coordinator indicating that they did receive the referral and that it is a done deal. Once that is confirmed, we close that case, in terms of new patient input. We are then able to track the time they called and the date they called, the time of the appointment they're offered, and the time and date that the appointment was accepted. If that falls outside of that 72-hour guideline, the clinician must make contact with that new patient prior to the scheduled appointment and gather basic data. Most of this involves risk assessment. This is documented on a special form and this information is kept in the chart.

STEENBARGER: How is billing handled in your group?

SMITH: Billing is handled in two different ways. For most of the accounts we have, these are just individual provider relationships. Each provider is responsible for inputting [his or her] own computer data. [Providers] can print out statements and they can print out claim forms. Each provider is responsible for [his or her] own billing. How they do it, how often they do it, how they track it—that's up to them. The computer system is fairly easy to learn and easy to manipulate. With a computer in their office, [providers are] able to log in any time, day or night, and download or print claim forms.

One thing that we do for our main contracts, however, is that the management company will provide the billing services. . . . We do that simply because we need to print and handle these claims in bulk. Most of the time we do our billing on a weekly basis for larger contracts. These may involve hundreds of HCFAs [forms from the Health Care Financing Administration], each time we send out a billing. With some companies, we are able to transmit claims electronically. This way we can generate the income back into the practice as expeditiously as possible.

STEENBARGER: Sounds as though you need a powerful system to handle all of these information needs.

SMITH: As far as our information system . . . I did a lot of research and previewed a lot of the software that was available at that time. . . . Our consultants recommended wholeheartedly that we start off with a Novell-based network. This provides the basic framework for any expansion we needed to make. This additional investment was basically handled via our line of credit with our bank. We sat down with our bankers and said, "Here's what we need. Here's how much money they predict we'll need to do it." We then secured the financing and invested in the system.

Initially we just started off with a local area network, Novell-based, with our client software. The software that we were looking at was always limited by whether it would work on a network. . . . We found at the time there was only one piece of software—this is the one we now use by Brand Software—which was network-capable. This was a big determining factor for us. There was a lot of independent-based software and PC-based software out there, but it was not set up to work on a network. We knew that was something we had to have.

We invested in our basic network software and computer system for our four facility offices and that ran somewhere around the $40,000 range. . . . We did this in 1994. By mid-1995 we made a second upgrade to enhance our wide area network capabilities. This is all basically software and computer systems that we add to our network. We added a new server, bringing us up to Pentium level, to give us the speed and file handling. It has the ability to handle up to 64 incoming phone lines, modem-based and digital (ISDN), so that all of our providers could be online simultaneously into the database. That's one of the advantages we have: 24-hour accessibility. They can log in and have access to all clinical data on their clients. We are able, via passwords and network security, to allow providers access to only their clients or to clients within their office based upon their log-in restrictions.

[Digital phone lines allow for a much more rapid transfer of information than is possible with conventional telephone lines and modems. They are also much more expensive than conventional lines and represent a meaningful investment in communications by REC.]

So far, to date, our computer system has probably cost somewhere in the vicinity of $80,000 with all the upgrades we have made. This has probably been the single most expensive component of our group practice. Reality is, it continues to cost money. The cost of maintaining a computer system is astronomical. It is like "the money pit"! That's where most of our funds tend to go. Because if the computer system is ever down, we're in essence out of business at that point. So that and our phone system are probably our two most critical components, because those are our lifeline.

Managed Care Contracting

STEENBARGER: If I could just switch gears quickly and ask you about managed care contracting in the greater Atlanta area: How much of your business is straight fee for service, how much is on a risk-sharing basis?

SMITH: Of course, you know we are a little unusual for the rest of the city. Are you wanting to know where Atlanta is or where we are?

STEENBARGER: Let's talk about your practice.

SMITH: OK. We have one fairly large contract that is for a modified case rate. I guess that's the best way to describe it. Instead of receiving a lump sum in the first session, it's spread out over the first three sessions, which is kind of a safety factor built in for the MCO. That way, if the patient only comes in one time, the [MCO is] not out a ton of money. . . . Probably 40% of the case rate is paid out after the first session and 60% is paid out after the second session.

STEENBARGER: And what does the case rate cover?

SMITH: The case rate basically covers full care and treatment for that patient.

STEENBARGER: Everything?

SMITH: Less the copay. The patient still has a copay.

STEENBARGER: When you say full treatment, you're talking . . .

SMITH: Outpatient mental health.

STEENBARGER: Chemical dependency?

SMITH: Yes, it covers all treatment for that episode of care including medication management, which we are at risk for. It does not cover any type of rehab or IOP or inpatient, just the standard outpatient treatment.

We have probably three other contracts that are standard case rate. That represents probably 65% of our business. Ten percent of our business is fee for service [managed care]. About 15% is full fee and the rest would be sliding scale. Most of those would be noninsurance coverage.

STEENBARGER: What are some of the challenges you've experienced in the process of negotiating these case rates?

SMITH: One is the fear of going at risk. Not so much from the clinical side, from the REC side, but the fear we're hearing from the MCOs who are concerned that, by going case rate and delegating risk or delegating care management, patients will be hurried through therapy in order to earn the greatest amount of money in the shortest period of time, that care will be compromised.

STEENBARGER: So, do you have some MCOs that absolutely *don't* want to work with you on this basis?

SMITH: Absolutely. That is correct. There are many of them that come in and say, "We want to work with you. Let's start with fee-for-service, let's track our outcomes, let's track your ability to respond, and then—as we develop that relationship—we'll get an idea over time as to utilization and, from that, we'll have a better idea of looking at aggressive cost pricing." The door is always open, they're always interested in finding a better mousetrap. But they're not very quick to jump right in to an aggressive risk sharing. In this day and age, you have to be very careful who you sleep with.

STEENBARGER: When you do have a company that wants to do the risk sharing, what have been some of the challenges you've faced?

SMITH: The biggest challenge for us is being able to find a company that really suits what we're looking for as a behavioral health partner. I feel real confident in our ability to respond. We have a pretty solid track record and currently have about a 98% patient satisfaction rating across the board with all companies. We don't distinguish patients by their insurer. Every patient that comes in is viewed as an individual.

But one of the concerns that we have is that we know what our cost to deliver service is, per unit of service, and we know how much it costs to treat a patient. Our concern is finding a company that will respond to us when we have a problem and one that will pay us in a timely manner. That's what we have found to be the biggest frustration to date: the filing systems and claims adjudication aspect of many of the managed care companies. Many of them are *horrendously* slow at paying and, unless you have an extremely solid financial backer, you can find yourself bankrupt in just a couple of months.

It has cost us . . . on the average, to bring on a contract of 100,000 lives about $12,000 to $15,000. That's not including salaries and time expended. Just actual cost . . . from the day we get the RFP to the day the contract is signed. That is quite costly.

STEENBARGER: What is that money going toward?

SMITH: Many are hidden costs. Travel fees, time to consult with attorneys, time involved with consulting with some of the consultants we used, time spent in negotiating with them, running surveys, running outcomes, running statistical analysis. All of this is involved in going into any type of contract that involves risk. You don't enter into those lightly.

STEENBARGER: Can I assume that, because of your problem with reimbursement, you would welcome a fully capitated arrangement with the right partner?

SMITH: To be honest with you, probably we'd be interested in going subcap initially, as opposed to a fully capitated arrangement. Until we have a real solid history of penetration with any company, we would want to at least go subcapitated until we have a good understanding of what our costs are going to be.

We already self-manage the practice. We monitor outcomes by therapist now and we have a real good idea of our clinical abilities and our clinicians' training. We also provide our own training to our clinical group. We offer quarterly trainings which we offer CEUs [continuing education units] for . . . in the goal of trying to continually monitor and improve our quality.

Clinical Training

STEENBARGER: Maybe you could talk a little more about the training that you offer. What are the areas you find the clinicians need the most assistance with?

SMITH: Primarily in terms of diagnosing accurately through DSM-IV training and probably solution-focused techniques. We have found that, to get beyond just the basic techniques of solution-focused, we need to bring in our people and hire our own professionals to come in and do the training.

STEENBARGER: And is that a major investment for REC?

SMITH: Actually it's not. Our cost per unit to bring in a consultant to train is much more cost-effective than having each of our clinicians individually come out and have to secure training on their own. If they take a day to go to a CEU and get training, they're not seeing clients that day. They're not generating revenue. . . . If we train everybody in one fell swoop in a half-day training, then basically I save money over the long haul. There's a break-even point in there somewhere in terms of how many clinicians are in a group. We couldn't do that if we were 5 therapists, obviously. Once we broke the 20-clinician barrier, the practice took on a whole new character . . .

STEENBARGER: In terms of the size of your practice, it sounds as though you've grown recently.

SMITH: In fact . . . we're now at 35 clinicians in 30 office locations. . . . It marks the first time that REC has opened offices outside the metro Atlanta area. We currently have offices in about 20 different cities in the metro Atlanta area.

STEENBARGER: So that poses some new management challenges.

SMITH: Yes it does. But in terms of communications—management information transfer—predominantly what it means is that we've had to pick up toll-free phone lines for modem connections. Basically the clinician now calls in via an 800 number to log in to our computer system, as opposed to it being a local call!

STEENBARGER: So you're covering a good part of the state now.

SMITH: Right. Also, it's a little easier as far as communication of information because everything is already streamlined now with faxes and e-mail. [It] is as if [those clinicians are] next door to us. They can log in, fill in electronic forms, they're on our system-wide e-mail, and we can fax information to these offices on a daily basis. We also have an 800 voice number for that clinician that we provide. That helps keep our costs down.

Summary of the Case Study

One of the first things that comes across when speaking with Bret is his ability to transcend the dichotomy between cost-consciousness and quality-consciousness. He is as proud of the fact that his group averages 4.6 sessions per client as he is of the group's 98% client satisfaction rating. He very sincerely believes that "placing clients' needs first" and keeping health care costs down are not contradictory.

A second outstanding factor behind REC's success is the group's devotion to technological innovation. By linking providers in multiple locations and towns, REC can cover a wide geographic area, rapidly expand to new markets, and collect outcome data on the fly, so as to manage the practice with up-to-date information. Even a cursory look at REC's Web page (http://www.recmgmt.com) suggests that this group is an innovator in its development of communications and information systems.

[The REC Management Web page is an excellent example of the uses of technology for marketing.]

Finally, it is clear that REC has arrived at a most innovative structure to meet the needs of clinical staff and management. Clinicians are independent contractors and thus can maintain their own offices and practices. At the same time, they become partners in the REC limited liability company. A willingness to invest resources in clinical staff development and facilitate intragroup communications through fax and e-mail capabilities sets REC apart as a true collaborative practice.

CASE STUDY II: VALUE BEHAVIORAL HEALTH, INC.

Value Behavioral Health, Inc., headquartered in Falls Church, Virginia, is one of the largest specialty managers of behavioral health services in the country. Starting as American PsychManagement, Inc. (APM), the company merged with Preferred Health Care, Inc., and became a division of Value Health, Inc. It now manages "carve-out" programs for large employers and health plans, as well as several states. All told, the VBH provider network has 38,000 individual practitioners, 2,500 programs and facilities, and 2,500 EAP affiliates.

Julie Bigelow, chief operating officer for public sector programs, has also served as executive vice president for provider relations. In those roles, she has worked closely with group practice development in the VBH network. She spent a morning with Brett Steenbarger to discuss VBH's new model of collaborative practice, which has already been implemented in 20 markets.

Models of Collaborative Practice

STEENBARGER: Perhaps you could talk a little bit about your model of group practice.

BIGELOW: We have two types of group practices. One is called regional care groups—and there's about 100 of those—and there's probably about 20 clinical groups at this point.

STEENBARGER: Could you differentiate the two: regional care and clinical groups?

BIGELOW: Regional care groups [RCGs] came out of the old APM anchor group model and primarily is the psychiatric component of care. Many of the benefit plans that we manage require patients to go through the regional care group for the highest level of benefit . . . for any type of program-based care. The psychiatrist conducts the evaluation to determine the appropriate level of care. We have a fairly broad continuum of care in our network, even including levels of care, such as group homes and recovery homes. . . . Historically I think we were the first company to look at alternative levels of care that were more community-based than facility-based. We continue to expand that approach, particularly for public-sector programs.

There's usually at least three psychiatrists [in a regional care group], but there's not a requirement that there has to be three. The requirement for the group is that it provides 24-hour availability to us over the phone, as well as response to our clinicians over an 800 line within 20 minutes of the contact. We typically have sold to clients that emergencies are caller-defined, so that if we have a mom with an adolescent locked in the bathroom being hysterical, it may not be truly a psychiatric emergency from a clinical point of view. But that family is in crisis and we call it an emergency. At that point, we call the regional care group. The psychiatrist calls us back and we provide him or her with the care information. The psychiatrist then responds to the family immediately. This occurs within 30 minutes of VBH's call to the psychiatrist.

Now that's in a situation where the family or the patient can wait by the phone. If it's truly life-threatening, we intervene and get [the patient] to the nearest hospital and then get the regional care group involved at the first reasonable opportunity.

RCGs are required to cover adult and adolescent psychiatry and chemical dependency and provide 24-hour availability. They also provide . . . medication evaluation and med management for us. They're assigned to a catchment area. These groups are typically in urban areas, where we have concentrations of numbers/beneficiaries.

STEENBARGER: And clinical groups?

BIGELOW: One important aspect is that we don't have [an RCG] in the same geographic location as we have a clinical group because clinical groups are an expansion of the [RCG] model. It includes all those components I just mentioned. It also includes the outpatient component. Clinical groups are assigned a catchment area by ZIP code. They are required to be multidisciplinary; it's a much more formalized model than the regional care group.

As we developed the model, we went back and looked at the community mental health center during the Kennedy era. We're really trying to develop something that is more well funded. So the clinical groups are multidisciplinary. They are also required to have a formalized intake and referral system. There are some differences for us operationally as well as for the groups. . . . We call the regional care group and Dr. Smith calls us back. That patient becomes Dr. Smith's. When we call the clinical group, we refer the patient to the group [as a whole]. We do provide them with more information initially than we do during the normal referral process to an outpatient practitioner. And they refer within their own groups to the practitioner that matches the patient's needs, requests, and our identified needs.

They need to have a formalized case management/utilization review system. We typically delegate the utilization review function to the group, which means that they don't have to turn in outpatient treatment reports to us. The group submits a claim; we pay it. The group needs to have an internal, formalized quality management plan and we also do a lot of monitoring of utilization. . . . In a monthly report, the group will be provided with information regarding how it is doing on all the quality monitors and there's quite a lot of them.

Quality Management

STEENBARGER: That's fantastic!

BIGELOW: They will see how they're doing on utilization. They will see how they're doing on [feedback]. If we get calls from members or providers in our system, we code all those calls and the groups get feedback on anything that comes in related to them. Of course, we're more concerned about quality of service and quality of care, but if there were administrative concerns around claims submission or they had a problem with us, that will also be included in the monthly report.

[When Ms. Bigelow says that VBH provides a lot of information to Clinical Groups, she is quite serious. She forwarded a copy of the forms from a typical monthly report. In all, there were more than 50 pages of feedback, covering such domains as "clinical indicators," "medical records," "response time/access standards," "patient satisfaction," and "quality of care and quality of service." An interesting facet of the feedback is that each clinical group's results are statistically compared to those of other clinical groups to identify outstanding or deficient performance. Clearly, VBH is investing considerable resources in the monitoring of quality.]

STEENBARGER: Julie, I'm hearing the word "quality" again and again. How much has this clinical group arrangement been designed to meet the demands and needs of NCQA?

BIGELOW: A whole lot of it.

STEENBARGER: Because there's a huge overlap.

BIGELOW: There *is* a huge overlap. The quality indicators, I think are unique to us. They are things that most people in the healthcare world would be concerned about. They have to do with [such things as] access. We have an external firm that we retained that [does access audits]—this is usually an issue with the groups, but it's been pretty fascinating: [It is] one of the tools that we've seen the groups use and make internal changes to do better with. We have clinical scenarios that we've developed. Lay people at this external firm call up and pose as patients.

STEENBARGER: That's really interesting!

BIGELOW: They rate the call according to criteria. We share all the criteria with the group ahead of time. There's nothing that's a secret. Those scenarios are routine, urgent, and emergent. They go so far as to make the appointment. If it's an emergency scenario, then they call *right* back and say that it's a test call and then the routine appointments are canceled within an appropriate time period, so the group can use that time for a patient. That's been a fairly contentious component of working with new groups; however, the information has been *extremely* valuable and we continue to do it. As they do well on the audits, then we back off on the frequency of those calls. They know what the parameters of that are, so they try to get themselves up to speed.

STEENBARGER: Do you have among your quality indicators outcome assessments? Are you looking at change on clinical dimensions?

BIGELOW: We have a couple of things. One is called the Life Role Function Scale.

It's a scale that a patient and the provider evaluate. It's a Likert scale: How am I doing with my occupation, my marriage, with school, et cetera. That's done by the provider and the patient at the beginning and the end of treatment, so we can begin to see some comparisons. We are beginning to roll out a more formalized outcomes program. We're going to pilot it with one of our groups out in California very soon.

We also do medical records audits. We're looking to see that the assessment is appropriate, that the treatment plan matches what the assessment is finding. We focus a whole lot on assessing chemical dependency issues. We've found over time and have seen in internal and external audits that mental health practitioners often don't pick up substance abuse issues . . . so we focus very heavily on that.

The other thing is coordination of care with the primary care doc and internal to the group. One of the advantages with the group is they have a core of psychiatrists with various types of expertise. The outpatient practitioners can quickly refer, they can get a psych consult, they can get a [medical evaluation]; when it's working well, it's a very collegial atmosphere, a multidisciplinary approach to care. So patients aren't having to get bumped back and forth to us for another referral to another practitioner. There's much more continuity of care between inpatient and outpatient and between practitioners than we can facilitate.

STEENBARGER: And I'm hearing a lot more delegation on your part, with the utilization management functions, with the coordination functions. You're delegating to the multispecialty groups and you're functioning in the auditing role.

BIGELOW: Yes.

STEENBARGER: And in a developmental role, in terms of giving feedback to these groups and keeping a scorecard.

BIGELOW: Yes. It has really worked well. I think there *are* areas where it doesn't work and those tend to be smaller communities . . . where the community hasn't gotten to a group model yet. And for certain kinds of practitioners [who] went into the field because they wanted to have an independent practice and they have certain ideas about what is appropriate care—it doesn't work for people like that. But people who have been trained in a background where they worked within a team atmosphere, they love it and they see the benefits of it.

Group Practice Finances

STEENBARGER: One question I have in terms of the delegation is: Are you also trying to nurture these groups along toward greater levels of risk sharing, financially?

BIGELOW: In California, we have some creative financial models. We capitate the groups for inpatient professional fees and the medication evaluations and med management. Part of that is when . . . the groups perform that regional care group function, those are pieces we can predict and control in a catchment area. . . . On the outpatient side, we've typically sold really, really, open access, so patients don't have to go to the group, they don't have to go to any particular place based on where they live. They don't choose a group or choose a catchment area. In some cases, they don't even need to call us for a referral. As long as they go to a network provider, it would be covered. . . . That way, it's been a "leaky" referral system and we haven't been able to capture that whole catchment area or that whole group. But we have been able to ramp up the referrals to the group over time and really provide a choice to the patient within a group. . . .

In California, we do set utilization targets and quality targets. That's the other piece of this. When we set utilization targets, there is a chance to get a bonus, but you can't get your bonus unless you do well on the quality.

STEENBARGER: I see. So it's a withhold kind of arrangement.

BIGELOW: Well, it's not even a withhold. We just cough up money! (*Laughs.*) We don't do withholds. So we do that in California even on the outpatient side. We're beginning to run into much more HMO business, where a model like this fits very nicely.

STEENBARGER: In terms of this issue of getting patients to the group, the issue of open access, and working more exclusively with the groups, in general, what percentage of patients would you say in a given catchment area would end up in the clinical group, as opposed to the individual provider network?

BIGELOW: Yeah, that's a great question and it's a little bit of a squishy number. I don't know the current number. I know that when we implement a group, there are, of course, a lot of patients already in treatment and maybe in treatment within the group. Those cases we don't do anything with. We let them run out; we let them be managed however they need to be managed. If a practitioner in the group has a current case, we tell the group that they can start to manage that, but they need to honor absolutely any previous certifications and we have to have absolutely no complaints about that case, about that provider, or from the patient's family. That's worked pretty well.

So those cases run out and then, as we have the opportunity to make new referrals, we try to get those into the group. There's a couple of issues around that. First thing is, we let callers know that we have a multidisciplinary group that really can meet all their needs that they have specifically about when they're going to be seen and what kind of background of practitioner they want to see and what they think their needs are. When we make the referral to the group, we tell them all of that and that's one of the things we measure around access. So if [a group] can't meet that need, [the group has] to give the patient back to us and we find somebody in the open network that can meet that need. . . . It took us in California, where the model's been going about 3 years, a *very* long time to ramp up the referrals—much longer that we had hoped. And I would imagine we're probably at about 40%. That's a real guess.

STEENBARGER: That's very significant business, if you're working with some large employers or you're working with a state.

BIGELOW: Yes, absolutely. We figured out that we have probably the opportunity to make a referral about 50% of the time, because of . . . the open access issue. The business is beginning to change and the employers are saying, "How could we get better control over utilization and quality?" and we say, "Well, we could provide this to you, but we're going to limit the number of providers that are available." We're beginning to see that trend. So we're hopeful we can ramp up more referrals.

STEENBARGER: What's your thought on the vertical integration issue? We have some behavioral MCOs that are actually going out and either forming or buying behavioral group practices. Is that something VBH has contemplated? What are your thoughts and feelings about that?

BIGELOW: We have contemplated buying groups and we have decided that that's probably not a good idea. . . . We do a clinical group contract that has different requirement. It's a much closer relationship, much more frequent communications, than an individual practitioner or even an independent group . . . could ever hope to have from a big organization. So I think it's a very collegial relationship we try to foster and we think we're getting the benefits without owning the group. We also think, at this point anyway, that the group needs to have other business and not be locked into us.

As far as the facility and program components, we historically contract separately with programs and facilities in a catchment area. We do that usually on an all-inclusive basis or per diem. Some case rates where it makes sense, or maybe per diem up to a max: that sort of thing. We think it creates a sort of healthy tension.

[Some behavioral health care companies have attempted to form or buy their own clinical practices. These schemes have not gone very well. The major problem is that when a practice is "owned" by a managed care company it becomes identified with that company and other MCOs do not make referrals to them. From our point of view such an arrangement (i.e., linking group practices and managed care companies) is probably untenable. A possible exception would be group model HMOs, in which an HMO with a strong regional business can secure an adequate referral base.]

STEENBARGER: So is that continuing with the clinical groups, separate contracting with facilities and outpatient groups?

BIGELOW: Yes. Groups manage their own patients within a facility, but the facility has a recourse to come back to us if the group wants to discharge somebody too soon. So we . . . look at their utilization and how we could guard against that. . . . I think probably in an HMO environment, we're going to have to figure out how to contract with an entire system.

Group Development

BIGELOW: There's another piece of this that I want to talk to you a little about, because I think it's one of the components that really makes this a go: We assign a field case manager to the group. This is somebody who's not on the phone conducting traditional UR [utilization review]. This is somebody who's out and about in [his or her] catchment area, pretty much full-time. [These field case managers] come into the office for meetings and clinical rounds and that kind of thing, but for the most part work out of their homes. We set them up with a system inside their home and confidential filing cabinets. Typically, they are very seasoned in the mental health field, ideally [people] who live in the community that they're serving. They act as liaisons between the facilities and group. . . . The field case manager meets with the group and says, "What facilities are you using now? Where do you think you have some needs?" They go out to our contracted facilities in the catchment area and meet with the UR staff and make sure they know our policies and procedures, explain the clinical group model and how that might be a change from what they're used to. The group may identify, "We don't have enough structured outpatient programs and we heard about this one over here." The field case manager will do a site visit and initiate provider relations to do the contracting and credentialing if it seems appropriate.

They also—and this is one of the biggest pieces—teach the group how to do its own UR. A lot of the providers, although they've worked with managed care for a long time, if [they] look at internalizing this process, it's somewhat different.

STEENBARGER: *Very* different.

BIGELOW: The groups are required to use our clinical criteria. The field case manager attends the UR meetings that the group holds in order to provide technical assistance. As the model evolves, the group doesn't require nearly as much technical assistance in the UR area. The field case manager also helps identify high-risk cases and, ideally over time, the group is identifying their own high-risk cases and notifying us, which we're beginning to see happen. It becomes much more of a collegial atmosphere. Peer review pretty much goes away. At times for the high-risk cases, the group requests peer review because they're wondering what options might be available. The field case manager typically knows more about community resources than our phone people and offers community-based options as integral components of the treatment plan.

☞ LOOKING AHEAD

Can there be a collaborative spirit between managed care firms and practitioners?

    Martin Klein, PhD, offers his views in Reader's Resource 7.1 at the end of this chapter.

STEENBARGER: What I take away from this is that you are working with the groups in a mentoring function and really trying to get away from some of the adversarial relationships that providers perceive with managed care organizations.

BIGELOW: And we're trying to get away from micromanagement. Our goal is to meet NCQA requirements, and it is very difficult. But we're not micromanaging each case. We're letting the practitioner and the group be much more independent in their decision making around the treatment plan. They don't have to deal with Suzy today and Jane tomorrow and another person the next day depending on the case they have. They have much more administrative support and clinical support in the field case manager, with someone they really know.

    One of the stories I like to tell [is about] one of our field case managers in California [who] is an absolute delight. I wish I could clone her. One of her groups called her up and said, "This isn't a VBH patient, but I know you can really help us! Could you just spend five minutes and tell us what you'd suggest for this patient?" And I thought, "That says a lot."

Becoming a Clinical Group

STEENBARGER: In terms of what a group needs to do to be one of these clinical groups, how multispecialty is multispecialty? Does the group need to cover all the pieces: child, adolescent, adult, multiple levels of care like IOPs?

BIGELOW: All of the practitioners, yes. We look at . . . the ratio of providers. It's kind of a moving target; very difficult to predict how many social workers you'll need, how many bilingual people you're going to need, that kind of thing. So we do an analysis of what the group has, the locations [the group is] in. We meet with and work with the [group members]. We look at the cultural needs of the given area. One group may have a lot more need for cultural diversity than another, depending on our population and, in general, the population in that region.

    As far as the levels of care, when it gets into structured programs, we're basically contracting separately for those programs. Some of our groups are developing internal IOPs, but what we try to do is support them with the right program-based network in place in their catchment area. We give them information as to what's out there in the network and they give us feedback about their needs. So we work together.

On the practitioner side, they need to have 24-hour availability; they need to have people in the right locations. If we want to use the group and [it doesn't] have a broad geographic area, then we probably won't give the group as big a catchment area, because access is an issue.

[Groups] need to be a formal legal entity and, to the extent that we're delegating case management . . . they need to have case management insurance that covers them for that. That's usually a significant expense for them, the biggest initial expense.

STEENBARGER: Do you have a ballpark on what that will run a typical group?

BIGELOW: Typically, it depends on how many practitioners you have, so it varies a lot. I'd say $20,000 to $30,000.

STEENBARGER: How large would you say your average clinical group is in terms of the number of providers?

BIGELOW: I'd say anywhere between 30 and 100 providers.

STEENBARGER: 100! So you're dealing with some mega-entities.

BIGELOW: Yes. Typically our groups have been IPAs. We don't make that mandatory, but it seems to be what's evolved.

STEENBARGER: So they might be structured as networks themselves to get the diversity by geography.

BIGELOW: Yes. The other piece besides the centralized intake and referral [is that] they need to do centralized billing. Bills come to us. We have those practitioners all coded as clinical group providers. That's how we know we're going to pay them, even though we didn't do the review.

Demands and Challenges for Practitioners

STEENBARGER: One of the things I'm hearing between the lines is that the demands that NCQA places upon you inevitably become demands upon the groups.

BIGELOW: Absolutely.

STEENBARGER: Because the groups have to work with you to achieve those goals.

BIGELOW: Yes, absolutely. And I would say that's true in general. Providers are concerned about their reimbursement rates. They feel in general, aside from groups—but groups too—that they're having to do more for less, that things are getting to be a pretty tight squeeze and it's true for managed care as well. It's not only NCQA, although that's a big piece of it. The employer groups, the consultants that bring these contracts to us, are demanding more and more and more for a lower price. Things go out to bid just based on price.

The whole industry is feeling that and I think it's important for providers to understand that they're a component of this whole thing and, yeah, they are. They're going to experience this.

STEENBARGER: What would be your advice to behavioral providers who may be thinking about forming groups or expanding the groups they already have to better position themselves to work with organizations like yours?

BIGELOW: Well, the first thing, I think, is to recognize that the historical way of doing business is changing for all of us and that the requirements are going to be a little steeper. Recognize that they need to develop a formalized model. That's not just sort of getting together as a group and saying, "We can give you 24-hour coverage." That approach isn't going to work any more.

Providers really have to decide if they're in this for the long haul and whether or not they can sign up for something that is much more interactive at their level with each other. If they want to be independent, then they shouldn't even think about this, because this isn't an independent way of working. . . . This is my feeling. To the extent that they develop a formalized model and they can demonstrate value, they're going to be around for a long time. They're going to be the providers of choice. It's a huge paradigm shift for a lot of providers. That means you have to invest in it and realize that you might not get your investment back for some time.

Summary of the Case Study

At the time we scheduled this interview, we did not anticipate making it one of our case studies, especially as it did not feature a practice organization per se. Several minutes into the talk, however, it became clear that the VBH clinical group model is a signal event for collaboration. It is significant, because—for the first time—it places quality on a par with cost in the management of care. Furthermore, it does so in a manner that is data-based and collegial.

The clinical group model is also noteworthy in its removal of the managed care organization from the "micromanagement" mode. The idea behind the model is that clinicians should manage the care of individual patients while the MCO assists with the management of overall quality and efficiency. This is a major philosophical shift. For the first time, it appears possible that behavioral health can be managed by data, not solely by the subjective impressions of clinicians or cost concerns of MCOs.

Finally, the clinical group model is significant in its attempt to establish collaborative working relationships between providers and managers of care. The innovation of the field case manager suggests that VBH is willing to devote real resources to helping groups learn how to manage care and document quality. Julie clearly articulated the "team" nature of the work demanded by the model. It is meaningful that she considers providers to be part of the VBH team—not opponents!

CASE STUDY III: CPG BEHAVIORAL HEALTH RESOURCES

Jeff Zimmerman, PhD, is one of three principals for Connecticut Psychological Group, PC, which recently expanded its name to CPG Behavioral Health Resources. The group began in 1985 as a two-person practice covering two cities in Connecticut and has rapidly grown into a statewide collaborative practice, with 17 full-time staff covering seven locations. Dr. Zimmerman recently took a Friday morning to speak with Brett Steenbarger about his group, its evolution, and its unique approach to practice management.

CPG's Model of Group Practice

STEENBARGER: How are your offices structured? Are they offices or buildings that you acquire or do you have the practitioners setting up their own practices in their own offices and then linking to the group somehow?

ZIMMERMAN: They are wholly owned by the group—wholly rented by the group. When we began the practice in 1985, one of our visions of the future was the practice was going to be what we call a "true group practice." There are many ambulatory practices in mental health and in medicine that really are a conglomeration of either subcontractors or . . . separate, individual practices under a common name. That was something that we were very much looking to steer away from. So these seven offices all function as part of the practice, participate in our outcome studies, and are all part of one mental health delivery system. It's really a decentralized practice model, as opposed to a centralized practice model.

STEENBARGER: Maybe you could talk more about your reasoning in wanting to be what you call a "true group practice," as opposed to a network-style practice.

ZIMMERMAN: Well, in 1985 our feeling was—and still is—that, in terms of trying to enhance outcome and ensure quality, there needed to be consistency built into the practice. . . . Everything we've learned and experienced tells us that, just like in any profession, quality assurance is a very important aspect. To provide quality, and especially to provide quality in multiple locations, where there are going to be times when the supervision is lighter, you need to have some basic level of consistency. To hire a number of people who have as many different ways of doing things because they have different practices with different philosophies about treatment and outcome would not create a culture and environment that was consistent with our long-term goals.

Compensation of Clinical Staff

[The compensation model used at CPG is one of the most sophisticated we have seen. Clinician compensation represents an enormous issue at many of the group practices we

have visited. On the one side, many practices operate on a straight salary arrangement. We have some concern about this model in that there are no particular incentives for productivity. Most of these programs become highly expensive over their lifetimes and non-competitive in the current environment. On the other side are models where the clinician is paid a percentage of what he or she brings in. Usually this percentage is between 40% and 60%. The problem with this model is that compensation can be very low and there is no clear cash flow for the clinician. The model described here by Dr. Zimmerman seems to have some of the useful elements of both models. We have seen some similar creative thinking about this issue in several other programs to which we consult as well.]

STEENBARGER: That makes a lot of sense. In terms of how your staff is connected to the group, are they paid on a salaried basis or are they paid on a per-unit-of-work basis?

ZIMMERMAN: Both and neither. . . . We've instituted a system where we wanted to keep a little bit of the best of both worlds. The best of the world where you know your income is relatively stable, as opposed to a percentage split, which you see in many practices, where—especially for a new person coming in—the first week you make $1.98! . . . That [wasn't] a model we wanted to pursue either. It also, we think, leads to a lot of intragroup competition, in the sense that "every referral that comes in, I've gotta take no matter what." And there are times when it really makes sense for a certain clinician *not* to take a referral and to pass it to another clinician who is perhaps more skilled in that area, who may do a better job with that patient. That's good for the whole practice.

So we've instituted a system where there's a base salary—actually it's a base draw, that would be more appropriate. There's an expectation each clinician sets for himself or herself in terms of what the target for the year will be.

STEENBARGER: Target, in terms of billable hours?

ZIMMERMAN: No, dollars collected. Number of billable hours is becoming more and more meaningless. For example, here in Connecticut, the range of what you would collect, probably on the lowest side, is between $35 and $45 for an hour of psychotherapy up to whatever your maximum fee is. Anywhere in between. That's a pretty large range. Billable hours, if you're not collecting copays, if you're not submitting your weekly billing logs or what have you, can be very distant from what you actually bring in.

STEENBARGER: Good point.

ZIMMERMAN: So what we look at is the actual income that someone brings in. Instead of negotiating salaries every year . . . now each clinician sets [his or her] own target. They say, "This is how much I anticipate bringing in." The target is based essentially on three numbers. It's based on what they want their draw to be, what the FICA/Social Security match would be to that draw . . . and what their expense share would be.

Each year we have a budget. We figure out, not only what our expenses are expected to be, but how many clinical FTEs we anticipate having over the course of the year. We then divide and are able to have a number that represents the cost of running the practice per FTE. Those costs are rents and phones and malpractice insurance, profit-sharing contributions, as well as administrative and secretarial salaries. The only numbers that aren't in the expense share are the clinicians' salaries, because those are the draws. So each clinician can determine how much income [he or she wants] to make.

STEENBARGER: I see. And is each clinician actively engaged in drumming up business then?

ZIMMERMAN: Some more than others. We have a system where, if you bring in more than your target, you get a bonus every quarter. If you bring in less than your target, there's a reconciliation. So some people are really excited about drumming up business and are very active in being out there, looking to build their caseloads and other sources of business besides caseloads, while other clinicians say, "Look, all I want to do is see patients." The practice in many of our locations is at the point where the community knows us by name, not just by clinician. . . . There are many referrals that come to the group at large which can, if clinically appropriate, go to a clinician [who's] not out there marketing aggressively.

In terms of origination [of referrals to the group as a whole], we began with some very complex formulas for establishing bonuses. They were close to correlation equations, where there were weightings on different factors related to performance. . . . What we found each year was that the equation never seemed to fit and that using the system that we had in place never seemed to feel right in terms of recognizing enough of the contributions of a particular staff person relative to the others. . . . So we went to the other side of the continuum and decided that we would give a discretionary bonus each year if the practice was successful; that is, if there were monies left over at the end of the fiscal year to allow for a discretionary bonus. And that would be based on a number of factors, but it would be more subjective and less an illusion of objectivity! So somebody who has built a caseload in an office, for example, and developed a significant referral base, well that would obviously be looked at as a valued behavior and, if there were monies left for a discretionary bonus, that would certainly be something to consider. But there are other things to consider as well in the discretionary bonus that may not be directly measurable in terms of revenue that was immediately generated.

STEENBARGER: Would one of the bases for the discretionary allotment be performance on quality measures?

ZIMMERMAN: Yes, absolutely. If somebody was alienating half [his or her] caseload, that would outweigh a lot of other things that [he or she] might have done that were pretty good!

STEENBARGER: So it sounds like the discretionary payment would really be a profit-sharing mechanism.

ZIMMERMAN: It *is* a profit-sharing mechanism. I'm not saying profit sharing in terms of IRS types of profit sharing—we do have a profit-sharing plan as well. And we also have a 401(k) [retirement plan] that we initiated for voluntary contributions. Additionally, at the end of the fiscal year, if there's money left over, there's 3 ways that money gets distributed: 1 is the discretionary bonus, 2 is the partners [shareholders] determine how much of the monies left over are going to go into the profit-sharing plan and three is how much is going to profits for the partners. . . . The profit-sharing plan is not at all based on performance. It's based on income—salaried income, the draw—and it's based a little bit on age. It's weighted so that people who are closer to retirement are able to get a little bit more of a percentage than people who are further away from retirement. You also have to qualify in terms of years of service. It's not at all based on performance.

The distribution to the partners is based on years of service in the firm. We had given that a lot of thought as well. Should it be based on how much income each of us brought in, should it be based on our own caseloads, on our own performance statistics? The principals are not on the clinical compensation system. They're on a straight salaried system. We distribute the profits based on length of tenure in the firm as a partner. The rationale is to avoid competing with each other. We made the assumption that all of us were doing professional activity that was in the best interests of the firm and that we wanted to share in that equally.

STEENBARGER: You've obviously placed a lot of time and effort in the human resources aspect of your practice.

ZIMMERMAN: Yes we have. We bought our own consultation over the years and we've consulted to other practices, which is always a learning experience in itself. We've talked to many, many other practices over the years and have also worked in other places. Most of us of have been frustrated significantly in other places where we worked and that's why we don't work there any more! We've tried to incorporate some of the best elements of a private practice environment with the best elements of an institutionally affiliated environment.

[When, in a separate interview, I (S.H.B.) asked Dr. Zimmerman what he thought the most important key to success was in developing a group practice, he indicated: "Get consultation when you need it. Don't try to reinvent the wheel." This is obviously what he and his colleagues have done in developing their compensation system.]

The Economics of the Group Practice

STEENBARGER: Do you find that this compensation system gives you a cost structure that might be meaningfully higher than in a network practice, where folks are independent contractors and where you wouldn't be paying the fixed salary, FICA, et cetera?

ZIMMERMAN: Yes! In terms of bringing people into the practice. That is often an issue. I would say there are two issues if someone were looking to join our practice . . . compared to having your own solo practice or being networked in a network type of affiliation. One is the expense share. Our expense share *is* higher than it would be if you were running your own solo practice. However, you get a lot more. You're not doing your bills on Saturday morning on your kitchen table. You're in a structure that is growing, that is well recognized in the communities that it serves, that has the ability to get contracted work in managed care . . . and that has a level of security and growth potential. It costs more to operate that and maintain it.

STEENBARGER: Roughly how high would you "guesstimate" the expense share to be?

ZIMMERMAN: We've had this system in place for two full years and it's run between $60,000 and $63,000 per FTE. It went down last year. I don't know what it's going to be this upcoming year.

The other downside to someone joining our practice is the issue of autonomy . . . because you give up autonomy to be part of the team.

STEENBARGER: Let me reframe my question about competitive advantage and disadvantage, because I really had something different in mind. Let's say a managed behavioral health care organization comes to your region and puts out an RFP. They're writing a large book of business [obtaining business] in your region and they want to work on a case rate basis or a subcap basis. They're going to ask you to bid on that contract and you will be bidding against other groups. Those other groups may be organized in ways that don't require them to pay fixed salaries and FICA, if they're working with independent contractors.

ZIMMERMAN: We have a competitive advantage.

STEENBARGER: How do you see that?

ZIMMERMAN: Because it's a draw more than it is a set salary and there's a reconciliation against when a target is not met, the practice itself is at less risk than if it was all a straight salary. We believe we're at a competitive advantage as opposed to a network because of the way we're structured. When an MCO looks at us, they are looking not only at managing our 17 clinicians, but we also have a joint venture with a major psychiatric practice that has approximately 30 clinicians. So between us, we're approaching 50 clinical staff. The networked group that comes in has to manage 50 clinical practices with perhaps separate forms, with perhaps separate call procedures . . . and with perhaps 50 different ways of providing clinical care. When we do an RFP with our joint venture partner or we do an RFP on a smaller project ourselves, it's one. Even in our joint venture, we have one set of clinical forms that we use so the charts are all going to look the same. We are building a management information system and our plan is, down the road, we'll be able to be computer-linked in any office—theirs and ours—so that if a patient is seen through the system in one town by a psychiatrist and then 10 or 15 miles away by a clinical social worker, they'd have access to each other's information. That's how it should be done, with, of course, appropriate releases or informed consent. One of the places where treatment falls apart is in communication, especially with difficult patients that you're trying to keep out of the hospital. The management of the clinical information becomes important.

Staff Development

ZIMMERMAN: One of the hallmarks of our practice, since we began, has been our clinical staff meetings. That's a tremendous investment financially, in terms of having a meeting that's an hour and a half or two hours long every week that everybody attends. We do that regionally, so not everybody is driving across the state. Those meetings, besides handling some administrative issues that come up in the course of a week, are focused on clinical care and are opportunities in a safe environment—a no-rank environment, if you will—to get input on cases and sometimes to brag about a case!

STEENBARGER: Each of your sites has its own clinical staff meeting?

ZIMMERMAN: We do it regionally, since some of the sites are staffed less intensively than other sites. . . . That's another competitive edge: the exchange of information about cases. . . . We can staff the case, come up with a treatment plan, get input from our colleagues. It's wonderful to have seven or eight people sitting with you while you discuss a case.

STEENBARGER: That's a wonderful point you're making. It's interesting to me how you perceive it and how different that is from other groups I've talked to. You're dedicating a good amount of staff time when you multiply a couple of hours by the number of staff that you have.

ZIMMERMAN: It's about one person for the whole year. It's like hiring a psychologist or a clinician and just saying, "Sit here!"

STEENBARGER: Exactly. That's a very significant investment, and you see that as a competitive advantage. I think some other group would say, "Oh, my gosh! Here's a needless cost center we can eliminate!" By dedicating resources toward quality, you see yourself as being in a better competitive situation.

ZIMMERMAN: Yes we do. . . . In fact, one of the managed care companies wants to come in periodically and do clinical staff meetings with providers. So? (*Laughs.*)

STEENBARGER: Right! Been there, done that!

ZIMMERMAN: One of the little examples that we've often used when somebody new comes into the practice—even before managed care was so strong in Connecticut—was, "Pretend that you're writing a check for the work you just did out of your personal checking account. Based on the note that you just wrote for the work you just did, can you justify in your own mind the value of the work? Was it worth the full fee that you just wrote out of your personal checking account. . . . Am I aware of what I'm doing and why I'm doing it?"

Joint Venture

STEENBARGER: Maybe you could describe a bit more about your joint venture and how that came to be?

ZIMMERMAN: Sure. It's been almost 4 years now that we have been working on this. Quite some time ago, we were approached by a major psychiatric hospital in the area. . . . They had come to us after having researched us and a number of other practices to begin a dialogue about working together. And through that dialogue, we determined that it made sense for us to try to position ourselves in a way where we could obtain managed care contracts to provide a full spectrum of services that neither of us could provide individually. They couldn't provide the outpatient care in as diverse a way throughout the state as we had been [doing] and, of course, we couldn't provide all the programming—especially for the more seriously impaired patient—as they could. . . . They also introduced us to [their] medical group, which is the private practice of psychiatrists that are affiliated or do much of their work with the hospital. They entered into the dialogue as well. It became clear at a point that really this was not a venture that should directly involve the hospital, that really the medical group and Connecticut Psychological Group, PC, should be the participants in this joint venture. The hospital, while still being supportive, doesn't make a financial contribution to this venture in any way.

STEENBARGER: And the reason for that is?

ZIMMERMAN: I think there are a couple of reasons for that. One, is that they don't own it. Two is, we wanted to be able to make it clear that PsychSystems of New England, which is what we call this joint venture, was not a feeder for the hospital.

STEENBARGER: A lot of MCOs would be concerned about that.

ZIMMERMAN: Of course they would be. They should be. . . . We wanted to make it clear that this was a venture of two private practices. Yes, we are on staff of and affiliated with the hospital and the psychiatrists are attendings at the hospital, but this venture is not owned or funded by the hospital . . .

[Group practices run out of hospitals are constantly needing to demonstrate their independence from the hospital. If your practice is allied with a hospital, remember that this can be a major area of concern to potential referral sources.]

We have worked over these years in moving our relationship closer together. . . . That's really a major developmental milestone. To try to do it in a way that works, where you're blending or intersecting two cultures, is very challenging. We have spent much of the time not only building the clinical programs and procedures and infrastructure but also trying to build our relationship. That is a major challenge. . . . You have people that are working clinically for each other but that organizationally don't have anything to do with each other in terms of who pays whose salary.

Working with Managed Care

STEENBARGER: Just a couple of questions about managed care in your regions: How the level of penetration has progressed, how that's affecting your group and its practices, how that's affected reimbursement rates?

ZIMMERMAN: Managed care 5 years ago was not very significant. Now it is *very* significant. I want to say that probably 70% of the income to this practice is managed care based—maybe 85 or 90%, because you have many indemnity plans that are managed either directly or indirectly. . . . Some of the management is not very intensive, anywhere from no OTRs [outpatient treatment reports] and self-referral to MCO referral and OTRs every four sessions to physician gatekeeper. You talk about overhead costs, it has certainly increased the administrative costs. We were figuring recently that any one visit is approximately six or seven transactions on the computer. . . . That's an incredible amount of administrative overhead . . . and I didn't even talk about generating HCFA forms, electronic claims submission, and all of that!

STEENBARGER: Or collecting any of the quality-related data.

ZIMMERMAN: Right! So it has increased the administrative overhead: the filling out the contracts and agreements, reading them and understanding them, and negotiating around them, as well as our clinicians completing their OTRs in a timely way.

STEENBARGER: It sounds like the vast majority of business must be fee for service, then.

ZIMMERMAN: Yes, and even the contracts that we are signing now are going to be fee for service at this point. Connecticut, unlike some other states, is not really doing much in outpatient case rate work or capitated work. We're in the midst of negotiating a case rate on an EAP. Certainly in the other EAPs that we hold the contracts for . . . those are virtually all capitated. So we're used to operating in that environment and being at risk. And actually I welcome that. I know that we do high-quality work, I know what our average length of stay is. We manage the work anyway. I'd just as soon get paid for managing it! I'm happy to take the risk to manage the work I manage already.

STEENBARGER: What would you say is your greatest challenge so far in working with MCOs?

ZIMMERMAN: That's a good question. . . . One greatest challenge is understanding and recognizing the business aspects of the relationship. When we're negotiating, we're not just negotiating around quality and outcomes. This is a high-level corporate business relationship. . . . Quality and outcome are critical and important, but issues around cost and payment are going to be negotiated . . . as they would be in another [e.g., manufacturing] arena. . . . I think much of our training doesn't prepare us for that. Part of the challenge is getting up to speed on the business aspect of practice.

Information Systems

STEENBARGER: There are a couple of areas I wanted to touch upon. The first one is information systems and what your group's evolution has been and what kind of system you're currently working with.

ZIMMERMAN: We began as two clinicians [managing financial information with a checkbook]. . . . Pretty quickly, though, we moved to putting our accounts payable on computer. That was with fairly great ease, given the relatively inexpensive software that's available. We happen to have been using Quicken for many years and it's just a pleasure. We get upgrades—pretty much every other upgrade. It's inexpensive, easy to use, and doesn't require a lot of maintenance on the software side. It really takes care of accounts payable and gives our accountant most of the information that he needs at the end of the year.

Clinical information and accounts receivable are more challenging. When we first began, we were not doing outcome studies. We began doing outcome studies in 1989, which in Connecticut was long before anybody asked us for them . . . tracking things like length of stay by diagnosis and other demographic aspects of the patient. . . . We began tracking time between telephone call and first appointment, wanting to make sure that we were bringing people into the office in a timely fashion. . . . We began doing that on a rather old computer—it was an XT—with a rather labor-intensive database that was available at that time. It took an awful lot of energy. . . . Accounts receivable back then were also still being done by hand.

The next level was to go out and purchase a mental health software program to do our accounts receivable . . . after researching many of them. We really weren't too happy with it over the many years that we used it. . . . We upgraded our computers over the years. Recently, we have gone to a new system which we are much more happy with and have a network of computers in our billing department to handle our accounts receivable—but that's not enough. . . . Each time that we upgrade and think that we're going two steps out ahead, by the time it's all in place, we're one step behind again!

STEENBARGER: Do you have one central billing office for all the locations?

ZIMMERMAN: Yes we do.

STEENBARGER: And each of your clinical sites, I assume, is on some kind of wide area network or has some way of connecting—

ZIMMERMAN: I wish. Right now they're connecting with paper. Each clinician keeps a weekly log of all his or her visits and copayments received by that clinician or by the secretary in that office. The weekly logs and the face sheets for new patients are sent in weekly or faxed to our billing office, which then enters all the information in the system. So we have centralized billing, while we have decentralized patient care.

STEENBARGER: So it doesn't sound as if the individual clinicians are online.

ZIMMERMAN: Not yet. And maybe never. For two reasons. One is the time it takes them to enter the information and what's the quality of the information they're going to enter? With all due respect to all the clinicians out there, some of us are better with computers than others of us and some of us have better typing skills than others. Some of us are more obsessive than others! . . . So maybe never in terms of billing information. But the idea of clinical information being online is something that's very interesting.

STEENBARGER: How much would you say you're investing in computer resources, upgrades, your whole information platform?

ZIMMERMAN: That really depends on the year. This fiscal year was a much greater investment than last fiscal year. Probably next year will be like this year because of the growth we've seen.

STEENBARGER: Could you give me a ballpark?

ZIMMERMAN: Last year, we bought a couple of PCs, so maybe that was $5,000. . . . This year, it's probably about triple, between $15,000 and $20,000. That's really a drop in the bucket compared to what we really could do ideally.

STEENBARGER: When you start talking about $20,000, though, that's a meaningful fraction of an FTE.

ZIMMERMAN: Absolutely. It's also not much different if you have a 3- or 4-person practice or if you have a 20-person practice. You still have to have the software, you still have to have the ability to access the data, you still have to have maybe a laptop or something if you want to call in from home, you still have to have a network if you have more than one person inputting data.

STEENBARGER: Do you finance all of this growth and expansion internally or do you have external financing?

ZIMMERMAN: We have a credit line which we are personally at risk for. . . . That gets a little anxiety producing when the credit line is up at $40,000.

STEENBARGER: And it's your house that's securing the line!

ZIMMERMAN: Nowadays, in the business environment, that's part of it; $40,000 in today's business world is nothing. But it's more than some people make in a whole year in salary. . . . When you're talking about MIS or other kinds of investments, if you're going to be competitive in the marketplace with billion-dollar companies and hundred-million-dollar companies which are going to be contracting with you, then you have to be able to provide a level of service and organizational infrastructure that is appealing to them and that they're used to.

[A major problem for many of the group practices to which we consult is undercapitalization. (This has long been known to be a problem for small businesses in general.) Running a group practice, one is often torn between feeling that you would like to upgrade systems and improve the company in general and feeling that you have to pinch pennies. The Small Business Administration (SBA) has some excellent loan programs available to small business owners. If you are needing capital for your group practice you should check with the SBA, which has regional offices around the country.]

Data Collection

STEENBARGER: What sort of information are you currently gathering to help you manage utilization and then to help you collect the quality data? You mentioned outcome studies.

ZIMMERMAN: Pretty much along the lines of what I've already described. We haven't necessarily changed too much with regard to the variables that we're looking at, although we also now use a screening inventory which we administer at intake, at session 6, and, if there's a session 12 and every twelfth session thereafter. We've begun tracking those data to see if there are consistent changes within patients and also across caseloads and across the whole practice.

STEENBARGER: Is that all being done manually? The patients fill it out, pencil and paper, and then the paper goes over to some clerical staff who inputs in into the PC?

ZIMMERMAN: Right. [We send our patient satisfaction] about a month after discharge, seeking anonymous return from the patient. We give [patients] a metered envelope to send it back to us. The only identifying information we ask them is who the clinician is that they saw and whether the treatment was for them or their child.

STEENBARGER: You're using something like a CSQ for your patient satisfaction?

ZIMMERMAN: We developed it ourselves.

STEENBARGER: In terms of your clinical triage, do you work off any kind of formalized system? Do you have any protocols?

ZIMMERMAN: We do have some protocols in place that we've developed. But it's really very customized to the caller at the time. One of the things that we have found is that the callers do not want to spend much time talking to a secretary. We have the calls all come directly to a live person. We don't use voice mail at this time. . . . The calls come initially to a secretary who makes sure at least that it's not urgent. We don't ask that she do a clinical assessment, but if the person sounds very distressed or says to her it's urgent, then she goes down another decision tree. The routine call is then either returned by our clinical director or, based on the questions we've instructed our secretary to ask, routed directly to a clinician who seems appropriate for the case. The clinician then returns the call and will do more of a brief phone assessment at that time.

STEENBARGER: In terms of numbers, roughly, the number of patients seen within your group during a year?

ZIMMERMAN: In 1990, we saw 450 new patients. In 1995, we saw 1343 new patients.

STEENBARGER: Roughly, what is your average length of outpatient treatment across diagnoses?

ZIMMERMAN: Our average length is about eight sessions. This is over approximately 2,500 patients from 1989 to 1995. Approximately 60% are seen in five visits or less; approximately 20% . . . are seen in 6 to 10 visits; 11% in 11 to 20 visits; and about 9% in 21 or more visits.

STEENBARGER: Do you also track your hospitalization rates?

ZIMMERMAN: Hospitalization rates are *so* low that there's almost nothing to track.

Clinical Services

STEENBARGER: That really says something. Do you have special clinical programs in place, IOPs or the equivalent, to keep people out of the hospital?

ZIMMERMAN: We are building some intensive outpatient programs. We have an anxiety management program in place . . . we have a number of group therapies that we're running, and that's also helpful. But I'd say one of the things that keeps the patients out of the hospital is our willingness to combine a psychotherapeutic approach with a psychopharmacological approach. We also focus on early intervention, as opposed to just managing the crises. We also don't just do weekly visits and then stop. We fade out our treatment as quickly as the patient can tolerate it. . . . We find that this is tremendously useful in avoiding relapse and avoiding crises. It means you have more active cases in your caseload, which is a little bit more difficult to manage administratively, but you have far fewer hospitalizations.

The average clinician probably sees between 1,400 and 1,500 hours of clinical work a year. It gets difficult to talk about how many cases, because if you have six or seven people in a group, how many cases is that? They do about . . . 32 hours a week of clinical care on the average per FTE.

STEENBARGER: How is your IOP structured, this anxiety program that you mentioned? And how is it reimbursed?

ZIMMERMAN: Right now it's being reimbursed on a fee-for-service basis, not on a programmatic basis. We hope that it can eventually be reimbursed on a programmatic basis.

STEENBARGER: So you have to get separate authorization for each component of the IOP?

ZIMMERMAN: For each component. There's an educational component incorporated throughout, there's individual treatment that's often necessary, and there's a heavy weighting on group and then med management as appropriate for each patient.

   We also do our own internal chart reviews. Every twelfth session, we do a chart review and we also do retrospective chart reviews on every single closed case that goes through the practice.

STEENBARGER: Wow!

ZIMMERMAN: That's another major investment.

STEENBARGER: What are you looking for in these chart reviews?

ZIMMERMAN: A couple of things. . . . One is we are looking to make sure that the chart is intact, structurally, that releases of information were signed, are appropriately updated and extended as needed, that requests for authorization and OTRs have been submitted and how those are written and what they say. We check that progress notes are written in a way that provides a sufficient level of documentation and are signed and dated and [have] the patient's name on the paper. We're also looking from a clinical perspective at the treatment plan and the course of treatment. Is this patient progressing? [Does he] need to get a medication evaluation? [Does she] need group therapy? Can treatment be discontinued or reduced in terms of intensity? So we'll look at both sides of it: the structural aspects of the chart and also the clinical care that's being provided.

The Group's Management Structure

STEENBARGER: How are the management responsibilities divvied up among the three principals . . . ?

ZIMMERMAN: I'm the managing partner. I take care of most of the financial management, such as the profit-sharing plan, and work with our office manager in terms of all the administrative issues related to the practice. . . . Another one of our partners, Arnie Holzman, PhD, is in charge of our networks and contracted activities. So he's the one who is spearheading the PsychSystems of New England joint venture . . . and is the one who works on maintaining most of our relationships with the MCOs that we work with. Liza Thayer, PhD, is one of our clinical directors and, as a partner, she oversees the clinical operations of the practice. She will work with the other clinical director who we have and with other staff that have clinical issues that need tending to. She puts into place and oversees our internal quality assurance activities [the chart reviews].

STEENBARGER: What percentage of your time is spent administratively in management and what percentage clinically?

ZIMMERMAN: That's a little hard to say, because the total amount of time is over 100%! But I would say I do about 15 to 20 hours of clinical care a week and about every other waking hour [on management]! (*Laughs.*) I'm trying to work on adding in more personal time, which is very difficult. I have a family and two children and I find that the practice will take as much or more than any one of us could give. . . . I'm usually here 7:30 A.M. to 6 P.M., 10 to 11 hours. And then I probably work about another 2 to 3 hours in the late evening. I try not to do much work in the weekends, but invariably I put in another 2 to 3 hours.

[As you can see from both Mr. Smith's and Dr. Zimmerman's comments, running a successful group practice is not a 9 to 5 activity. Are you willing to make the business of the group practice a very central piece of most of your waking hours? If you are not, you might consider working *for a group practice.]*

In terms of our structure, we have a board of directors, which is the three of us. We also have a management team, which is probably close to half of us. . . . The management team is broken into two areas. One is professional services and the other is operations. Under each of these areas is a number of, for lack of a better word, committees . . . that have different focal points. Marketing is one of them. Program development would be another one. Quality assurance, administrative, and all the clinical areas. . . . The management team is charged with carrying out the strategic plan for the year. Marketing is done at a number of different levels. There's marketing certainly to the managed care companies, looking to get contracts and building the PsychSystems of New England joint venture. There's also community-based marketing, which is really the bread and butter of the practice. On the one hand, contracts and being providers on a panel allow reimbursement for the patient, but if you don't have a strong and positive presence in the communities you serve, you don't have access to the patients!

That's something that we try to impress upon everybody in the practice. Marketing is something they're doing all the time. If they're taking to a referral source, if they're talking to a patient, if our secretary is keeping a patient waiting at the window, if a secretary is keeping a patient on the phone on hold for too long, if a clinician hasn't returned a phone call in a timely way . . . then all of this is negative or positive . . . marketing of the practice. We all are marketing the practice constantly.

Summary of the Case Study

Perhaps the most outstanding feature of CPG is its embodiment of a vision charted by the founders, and its dedication to the fulfillment of this vision. Dr. Zimmerman and his colleagues have obviously thought a great deal about the culture they want to create in their practice. This collaborative culture is expressed in a multitude of ways, from ongoing clinical staff meetings to a broadly participative management team to an innovative compensation system that includes bonuses and profit sharing.

A second noteworthy feature of CPG is its blending of centralization and decentralization. In one sense, the practice is very controlled and centralized, with clinical protocols, centralized billing, and a common treatment philosophy. In another sense, the group is decentralized, with locations across the state and an active joint venture with another practice. There is considerable management of both clinical and administrative aspects of the practice, but—through such mechanisms as case conferences and committees—this is accomplished in a highly collegial manner.

Finally, it is clear that CPG has its eye on the quality ball. Many of the innovations described by Dr. Zimmerman, including the case discussions and outcome studies, predated the group's involvement with managed care. It is clear that this group is very concerned with offering true value to consumers. Jeff's admonition to ask yourself whether you would be willing to pay full fee for the service you've just rendered is a pointed example of this commitment to quality and value.

LESSONS BEHIND THE TRIUMPHS

Our case studies illustrate several key ingredients of success in mental health's future. These are the features that define any collaborative practice that you would want to join or establish. Most of the factors underlying the triumphs we have observed strike us as a reconciliation of seeming opposites. That is, the successful practice is able to balance opposing forces in such a way as to generate a constructive equilibrium. Several factors highlight some of those forces and their syntheses.

Dedication to Work/Preservation of Self

It is clear that the leaders of group practices live and breathe their business. They belong to numerous professional organizations, read voraciously, participate on

Internet lists, and network with professionals continuously. This is true continuing education! The successful practice leader *has* to be immersed in the field if he or she is to keep up with fast-paced developments.

As our studies underscore, success cannot be achieved in collaborative practice on a 40-hour-a-week basis. Dr. Smith and Dr. Zimmerman spend 60+ hours on the job and often take work home. Much of this time is spent in dealing with day-to-day problems—on top of handling a half-time caseload. Despite this load, Dr. Smith and Dr. Zimmerman sound remarkably easygoing in the ongoing conversations we've had. It is clear that they have learned to delegate responsibilities where possible, focus on essentials, and pace themselves so as to not burn out.

Pride in the Staff/Managerial Firmness

The organizations' pride in their professional staff was evident throughout the interviews. They strongly believe that their professionals do good work and revel in the positive patient satisfaction rate and community goodwill the practices are able to maintain. All the firms are very concerned with communications among staff and have devoted significant resources to maintaining a flow of information to and from clinicians at distant locations. Considerable time and effort are also spent on the ongoing support and training of clinical staff. This view of staff as resources rather than cost centers permeates all of our profiled practices.

At the same time, the practices are very active in managing the activities of clinicians. They acknowledge that a collaboration is more than a collection of individuals, each out for him- or herself. All of the profiled groups have very explicit standards and expectations and devote significant resources to ensuring that these are being achieved. All are also quick to intervene if clinicians are falling short of the norms with respect to client satisfaction, outcomes, or utilization. Each practice acknowledges and rewards superior performance—with additional referrals, public praise, monetary bonuses—and each is committed to correcting problems collegially when these arise. Fondness, fairness, and firmness are found in equal measure.

Computerized/Personalized

Much has been made in recent years of the need for organizations to combine the advantages of technology with personalized service. As business increasingly rely on technological solutions, they can find themselves precariously distanced from their customers. The organizations included in our case studies have made a major commitment to computer systems and the linkage of clinicians. They have also made use of technology in ongoing data collection, ensuring that they can triage clients efficiently and effectively and monitor their progress as treatment progresses. This management-by-information approach starkly contrasts the leadership style of other practices that make no effort to ascertain their success.

Nevertheless, even technologically savvy firms recognize the need to maintain the human touch. Phones are answered by people, not voice mail systems, in order to place patients and referral sources at ease. Service takes priority, with a commitment to see patients within hours of their initial call. The system is designed with user-friendliness for patients and referral sources firmly in mind. The goal is to create a system that works, not simply to press one's short-term agendas.

Willingness to Invest/Minimizing of Overhead

This was perhaps the most outstanding feature of the organizations profiled in the case studies. They have not hesitated to make major investments in their success. From the inception of the groups, they have spent significant money on high-quality consultation from attorneys, accountants, and computer experts. They continue to invest in the training of clinical staff and upgrading of computer resources. Staff time and resources are devoted to maintaining and extending the integrity of the administrative and clinical systems. VBH's creation of the field case manager position is a perfect case in point. This person works full-time, simply to make clinical systems work better within a region—not to sell new accounts. To these organizations, *quality matters*.

On the other hand, these are also organizations with a keen eye for the bottom line. They are careful to minimize overhead wherever possible. They find time-effective ways of delivering clinical supervision and consultation and collecting needed data. They do not pay staff in fixed salaries but create compensation systems that reward effort and productivity. All are aware of the pricing pressures within the marketplace and have figured out efficient ways to expand geographically. Indeed, each organization has articulated a clear model of operations and is dedicated to building a culture around this model. To no small degree, the model is that organization's response to the need to blend expansion and growth with cost containment and quality enhancement. These are not hastily patched together entities. They have spent considerable time in strategic planning and have been proactive in revisiting and revising their plans.

CONCLUSION

Although there is no recipe for success in any complex field of endeavor, there are common elements that can guide those seeking personal and professional triumphs. Health care is undergoing changes of a fundamental nature, but our case studies suggest that much can be accomplished with initiative, business smarts, and a concern for cost-efficiency and quality. Those who expect to conduct practice as it has been conducted for the past several decades will find themselves severely challenged in the new climate of accountability. Those creative enough to

✔ SUMMARY

- Successful collaborations establish collegial working relationships within the practice, as well as between the practice and referral sources and payers.
- Successful collaborations operate in a data-intensive fashion, creating supportive structures for improving performance.
- At the heart of every successful collaboration is a mission and a culture that supports that mission.

establish high IQ, collaborative practice structures will be poised to survive and thrive over the next decade.

The moral of the story is that **you don't have to go it alone, even if your goal is to stay in solo practice**. Mandates for cost-effectiveness and quality are pushing mental health professionals toward greater collaboration and integration. Those same mandates will continue to nudge multispecialty practices toward even greater linkages with social services agencies, medical practices, and facilities. Now is the time to figure out who your partners will be in addressing the needs of the marketplace.

Whether you are interested in joining a group, establishing one, or helping an existing practice expand, we hope the preceding pages have helped you to think through the changes that are occurring and the ways in which you might address these. With a little luck, a lot of hard work, and a well-chosen collection of tools and tactics, may you find your personal and professional triumphs!

READER'S RESOURCE 7.1
Conversation with Martin Klein, PhD

"My role . . . is as a person who educates"

Marty Klein has had a diverse career as a private practitioner, academic psychologist, and managed behavioral healthcare reviewer. He has worked as regional clinical director for U.S. Behavioral Health, coordinating group practice development in the eastern half of the United States, and recently assumed the position of vice president of network development, East Division, for Merit Behavioral Care. In these roles, he has coordinated the development of contracts with groups and networks of practitioners. He recently took time from a busy schedule to talk with Brett Steenbarger about his perspectives on group practice. Below is a segment of that conversation.

STEENBARGER: What are the ingredients for success among behavioral group practices?

KLEIN: What I find most amazing about my position working with developing groups is that mental health workers are unusual. When I call them up and say I'd like to develop a group—a preferred group—and you can have this book of business and it seems like a no-lose proposition, they always need time to think about it. In any other type of business they would just grab the opportunity. That always seems a little strange to me! . . .

    I think the problem with most people in our field is that each discipline tends to stick together. They have a hard time developing an interdisciplinary group. The disciplines don't trust each other. Basically, it's like cats and dogs. . . . For the sake of what a group has to be, it has to be interdisciplinary. What most managed care companies are looking for are groups that are comprehensive, that can cover every aspect. . . . Basically, what we want from a group is to make sure that no matter what cases we refer to them, they can treat them and they can treat them in a timely, cost-effective manner.

STEENBARGER: I'm sure you've worked with groups that are a bust. I'm sure you've worked with groups that are exemplars. What differentiates them?

KLEIN: I'm actually someone who tends to develop groups. I believe that sometimes you have really good clinicians who are not really great business people. So I tend to develop groups, bring different small groups—maybe from each discipline—together. The positive about that is that they're generally the top clinicians. I get their names from care

(cont.)

managers and people I know in the field. The negative is that they're not business savvy and they're not always that sophisticated. We have a lot of problems on the administrative side because of that.

Then there are groups that are sophisticated and know the business side, and they tend to be very profit-oriented and tend to hire clinicians at a lower rate. So you try to balance between the two. You want a cost-effective group, but at the same time you want a group with top quality clinicians. . . . And that's a difficult combination. If the group is weak on either side, it will cause the managed care company problems.

We're also looking for members of the groups that are managed care friendly. So you tend to stay away from clinicians who don't believe in psychopharmacology or who only believe in long term work. . . .

STEENBARGER: So do you see some of your role as helping groups with the administrative/business side of practice?

KLEIN: Yes, and also clinical. My role, in all its aspects of managed care, is as a person who educates. Even in previous roles as a medical reviewer, I always saw my role as educating people I had to work with. I think ther's a lot of magazines out there and a lot of information out there that make clinicians paranoid of managed care. And a lot of it isn't warranted. I don't think we're some evil empire. We really want quality work. So I see my role as helping groups form and move into the 21st century. . . .

The Chinese have that one symbol that everyone refers to that stands for crisis and opportunity. I think this is a wonderful opportunity for clinicians to join forces and to go into the 21st century in a positive way. It's clear groups are the wave of the future. And you can either become paralyzed or victimized or you can join forces and prosper. . . .

STEENBARGER: In terms of folks who are just in the process of thinking about group development . . . where do you see the opportunities? What advice would you give them?

KLEIN: I think it's always important to contact a person like myself—a regional director in charge of the network—in the area, to find out what's going on in that area. There are many variables involved in whether we develop a group there, like how many lives we have in that area. If we don't have that many members, we're not going to need a group. . . .

STEENBARGER: Is there a threshold you look to?

KLEIN: There is no magic number, but usually if an area has about 10,000 lives, we might want to develop a group there. . . . And I think as we move forward, we start to look a different types of groups. Different areas have different needs and require different structures. For example,

(cont.)

READER'S RESOURCE 7.1 (*cont.*)

one area might require a group with walls, another area might need more of a group without walls. . . .

STEENBARGER: Have you had much experience with centralized versus groups without walls, and can you make any generalized statements about some of the promises and pitfalls of the different organizational models?

KLEIN: I have groups in both categories. I have a lot of groups that have mixed models. And especially when I help to create groups, you tend to have a larger group and then smaller groups joining that group. The smaller groups tend to be satellites without walls. There's pros and cons to both types of models. The pros of a with-walls is that they're tighter groups administratively. The pros of a without-walls is that you have more localized coverage.

[Over time] there will be more QA required. . . . We're going to want to know number of sessions [by patient characteristics], how quickly the member has been seen from the initial call, QA around diagnostic categories, relapse around inpatient care. The other thing we like to see is peer supervision and peer education. It's very important to us that these groups use each other as resources.

STEENBARGER: And have some structure programs around that?

KLEIN: Right. We want to make sure that these groups are the highest quality and up on the latest methods.

Resource List

There are few readings and resources specific to the development of groups and networks in behavioral health. Nonetheless, the materials below should prove helpful to readers interested in further exploration. All book and article references appear in the References.

ORGANIZATIONS

Institute for Behavioral Healthcare (IBH)—4370 Alpine Road, Suite 108; Portola Valley, CA 94028; 415-851-8411.

Medical Group Management Association (MGMA)—104 Inverness Terrace East; Englewood, CO 80112-5306; 303-799-1111.

National Committee for Quality Assurance (NCQA)—2000 L Street, NW, Suite 500, Washington, DC 20036; 202-955-3500.

PERIODICALS

Behavioral Healthcare Tomorrow—1110 Mar West Street, Suite E, Tiburon, CA 94920-1879; 415-435-9848.

Open Minds—10 York Street, Suite 200, Gettysburg, PA 17325-2301; 717-334-1329.

Practice Strategies—442½ E. Main St, Clayton, NC 27520; 919-553-0637.

BOOKS AND ARTICLES

Overview of Managed Care

Kongstvedt (1996); Finkel (1996); Korenchuk (1994); Lazarus (1996); Wilkerson, Devers, and Given (1997)

The Business of (Behavioral) Healthcare

American Psychological Association Practice Directorate (1996d); Cummings, Pallak, and Cummings (1966); Pavlock (1994); Yenney (1994); Younger et al. (1996); Zieman (1995)

Quality and Outcomes Assessment

Maruish (1994); National Committee for Quality Assurance, (1996); Ogles, Lambert, and Masters (1996); Steenbarger and Smith (1996); Vibberts and Youngs (1995, 1996)

Best Clinical Practices and Empirically Validated Treatments

American Psychiatric Association (1996); Barlow (1993); Bergin and Garfield (1994); Pollack, Otto, and Rosenbaum (1996); Roth and Fonagy (1996); Seaburn, Lorenz, Gunn, Gawinski, and Manksch (1996); Steenbarger (1994); see also www.recmgmt.com/psycoh/

Time-Effective and Brief Therapies

Budman (1994); Budman & Gurman (1988); Budman, Hoyt, & Friedman (1992); Cummings and Sayama, 1995; Steenbarger (1992); Wells & Giannetti (1990)

CONSULTATION AND TRAINING

Drs. Budman and Steenbarger, under the auspices of Innovative Training Systems (ITS), offer a variety of workshops and consultative services pertaining to the development and management of staff-model and network group practices. ITS also offers clinical training in time-effective therapy and a range of products and services aimed at primary prevention and outcomes assessment. ITS can be reached at 617- 332-6028 or at itsadmin@aol.com.

ITS is currently offering a Collaborative Consultation Program, which allows leaders from behavioral group practices to assemble in small teams and participate in hands-on consultative and training sessions. This allows for far more indepth learning than is usually possible in workshops and conference programs, yet it is considerably more cost-effective than traditional consultation. For more information on the Collaborative Consultation Program, please contact ITS or Dr. Steenbarger at 315-464-3120 or psycohnet@concentric.net.

MANAGEMENT SERVICES ORGANIZATION (MSO) DEVELOPMENT

Bret Smith, MEd, profiled in Chapter 7 of this book, has recently authored a volume on MSO development that is quite useful and practical. Its title is *Developing, Implementing, and Managing a Management Service Organization (MSO) for Behavioral Health Practices*. (1997; Atlantic Information Services, Washington, DC).

Ordering information and a wealth of continuing education information pertinent to group practice are available at: www.recmgmt.com/psycoh/.

CONTINUING EDUCATION

Brett Steenbarger, PhD, Bret Smith, MEd, and Jeff Zimmerman, PhD, have developed an interactive multimedia web site to support the continuing education of clinicians interested in collaborative practice management. The site is called *psycOH!* (www.recmgmt.com/psycoh/) and features an online newsletter, free practice management consultation, and archives of clinical and administrative best practices. Readers and browsers can e-mail Dr. Steenbarger at psycohnet@ concentric.net for more information.

References

Abrams, R. M. (1993). *The successful business plan: Secrets and strategies*. Grants Pass, OR: Oasis Press.

American Managed Behavioral Healthcare Organization. (1995, August). *Performance measures for managed behavioral healthcare programs*. Washington, DC: Author.

American Psychiatric Association. (1994). *Diagnostic and statistical manual of mental disorders* (4th ed.). Washington, DC: Author.

American Psychiatric Association. (1996). *Practice guidelines*. Washington, DC: Author.

American Psychological Association Practice Directorate. (1996a). *Models for multidisciplinary arrangements: A state-by-state review of options*. Washington, DC: American Psychological Association.

American Psychological Association Practice Directorate. (1996b). *Managing your practice finances: Strategies for budgeting, funding, and business planning*. Washington, DC: American Psychological Association.

American Psychological Association Practice Directorate. (1996c). *Organizing your practice through automation: Managing information and data*. Washington, DC: American Psychological Association.

American Psychological Association Practice Directorate. (1996d). *APA practitioner's toolbox series*. Washington, DC: American Psychological Association.

Attkisson, C. C., & Greenfield, T. K. (1994). Client Satisfaction Questionnaire—8 and Service Satisfaction Scale—30. In M. E. Maruish (Ed.), *The use of psychological testing for treatment planning and outcome assessment* (pp. 402–422). Hillsdale, NJ: Erlbaum.

Bangs, D. H. Jr. (1995). *The market planning guide* (4th ed.). Chicago: Upstart.

Barlow, D. H. (Ed.). (1993). *Clinical handbook of psychological disorders: A step-by-step treatment manual* (2nd ed.). New York: Guilford Press.

Beck, A. T., Rush, J. A., Shaw, B. F., & Emery, G. (1979). *Cognitive therapy of depression*. New York: Guilford Press.

Beebe, J. C. (1992). The request for proposal and vendor selection process. *Topics in Health Information Management, 13*, 11–19.

Belch, G. E., & Belch, M. A. (1995). *Introduction to advertising and promotion: An integrated marketing communications perspective* (3rd ed.). Chicago: Irwin.

Bergin, A. E., & Garfield, S. L. (Eds.). (1994). *Handbook of psychotherapy and behavior change* (4th ed.). New York: Wiley.

Bohlmann, R. C. (1991). Consultants: Selection and use. In A. Ross, S. J. Williams, & E. L. Schafer (Eds.), *Ambulatory care management* (2nd ed., pp. 383–397). Albany, NY: Delmar.

Briggs, J., & Peat, F. D. (1989). *Turbulent mirror: An illustrated guide to chaos theory and the science of wholeness*. New York: Harper & Row.

Budman, S. H. (1994). *Treating time effectively: The first session in brief therapy* [Manual and videotape]. New York: Guilford Press.

Budman, S. H., & Armstrong, E. (1992). Training for managed care settings: How to make it happen. *Psychotherapy, 29,* 416–421.

Budman, S. H., & Gurman, A. S. (1988). *Theory and practice of brief therapy.* New York: Guilford Press.

Budman, S. H., Hoyt, M. F., & Friedman, S. (Eds.). (1992). *The first session in brief therapy.* New York: Guilford Press.

Budman, S. H., Cooley, S., Demby, A., Koppenaal, G., Koslof, J., & Powers, T. (1996). A model of time-effective group psychotherapy for patients with personality disorders: The clinical model. *International Journal of Group Psychotherapy, 46,* 329–356.

Ciotti, V. G., Seitner, T. J., & Pagnotta, R. R. (1994). It's a jungle out there: Strategies for controlling information systems costs. *Healthcare Financial Management, 48,* 41–47.

Clifford, D., & Warner, R. (1995). *The partnership book* (4th ed.). Berkeley, CA: Nolo Press.

Corporate Agents, Inc. (1995). *The essential limited liability company handbook.* Grants Pass, OR: Oasis Press.

Cummings, N. A. (1977). Prolonged (ideal) versus short-term (realistic) psychotherapy. *Professional Psychology: Research and Practice, 8,* 491–501.

Cummings, N. A. (1996). Does managed mental health care offset costs related to medical treatment? In A. Lazarus (Ed.), *Controversies in managed mental health care* (pp. 213–227). Washington, DC: American Psychiatric Press.

Cummings, N. A., Pallak, M. S., & Cummings, J. (Eds.). (1996). *Surviving the demise of solo practice: Mental health pratitioners prospering in the era of managed care.* Madison, CT: Psychosocial Press.

Cummings, N. A., & Sayama, M. (1995). *Focused psychotherapy: A casebook of brief intermittent psychotherapy throughout the life cycle.* New York: Brunner/Mazel.

Dana, D. (1996). Measuring the financial cost of team conflict. In G. M. Parker (Ed.), *Handbook of best practices for teams* (Vol. 1, pp. 111–122). Amherst, MA: HRD Press.

Davanloo, H. (1980). *Basic principles and technique in short-term dynamic psychotherapy.* New York: Jason Aronson.

DeMuro, P. R. (1994). Management services organizations. *Topics in Health Care Finance, 20,* 19–27.

Derogatis, L. R., & Lazarus, L. (1994). SCL-90-R, Brief Symptom Inventory, and matching clinical rating scales. In M. E. Maruish (Ed.), *The use of psychological testing for treatment planning and outcome assessment* (pp. 217–248). Hillsdale, NJ: Erlbaum.

de Shazer, S. (1985). *Keys to solution in brief therapy.* New York: Norton.

Doherty, W., McDaniel, S., & Baird, M. (1996). Five levels of primary care–behavioral health collaboration. *Behavioral Healthcare Tomorrow, 5*(5), 25–29.

Doyle, O. (1990). Making the most of information system consultants. *Healthcare Financial Management, 44,* 34–44.

Egnew, R. C., Geary, C., & Wilson, S. N. (1996). Coordinating physical and behavioral healthcare services for Medicaid populations: Issues and implications in integrated and carve out systems. *Behavioral Healthcare Tomorrow, 5*(5), 67–72.

Eisen, S. V. (1995). BASIS-32. In S. V. Vibberts & M. T. Youngs (Eds.), *The 1996 behavioral outcomes and guidelines sourcebook* (pp. G127–G130). New York: Faulkner & Gray.

Elkin, I. (1994). The NIMH Treatment of Depression Collaborative Research Program: Where we began and where we are. In A. E. Bergin & Sol L. Garfield (Eds.), *Handbook of psychotherapy and behavior change* (4th ed., pp. 114–142). New York: Wiley.

Fink, P. J. (1996). Are psychiatrists replaceable? In A. Lazarus (Ed.), *Controversies in managed mental health care* (pp. 3–16). Washington, DC: American Psychiatric Press.

Finkel, M. L. (1996). *Health care cost management: A basic guide* (3rd ed.). Brookfield, WI: International Foundation of Employee Benefit Plans.

Frank, E. (1991). Interpersonal psychotherapy as maintenance treatment for patients with recurrent depression. *Psychotherapy, 28*, 259–266.

Freiman, M., Cunningham, P., & Cornelius, L. (1994, July). *Use and expenditures for the treatment of mental health problems* (AHCPR Pub. No. 94–0085). Rockville, MD: Public Health Service.

Garfield, S. L. (1994). Research on client variables in psychotherapy. In A. E. Bergin & S. L. Garfield (Eds.), *Handbook of psychotherapy and behavior change* (4th ed., pp. 190–228). New York: Wiley.

Gilligan, C. (1982). *In a different voice*. Cambridge, MA: Harvard University Press.

Gunderson, J. G., Frank, A. F., Ronnigstam, E. F., Wachter, S., Lynch, V. J., & Wolf, P. J. (1989). Early discontinuance of borderline patients from psychotherapy. *Journal of Nervous and Mental Disease, 177*, 38–41.

Gunter, P., & Abbey, F. (1996, August 19). PSOs: New entrant into managed-Medicare. *Business Journal of Central New York Health-Care Quarterly*, pp. 12b–13b.

Hanna, R., & Ritchie, S. A. (1992). Facilities design. In A. E. Barnett & G. G. Mayer (Eds.), *Ambulatory care management and practice* (pp. 488–505). Gaithersburg, MD: Aspen.

HMO enrollment continues to grow. (1995). *Behavioral Healthcare Tomorrow, 4*(6), p. 13.

How good is your health plan? (1996, August). *Consumer Reports*, pp. 28–42.

Howard, K. I., Kopta, S. M., Krause, M. J., & Orlinsky, D. E. (1986). The dose–effect relationship in psychotherapy. *American Psychologist, 41*, 159–164.

Howard, K. I., Lueger, R., Maling, M., & Martinovich, Z. (1993). A phase model of psychotherapy: Causal mediation of outcome. *Journal of Consulting and Clinical Psychology, 61*, 678–685.

IPRO. (1996). *Annual report: 1995/96*. Lake Success, NY: Author.

Jamieson, D. W. (1996). Aligning the organization for a team-based strategy. In G. M. Parker (Ed.), *The handbook of best practices for teams* (Vol. 1, pp. 299–312). Amherst, MA: HRD Press.

Katon, W., VonKorff, M., Lin, E., Lipcomb, P., Russo, J., Wagner, E., & Polk, E. (1990). Distressed high utilizers of medical care: DSM-III-R diagnoses and treatment needs. *General Hospital Psychiatry, 12*, 355–362.

Katzenbach, J. R., & Smith, D. K. (1993). *The wisdom of teams: Creating the high-performance organization*. New York: HarperBusiness.

Kongstvedt, P. R. (Ed.). (1996). *The managed health care handbook* (3rd ed.). Gaithersburg, MD: Aspen.

Korenchuk, K. M. (1994). *Transforming the delivery of health care: The integration process*. Englewood, CO: Medical Group Management Association.

Koss, M. P., & Shiang, J. (1994). Research on brief psychotherapy. In A. E. Bergin & S. L. Garfield (Eds.), *Handbook of psychotherapy and behavior change* (4th ed., pp. 664–700). New York: Wiley.

Kovacs, M., Rush, A. J., Beck, A. T., & Hollon, S. (1981). Depressed outpatients treated with cognitive therapy or pharmacotherapy. *Archives of General Psychiatry, 38*, 33–39.

Lambert, M. J., & Burlingame, G. M. (1995). *OQ 45.1*. Salt Lake City, UT: IHC Center for Behavioral Healthcare Efficacy.

Lazarus, A. (1995). A business plan for starting a behavioral group practice. *Behavioral Healthcare Tomorrow, 4*(4), 28–32.

Lazarus, A. (Ed.). (1996). *Controversies in managed mental health care*. Washington, DC: American Psychiatric Press.

Levit, K. R., Cowan, C. A., Lazenby, H. C., McDonnell, P. A., Sensenig, A. L., Stiller, J. M., & Won, D. K. (1994). National health spending trends, 1960–1993. *Health Affairs, 13*, 14–31.

Linehan, M. M. (1993). *Cognitive-behavioral treatment of borderline personality disorder*. New York: Guilford Press.

Littlefield, M. J., & Daily, S. (1992). Marketing techniques. In A.E. Barnett & G. G. Mayer (Eds.), *Ambulatory care management and practice* (pp. 385–394). Gaithersburg, MD: Aspen.

Malan, D. H. (1976). *The frontiers of brief psychotherapy: An example of the convergence of research and clinical practice.* New York: Plenum Press.

Mancuso, A. (1992). *How to form your own New York corporation.* Berkeley, CA: Nolo Press.

Mancuso, A. (1994). *How to form a nonprofit corporation* (2nd ed.). Berkeley, CA: Nolo Press.

Maruish, M. E. (Ed.). (1994). *The use of psychological testing for treatment planning and outcome assessment.* Hillsdale, NJ: Erlbaum.

Melek, S. P. (1993). *Research report: Mental health care reform—Can everyone win?* New York: Milliman & Robertson.

Miller, I. J. (1996). Managed care is harmful to outpatient mental health services: A call for accountability. *Professional Psychology: Research and Practice, 27,* 349–363.

Milling, B. E. (1995). *How to get a loan or line of credit.* Napierville, IL: Sourcebooks.

Milner, D. E. (1994). Topics in office management: Steps for selecting a computer system. *Journal of Medical Practice Management, 9,* 235–236.

Morrill, W. H., Oetting, E. R., & Hurst, J. C. (1974). Dimensions of counselor functioning. *Personnel and Guidance Journal, 52,* 354–360.

National Committee for Quality Assurance. (1996). *Draft accreditation standards for managed behavioral healthcare organizations.* Washington, DC: Author.

National Institute of Mental Health. (1994). *Caring for people with severe mental disorders.* Washington, DC: Author.

Nelson, D. C., Hartman, E., Ojemann, P. G., & Wilcox, M. (1995). Breaking new ground: Public/private collaboration to measure and manage Medicaid patient outcomes. *Behavioral Healthcare Tomorrow, 4*(3), 31–39.

O'Connell, D., & Velicer, W. F. (1988). A decisional balance measure of the stages of change model for weight loss. *International Journal of the Addictions, 23,* 729–840.

Ogles, B. M., Lambert, M. J., & Masters, K. S. (1996). *Assessing outcome in clinical practice.* Boston: Allyn & Bacon.

Panzarino, P. (1995). Report card indicators for managed behavioral healthcare: AMBHA begins efforts to define standards for accountability. *Behavioral Healthcare Tomorrow, 4*(3), 49–54.

Patricelli, R. E., & Lee, F. C. (1996). Employer-based innovations in behavioral health benefits. *Professional Psychology: Research and Practice, 27,* 325–334.

Pavlock, E. J. (1994). *Financial management for medical groups.* Englewood, CO: Center for Research in Ambulatory Health Care Administration.

Phillips, E. L. (1992). George Washington University's international data on psychotherapy delivery systems: Modeling new approaches to the study of therapy. In L. E. Beutler & M. Crago (Eds.), *Psychotherapy research: An international review of programmatic studies* (pp. 263–273). Washington, DC: American Psychological Association.

Piper, W. E., Rosie, J. S., Joyce, A. S., & Azim, H. F. (1996). *Time-limited day treatment for personality disorders: Integration of research and practice in a group program.* Washington, DC: American Psychological Association.

Pollack, M. H., Otto, M. W., & Rosenbaum, J. E. (Eds.). (1996). *Challenges in clinical practice: Pharmacologic and psychosocial strategies.* New York: Guilford Press.

Pomerantz, J. M., Liptzin, B., Carter, A., & Perlman, M. S. (1996). Is private practice compatible with managed care? In A. Lazarus (Ed.), *Controversies in managed mental health care* (pp. 17–28). Washington, DC: American Psychiatric Press.

Prochaska, J. O., Norcross, J., & DiClemente, C. C. (1994). *Changing for good.* New York: William Morrow.

Rakowski, W., Dube, C. A., & Goldstein, M. G. (1996). Considerations for extending the transtheoretical model of behavior change to screening mammography. *Health Education Research: Theory and Practice, 11,* 77–96.

Rating the HMOs (1996, September 2). *U.S. News and World Report*, pp. 52–63.

Ricks, D. F. (1974). Supershrink: Methods of a therapist judged successful on the basis of adult outcomes of adolescent patients. In D. F. Ricks, A. Thomas, & M. Roff (Eds.), *Life history research in psychopathology* (Vol. 3, pp. 275–297). Minneapolis: University of Minnesota Press.

Rogers, W. H., Wells, K. B., Meredith, L. S., Sturm, R., & Burnham, M. A. (1993). Course of depression for adult outpatients under prepaid or fee-for-service financing. *Archives of General Psychiatry, 50,* 517–526.

Roth, A., & Fonagy, P. (1996). *What works for whom? A critical review of psychotherapy research.* New York: Guilford Press.

Schafer, E. L. (1991). Financial management of medical and dental practices. In A. Ross, S. J. Williams, & E. L. Schafer (Eds.), *Ambulatory care management* (2nd ed., pp. 47–74). Albany, NY: Delmar.

Seaburn, D. B., Lorenz, A. D., Gunn, W. B., Gawinski, B. A., & Mauksch, L. B. (1996). *Models of collaboration: A guide for mental health professionals working with health care professionals.* New York: Basic Books.

Senge, P. (1990). *Fifth discipline: Mastering the five practices of the learning organization.* New York: Doubleday.

Shouldice, R. G. (1987). *Marketing management in the fee-for-service/prepaid medical group.* Denver, CO: Center for Research in Ambulatory Health Care Administration.

Solomon, R. J. (1991). *Clinical practice management.* Gaithersburg, MD: Aspen.

Steenbarger, B. N. (1992). Toward science–practice integration in brief counseling and therapy. *Counseling Psychologist, 20,* 403–450.

Steenbarger, B. N. (1994). Duration and outcome in psychotherapy: An integrative review. *Professional Psychology: Research and Practice, 25,* 111–119.

Steenbarger, B. N., & Budman, S. H. (1996). Group psychotherapy and managed behavioral health care: Current trends and future challenges. *International Journal of Group Psychotherapy, 46,* 297–310.

Steenbarger, B. N., & Smith, H. B. (1996). Assessing the quality of counseling services: Developing accountable helping systems. *Journal of Counseling and Development, 75,* 145–150.

Steenbarger, B. N., Smith, H. B., & Budman, S. H. (1996). Integrating science and practice in outcomes assessment: A bolder model for a managed era. *Psychotherapy, 33,* 246–253.

Stone, M. (1992). Borderline personality disorder: Course of illness. In J. F. Clarkin, E. Marziali, & H. Munroe-Blum (Eds.), *Borderline personality disorder: Clinical and empirical perspectives* (pp. 67–86). New York: Guilford Press.

Strupp, H. H., & Binder, J. L. (1984). *Psychotherapy in a new key: A guide to time-limited dynamic psychotherapy.* New York: Basic Books.

Sturm, R., & Wells, K. B. (1995). How can care for depression become more cost-effective? *Journal of the American Medical Association, 273,* 51–58.

Sullivan, K. W., & Luallin, M. D. (1992). Marketing in the managed care setting: Patient survey techniques and other factors in assessing patient satisfaction. In A. E. Barnett & G. G. Mayer (Eds.), *Ambulatory care management and practice* (pp. 395–424). Gaithersburg, MD: Aspen.

Suzuki, S. (1970). *Zen mind, beginner's mind.* New York: Weatherhill.

Tucker, L., & Lubin, W. (1994). *National survey of psychologists. Report from Division 39, American Psychological Association.* Washington, DC: American Psychological Association.

Umland, B. (1995). Behavioral healthcare benefit strategies of self-insured employers. *Behavioral Healthcare Tomorrow, 4*(6), 67–70.

Vaillant, G. (1977). *Adaptation to life.* Boston: Little, Brown.

Vibberts, S., & Youngs, M. T. (Eds.). (1995). *The 1996 behavioral outcomes and guidelines sourcebook.* New York: Faulkner & Gray.

Vibberts, S., & Youngs, M. T. (Eds.). (1996). *The 1997 behavioral outcomes and guidelines sourcebook.* New York: Faulkner & Gray.

Wells, K. B., Hays, R. D., Burnam, M. A., Rogers, W. H., Greenfield, S., & Ware, J. E. Jr. (1989). Detection of depressive disorder in prepaid and fee-for-service practices: Results from the Medical Outcomes Study. *Journal of the American Medical Association, 262,* 925–930.

Wells, R. A., & Giannetti, V. J. (Eds.). (1990). *Handbook of the brief psychotherapies.* New York: Plenum Press.

Whitman, P. A. (1994). Tax-exempt medical clinics. *Group Practice Journal, 43,* 42–44.

Wilkerson, J. D., Devers, K. J., & Given, R. S. (Eds.). (1997). *Competitive managed care: The emerging health care system.* San Francisco: Jossey-Bass.

Yen, J., & Goldberg, M. D. (1992). Creating a successful relationship with a bank. In A. E. Barnett & G. G. Mayer (Eds.), *Ambulatory care management and practice* (pp. 196–206). Gaithersburg, MD: Aspen.

Yenney, S. L. (1994). *Business strategies for a caring profession: A practitioner's guidebook.* Washington, DC: American Psychological Association.

Younger, P. A., Conner, C., Cartwright, K. K., Kole, S. M., Forsyth, J., & Marvin, D. L. (1996). *Managed care law manual.* Gaithersburg, MD: Aspen.

Zablocki, E. (1995). *Changing physician practice patterns: Strategies for success in a capitated health care system.* Gaithersburg, MD: Aspen.

Zieman, G. L. (Ed.) (1995). *The complete capitation handbook.* Tiburon, CA: CentraLink Publications.

Index